Supportive Care of
Children with Cancer

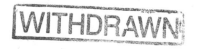

WITHDRAWN

NAPIER UNIVERSITY LIS
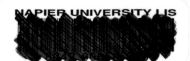

Supportive Care of Children with Cancer

Current Therapy and Guidelines from the Children's Oncology Group

Third Edition

Arnold J. Altman, M.D.

Hartford Whalers Professor of Childhood Cancer,
University of Connecticut School of Medicine

Head, Division of Hematology-Oncology,
Connecticut Children's Medicine Center

Hartford, Connecticut

WITH A FOREWORD BY

Gregory H. Reaman, M.D.

The Johns Hopkins University Press
Baltimore and London

618·92994 ALT
28 DAY COM

Drug dosage: The authors and publisher have exerted every effort to ensure that the selection and dosage of drugs discussed in this text accord with recommendations and practice at the time of publication. However, in view of ongoing research, changes in governmental regulations, and the constant flow of information relating to drug therapy and drug reactions, the reader is urged to check the package insert of each drug for any change in indications and dosage and for warnings and precautions. This is particularly important when the recommended agent is a new and/or infrequently used drug.

© 1993, 1997, 2004 The Johns Hopkins University Press
All rights reserved. Published 2004
Printed in the United States of America on acid-free paper
9 8 7 6 5 4 3 2 1

The Johns Hopkins University Press
2715 North Charles Street
Baltimore, Maryland 21218-4363
www.press.jhu.edu

Library of Congress Cataloging-in-Publication Data

Supportive care of children with cancer : current therapy and guidelines from the Children's Oncology Group / edited by Arnold J. Altman—3rd ed.
    p. ; cm.
Includes bibliographical references and index.
    ISBN 0-8018-7909-4 (pbk. : alk. paper)
1. Cancer in children.   2. Cancer in adolescence.
    [DNLM: 1. Neoplasms—therapy—Child.   2. Neoplasms—therapy—Infant. QZ 266 S9592 2004] I. Altman, Arnold J.   II. Children's Oncology Group.
    RC281.C4S94 2004
    618.92′994—dc22   2003017425

A catalog record for this book is available from the British Library.

Contents

Foreword

The Children's Oncology Group was organized in March 2000 as the result of the unification of the four pediatric cancer clinical trials groups: the Children's Cancer Group, the Pediatric Oncology Group, the National Wilms Tumor Study Group, and the Intergroup Rhabdomyosarcoma Study Group. These four multicenter cooperative groups have been designing and conducting clinical trials in the major cancers seen in the pediatric age group. In addition, they have developed and conducted trials of novel agents and innovative therapy regimens with the intent of improving outcome and decreasing the short-term morbidity as well as long-term toxicity associated with cancer and anticancer therapy.

Due to the significant improvement in outcome for children with cancer, it became apparent to clinical investigators that collaborating in this endeavor rather than continuing the healthy competition they once enjoyed would provide more opportunities for success, with a positive direct impact on children and families. The Children's Oncology Group is multi-institutional, with 238 pediatric cancer programs throughout the United States, Canada, Australia, New Zealand, and Switzerland, and a single site in the Netherlands. The Children's Oncology Group is composed of nearly 5,000 members from all clinical disciplines involved in the multidisciplinary management of pediatric cancer, including pediatric oncologists, surgeons and surgical subspecialists, radiation oncologists, pathologists, neurologists, nurses, psychologists, pharmacologists, neurologists, social workers, as well as clinical research support staff and laboratory investigators working in close collaboration on correlative biology studies.

Essential to multi-institutional clinical trials is uniform criteria for diagnosis, staging, eligibility determination, treatment, response criteria, grading of toxicity, and complications and measuring and determining outcome. Such policies and procedures are necessary to ensure that trials are conducted as uniformly as possible to ensure the quality and integrity of data submitted by each collaborating institution and guarantee that the data reflect protocol-specified variables and endpoints.

In addition to multidisciplinary treatment and the obvious concern for psychosocial support, caring for a child with cancer requires vigilant attention to the management of complications associated with therapy and, in many situations, ways to prevent such complications and toxicity. A significant contribution to the improved outcome for children with cancer has been the recognition of infectious, metabolic, and hemorrhagic complications associated with disease and treatment interventions.

The fine art of therapy and management varies considerably within institutions, particularly related to the management of complications and the provision of supportive care in the context of intensive multidisciplinary, anticancer treatment. An attempt has been made to provide guidelines for supportive care at the institutional level which will ensure some uniformity so that institutional and regional variations in clinical practice do not adversely impact clinical trial results.

Presented in this publication is a series of guidelines that have been refined over the past two decades for consideration of investigators participating in Children's Oncology Group clinical trials. As we learn more about the biology of cancer, we learn more about the biology of toxicities and complications; and as cancer therapy changes, supportive care management and therapy and prevention of toxicity change accordingly. The guidelines presented here are to be interpreted as recommendations and suggestions based on input from a series of clinicians from multiple disciplines in the Children's Oncology Group and are provided to lessen the potential impact of variability in toxicity management on clinical trial results. We recognize that all guidelines must be interpreted within the context of every individual clinical situation, which has distinguishing features and therefore potentially unique treatment requirements. These guidelines should be viewed, therefore, as suggestions or recommendations and are not meant to be interpreted as evidence-based standards by which clinical practice or care should be assessed in any single institution or by any single practitioner. These guidelines will continue to be evaluated and will change accordingly as new information becomes available to clinicians and clinical investigators involved in research efforts aimed at improving outcome in infants, children, and adolescents with cancer.

Gregory H. Reaman, M.D.
Chairman, Children's Oncology Group

Preface

The treatment of a child with cancer is not for the faint of heart. In our efforts to cure our young patients of the dread neoplastic diseases, we routinely expose them to toxic chemotherapeutic agents, invasive surgical procedures, and radiation oncology interventions that risk disfigurement, neuropsychiatric damage, and life-threatening organ toxicity. These potentially dire consequences have mandated that advances in cancer treatment go hand in hand with careful attention to supportive care measures that sustain patients through their therapeutic ordeal.

In an effort to derive guidelines to assist pediatric oncology care providers, the Supportive Care Committee of the Children's Cancer Group (CCG), under the leadership of Arthur Ablin, wrote the first two editions of *Supportive Care of Children with Cancer*. Now that the CCG, the Pediatric Oncology Group, the Intergroup Rhabdomyosarcoma Study Group, and the National Wilms Tumor Study Group have merged to form the Children's Oncology Group (COG), we have embarked on an effort to update the supportive care guidelines and to produce a document that reflects the experience and philosophy of these parent organizations. This edition has also recognized the extraordinary stresses on the men and women "in the arena" by adding a chapter on the emotional support of caregivers.

The recommendations published in this book are meant to assist caregivers in providing the best possible supportive care to their patients. However, it is not our intention to assert a dogmatic "standard of care," recognizing that individual patient needs are best assessed by those "on the spot."

I would like to express my gratitude to those members of the Supportive Care and Pharmacology committees of COG, as well as the outside reviewers who graciously provided advice and guidance during the preparation of this book: Ashraf Abdelmonem, M.D., Arthur Ablin, M.D., Susan Berg, Pharm.D., Helaine Bertsch, M.D., Gabriel Briones, Pharm.D., Betsy Bickert, Pharm.D., Charlton Davis, M.D., James Feusner, M.D., Kevin Graner, R.Ph., Darryl Grendahl, R.Ph, David Henry, M.S., BCOP, FASHP, Shirley Hogan, Pharm.D.,

Dean Jorstad, R.Ph., Michael Kellick, M.S., R.Ph., Steven Lipshultz, M.D., Barbara McCully, B.Sc.Pharm., Vicki Nussbaum, Pharm.D., Majid Rasoulpour, M.D., Kim Ritchie, M.D., Lillian Sung, M.D., Jean Schwab, L.C.S.W., Brad Sherburne, M.D., Mark Sorenson, Ph.D., Del Stringham, Pharm.D.

Abbreviations

ADH	antidiuretic hormone	cGVHD	chronic graft versus host disease
aGVHD	acute graft versus host disease	CMV	cytomegalovirus
AIDS	acquired immunodeficency syndrome	CNS	central nervous system
		CSA	cyclosporine
ALL	acute lymphocytic leukemia	CT	computed tomography
AML	acute myelocytic leukemia	CVA	cerebrovascular accident
ANC	absolute neutrophil count	CVAD	central venous access device
ANLL	acute nonlymphoblastic leukemia	CVC	central venous catheter
		CVL	central venous line
APCR	activated protein C resistance	DIC	disseminated intravascular coagulation
APML	acute promyelocytic leukemia	DLI	donor leukocyte infusion
APTT	activated partial thromboplastin time	DMOPA	depo-medroxy-progesterone acetate
ASCUS	atypical cells of undetermined significance	DMSO	dimethylsylfoxide
		DTaP	diphtheria, tetanus, acellular pertussis (vaccine)
BAL	bronchoalveolar lavage	EBV	Epstein-Barr virus
b.i.d	twice daily	ELISA	enzyme-linked immunosorbent assay
BMI	body mass index		
BMT	bone marrow transplant	EPO	erythropoietin
BUN	blood urea nitrogen	FDP	fibrin degradation product
CAM	complementary or alternative medicine	FFP	fresh frozen plasma
CBC	complete blood count	GFR	glomerular filtration rate

GI	gastrointestinal	OAE	otoacoustic emission
GVHD	graft versus host disease	OCP	oral contraceptive pill
HAV	hepatitis A vaccine	OPV	oral polio vaccine
HBIG	hepatitis B immune globulin	PBSC	peripheral blood stem cell
HBV	hepatitis B vaccine	PCR	polymerase chain reaction
Hct	hematocrit	PCV	pneumococcal conjugate vaccine
Hib	*Hemophilus influenzae* type B	PICC	peripherally inserted central catheter
HLA	human leukocyte antigen	PLT	platelet
HPV	human papillomavirus	PO	by mouth
HSCT	hematopoietic stem cell transplantation	PR	by rectum
HSV	herpes simplex virus	PRN	as needed
HUS	hemolytic uremic syndrome	PT	prothrombin time
Ig	immunoglobulin	PTLD	post-transplant lymphoproliferative disorder
IM	intramuscular	PTSD	post-traumatic stress disorder
IPV	inactivated polio vaccine	PTT	partial thromboplastin time
IV	intravenous	PUVA	psoralen with ultraviolet A
IV IgG	intravenous immune globulin	q	each, every
LMWH	low molecular weight heparin	q.i.d.	four times daily
MDS	myelodysplasia	RBC	red blood cell (count)
MEIA	microparticle enzyme immunoassay	RDA	Recommended Dietary Allowance
MMR	measles, mumps, rubella (vaccine)	rhG-CSF	recombinant human granulocyte-colony-stimulating factor
MP	methylprednisolone	RSV	respiratory syncytial virus
MRI	magnetic resonance imaging	SC	subcutaneous
MTX	methotrexate		
NPO	nothing by mouth		
NSAID	nonsteroidal anti-inflammatory drug		

SIADH	syndrome of inappropriate antidiuretic hormone	TFPI	tissue factor pathway inhibitor
		t.i.d.	three times daily
		TMP	trimethoprim
SMN	second malignant neoplasm	TPA	tissue plasminogen activator
SMS	superior mediastinal syndrome	TPN	total parenteral nutrition
SMX	sulfamethoxazole	UFH	unfractionated heparin
SVCS	superior vena cava syndrome	VOD	veno-occlusive disease
TAFI	thrombin-activated fibrinolysis inhibitor	VZIG	varicella-zoster immune globulin
TBI	total body irradation	VZV	varicella-zoster virus
TE	thromboembolic event		

Contributors

Edythe A. Albano, M.D., Associate Professor of Pediatrics, University of Colorado Health Sciences Center, Denver, Colorado

Dorothy R. Barnard, M.D., Associate and Head, Division of Pediatric Hematology/Oncology, Department of Pediatrics, IWK Health Centre, Halifax, Nova Scotia

Maru Barrera, Ph.D., Psychologist, Hematology/Oncology Program and Department of Psychology, and Associate Scientist, Public Health Sciences, Research Institute, Hospital for Sick Children, Toronto, Ontario; Associate Professor, Medical Institute of Sciences, Public Health Sciences, OISE, University of Toronto, Toronto, Ontario

Roger L. Berkow, M.D., Professor and Vice-Chair, Department of Pediatrics, and Assistant Dean of Clinical Education, University of Alabama at Birmingham, Birmingham, Alabama

Donna L. Betcher, R.N., M.S.N., CPNP, Pediatric Nurse Practitioner, Pediatric Hematology Oncology, Mayo Clinic, Rochester, Minnesota

Dana Bond, R.N., M.N., CPNP, Pediatric Nurse Practitioner, Center of Cancer and Blood Disorders, Children's Medical Center of Dallas, Dallas, Texas

Julia Cartwright, R.Ph., Oncology Pharmacy Manager, Vanderbilt Ingram Cancer Center, Vanderbilt University, Nashville, Tennessee

Claudia Deffenbaugh, Pharm.D., Clinical Staff Pharmacist, Lucile Salter Packard Children's Hospital at Stanford, Palo Alto, California

Kenneth De Santes, M.D., Associate Professor and Director, Pediatric Stem Cell Transplant Program, University of Wisconsin Comprehensive Cancer Center, Madison, Wisconsin

Sarah Friebert, M.D., Director, Division of Pediatric Palliative Care, Children's Hospital Medical Center of Akron, Akron, Ohio

Debra L. Friedman, M.D., Assistant Professor, Department of Pediatrics, University of Washington School of Medicine, Seattle, Washington

Connie Goes, R.N., Oncology Nurse, Children's Hospital of Oakland, Oakland, California

Kevin Graner, R.Ph., Pediatric Pharmacotherapy Coordinator, Mayo Eugenio Litta Children's Hospital, Rochester, Minnesota

Corin M. Greenberg, Ph.D., Executive Director, Pediatric Oncology Group of Ontario, Toronto, Ontario

Mark L. Greenberg, OC, M.B., Ch.B., FRCPC, FAAP, Medical Director, Pediatric Oncology Group of Ontario; Senior Staff Oncologist, Division of Haematology/Oncology, Hospital for Sick Children; and Professor of Pediatrics, University of Toronto, Toronto, Ontario

Paula K. Groncy, M.D., Associate Clinical Professor, Department of Pediatrics, Harbor/UCLA Medical Center, Torrance, California

J. Nathan Hagstrom, M.D., Assistant Professor, Department of Pediatrics, University of Connecticut Health Center, Farmington, Connecticut. Pediatric Oncologist. Connecticut Children's Medical Center. Hartford, CT

Gregory Hale, M.D., Clinical Director, Division of Stem Cell Transplantation, Department of Hematology/Oncology, St. Jude Children's Research Hospital, Memphis, Tennessee

Caroline Hastings, M.D., Associate Clinical Professor of Pediatrics, University of California, San Francisco, California

Joanne M. Hilden, M.D., Chair, Department of Pediatric Hematology/ Oncology, Cleveland Clinic Foundation, Cleveland, Ohio

Jeffrey D. Hord, M.D., Director, Pediatric Hematology/Oncology, Children's Hospital Medical Center of Akron, Akron, Ohio

Melissa E. Huggins, M.D., Clinical Instructor, Department of Obstetrics and Gynecology, University of California, Irvine, California

John Iacuone, M.D., Clinical Professor, Department of Pediatrics, Texas Tech University Health Sciences Center, Lubbock, Texas

F. Leonard Johnson, M.D., Robert C. Neerhout Professor of Pediatrics, Oregon Health Sciences University, Portland, Oregon

Anne E. Kazak, Ph.D., Professor and Director of Psychology Research, Department of Pediatrics, University of Pennsylvania School of Medicine, Philadelphia, Pennsylvania

Kara M. Kelly, M.D., Associate Professor of Clinical Pediatrics, College of Physicians and Surgeons of Columbia University, New York, New York

Wendy Landier, R.N., M.S.N., CPNP, CPON, Pediatric Nurse Practitioner, City of Hope National Medical Center, Duarte, California

Claudine Larson-Tuttle, M.A., CCC/Audiologist, Los Angeles County Public Schools, Los Angeles

Alan Lorenzen, Pharm.D., BCOP, Senior Clinical Pharmacist, Hematology-Oncology, Children's Medical Center of Dallas, Dallas, Texas

Karen Marcus, M.D., Assistant Professor of Radiology, Harvard Medical School, Boston, Massachusetts

Robert B. Marcus, Jr., M.D., Professor of Radiation Oncology and Pediatrics, Emory University, Atlanta, Georgia

Paul T. Monagle, M.B.B.S. Dept. Haematology Royal Children's Hospital Victoria, Australia

John S. Murphy, B.Pharm., Senior Oncology Pharmacist, Pharmacy Department, Princess Margaret Hospital, Subiaco, Western Australia

Elizabeth Nichol, R.N., Pediatric Consultant, Interlink Community Cancer Nurses/The Hospital for Sick Children, Toronto, Ontario

Robert B. Noll, Ph.D., Professor (Psychiatry and Pediatrics), Children's Hospital Medical Center, Cincinnati, Ohio

Richard S. Pieters, M.D., Clinical Associate Professor of Radiology, Boston University School of Medicine, Boston, Massachusetts

Karen Ringwald-Smith, M.S., R.D., LDN, Clinical Coordinator/ Research and Education Coordinator, Department of Clinical Nutrition, St. Jude Children's Research Hospital, Memphis, Tennessee

Zora R. Rogers, M.D., Associate Professor, Department of Pediatrics, University of Texas Southwestern Medical Center at Dallas, Dallas, Texas

Joan Ronan, R.N., Oncology Nurse, Sutter Medical Center, Sacramento, California

Nancy Sacks, M.S., R.D., CNSD, Clinical Nutritionist, Wallingford, Pennsylvania

Eric Sandler, M.D., Associate Professor of Pediatrics, Mayo Medical School, Jacksonville, Florida

Neil L. Schechter, M.D., Professor of Pediatrics, University of Connecticut School of Medicine, Hartford, Connecticut

Susan F. Sencer, M.D., Medical Director, Pediatric Hematology-Oncology, Children's Hospitals and Clinics, Minneapolis–St. Paul, Minnesota

Richard D. Udin, D.D.S., Director, Advanced Education in Pediatric Dentistry Program, University of Southern California, Los Angeles, California

Adrianna Vlachos, M.D., Assistant Professor of Pediatrics, Albert Einstein College of Medicine, Bronx, New York

Linda Waterhouse, M.S.W., R.S.W., Pediatric Oncology Social Worker, McMaster Children's Hospital, Hamilton Health Sciences, Hamilton, Ontario

Steven J. Weisman, M.D., Professor of Anesthesiology and Pediatrics, Medical College of Wisconsin, Milwaukee, Wisconsin

Lawrence J. Wolff, M.D., Professor of Pediatrics, Oregon Health Sciences University, Portland, Oregon

William T. Zempsky, M.D., Associate Professor of Pediatrics and Emergency Medicine, University of Connecticut School of Medicine, Hartford, Connecticut

Supportive Care of
Children with Cancer

1

The Prevention of Infection

Arnold J. Altman, M.D., and Lawrence J. Wolff, M.D.

Children receiving treatment for cancer are at increased risk of infection from bacterial, viral, protozoal, and fungal agents. Among the factors responsible are myelosuppression with decreased blood cell function, changes in humoral and cellular immunity, loss of integrity of physical defense barriers, hyponutrition, and changes in colonizing microflora. The following guidelines for care are considered to minimize the risk of infection and its associated morbidity and mortality in children with cancer who are undergoing treatment and to maintain the uniformity of care in a cooperative group study population to minimize treatment variables.

I. GENERAL MEASURES

A. Appropriate environment
1. Neutropenia alone is not sufficient indication for hospitalization; the exposure to antibiotic-resistant nosocomial organisms would put the patient at additional risk. If the patient is afebrile and has no other evident medical problems, hospitalization should be avoided, but careful attention should be given to total body (especially oral) and environmental hygiene.
2. Nonhospitalized children should avoid ill children and adults.
3. When hospitalization is necessary, place the patient in a private room or with another patient who has no active infection. The patient need not be restricted to the room but must avoid contact with patients who have active infections.

      4.   Hospital staff, families, and visitors should carefully wash their hands before and after contact with the patient.

B. Hygiene
1.   Dietary precautions
In view of the lack of evidence that dietary manipulation reduces the incidence of serious infection, the patient may eat a regular diet. The improvement in nutritional intake may compensate for any increased exposure to food-related organisms. Some prudent modifications to consider are:
a.   Have the patient avoid raw fruits and vegetables (especially salads).
b.   Have the patient avoid processed meats.
c.   Thoroughly cleanse the lids of canned foods and beverages before opening.
2.   Cleanliness
a.   Have the patient bathe and shampoo regularly.
b.   Have the patient and all who come in contact with the patient wash their hands with antiseptic soap.
c.   Pay meticulous attention to skin, and practice asepsis with Betadine or a comparable agent before venipuncture or finger prick.
3.   Dental hygiene (see Chapter 14)
4.   Catheters (in blood vessels, urethra, nose, and elsewhere)
a.   Use catheters only when absolutely necessary.
b.   Use meticulous care during dressing changes, flushing, and connecting.
c.   Change peripheral intravenous (IV) lines at least every 4 days (if possible).
d.   The care of central venous lines, external catheters, and implantable ports should be done by individuals who have been well trained. Fastidious care is essential.

C. Activities
The patient can attend school when the absolute neutrophil count (ANC) is $>200/\mu L$ and likely to increase. Neutropenia by itself is not a contraindication to attend school. The decision should be individualized. In all cases, teachers should be instructed to notify the parents of

children with cancer when epidemics or exposure to infectious diseases occur.

   D. Protection of the anal-rectal mucosa
1. Prevent constipation with age-appropriate diet and, if necessary, a stool softener (e.g., sodium docusate, 1–3 mg/kg/day PO; maximum dose 400 mg/day).
2. Avoid rectal suppositories to minimize the change of fissures and proctitis.
3. Do not insert thermometers into the rectum.

II. PROPHYLAXIS AGAINST *PNEUMOCYSTIS CARINII*

   A. Background
1. Patients being treated for cancer have a higher incidence of *P. carinii* infection. This risk can effectively be reduced by administering trimethoprim/sulfamethoxazole (TMP/SMX).
2. The low dosage suggested below does not appear to enhance bone marrow suppression from moderately aggressive programs of chemotherapy. However, this may not be true with more intensive cytotoxic regimens. When prolonged marrow suppression occurs in patients receiving TMP/SMX, consider substituting pentamidine.

   B. Dosage
1. TMP 5 mg/kg/day (150 mg/m^2/day—maximum daily dose 320 mg) and SMX 25 mg/kg/day (750 mg/m^2/day—maximum daily dose 1,600 mg) are given in 2 divided doses 3 sequential days a week.
2. TMP/SMX therapy should start with the initiation of chemotherapy and continue for 8–12 weeks after chemotherapy is stopped.

   C. Preparations
1. Tablet: TMP 80 mg/SMX 400 mg
Double strength tablet: TMP 160 mg/SMX 800 mg
2. Suspension: TMP 40 mg/SMX 200 mg/5mL.

   D. Intolerance of, or allergy to, TMP/SMX
For patients who are repeatedly unable to tolerate full doses of chemotherapy because of allergy or myelosuppression, omit TMP/SMX prophylaxis. Consider inhalation

or IV pentamidine or oral dapsone where the possibility of pneumocystis infection is high.

1. The prophylactic regimen for dapsone is 2 mg/kg/day (maximum 100 mg/day) as a single dose. (It comes in 25 and 100 mg tablets.)
2. The prophylactic regimen for IV pentamidine is 4 mg/kg (diluted to maximum concentration of 6 mg/ml in 50–250 ml D5W) infused over 60 minutes IV q4wk.
3. The prophylactic regimen for inhalation pentamidine is 8 mg/kg for children <5 years old and 300 mg for children ≥5 years old. It is administered q4wk via the Respirgard II Nebulizer.

III. PROPHYLAXIS AGAINST BACTERIA

A. Trimethoprim/sulfamethoxazole

Some evidence indicates that children have fewer serious bacterial infections; deaths related to infection; and episodes of otitis media, upper respiratory infection, urinary tract infection, cellulites, pneumonitis, and sinusitis when prophylactic TMP/SMX is given. The following recommendations are made to ensure uniformity in multi-institutional trials.

1. Patients on chemotherapy should receive prophylactic TMP/SMX *unless* they have
   a. Allergy to TMP or SMX
   b. Glucose-6-phosphate dehydrogenase deficiency
   c. Malabsorption
2. Schedule
   a. Patients should commence TMP/SMX prophylaxis at the time of the diagnosis whether or not systemic antibiotic therapy is also indicated.
   b. All patients should be given TMP/SMX 3 consecutive days each week.
   c. Patients should discontinue TMP/SMX 1 day before and for 4 days after infusion of high-dose methotrexate.
   d. Bone marrow transplant recipients should discontinue TMP/SMX 2 days before transplantation and then restart it when the ANC is >500/μL.
3. Dosage (see section IIB)
4. Preparations (see section IIC)

B. Other antimicrobial agents
    The quinolones, ofloxacin, norfloxacin, and ciprofloxacin, have shown promise in adult prophylactic studies. Ciprofloxacin appears to have the broadest antibacterial effect and should be considered as prophylaxis in the neutropenic young adult with cancer; however, ciprofloxacin is not approved by the Food and Drug Administration for use by children. The dosage usually used for ciprofloxacin in young adults is 500 mg b.i.d.

C. Prophylaxis against *Hemophilus influenzae* type b
    1. The use of *H. influenzae* vaccine for all children older than 2 months is recommended; however, remember that patients who receive very intense chemotherapeutic regimens may not form or maintain antibodies to *H. influenzae* (see Chapter 2, section IA2).
    2. Patients who have contact within the household or who have prolonged exposure to individuals with severe *H. influenzae* infection should receive rifampin prophylaxis regardless of their age.
    3. Dosage: 20 mg/kg/day of rifampin: (maximum 600 mg) PO for 4 days.
    4. Preparations
        a. Capsule: 150 or 300 mg. Powders can be pre-weighed by a pharmacist to give precise dosages.
        b. Rifampin suspension (1% in simple syrup) can be prepared by a pharmacist.

D. Prophylaxis against *Streptococcus pneumoniae*
    1. All children under 23 months should receive the 7-valent pneumococcal polysaccharide vaccine (PCV7).
    2. Children aged 24–59 months and receiving antineoplastic therapy should receive 2 doses of PCV7 (excluding bone marrow transplant recipients).
    3. Children older than 24 months and receiving antineoplastic therapy should receive the 23-valent pneumococcal polysaccharide vaccine 2 months after receiving 2 PCV7 injections.

E. Intravenous immune globulin (IgG)
    1. Many chemotherapy protocols and/or diseases are associated with low IgG levels. Bone marrow transplant patients are frequently deficient in IgG. It is recommended to measure IgG levels and use IV IgG.

Different institutional and cooperative protocols recommend various guidelines; however, if the IgG level is less than 300 mg/dl, use IV IgG.
2. Dosage: 200–400 mg/kg once a month.
3. Preparations vary. Listed are several:
   a. 5% solution (Cutter): 10, 50, or 100 mL vials
   b. Lyophilized powder (Sandoz): 1, 3, or 6 g vials
      Reconstitution fluid is provided to prepare a 3, 6, 9, or 12% solution.
4. Administer in a separate IV line. Initiate infusion at manufacturer's slowest recommended rate and titrate subsequent rate as directed in manufacturer's instructions. Also consult institutional guidelines for use.
5. Compatible with 0.9% saline.
6. Never use the intramuscular preparation intravenously.
7. Side effects
   a. Interstitial extravasation can result in local irritation, inflammation, and phlebitis secondary to the alkaline pH.
   b. Rapid IV infusion can result in reversible increases in serum creatinine concentrations.
   c. A small percentage of patients may experience nausea, vomiting, headache, diarrhea, and/or rash.
   d. Anaphylactoid reaction in agammaglobulinemic or IgA-deficient patients
   e. Inflammatory reactions: Fever, fatigue, shivering, local pain
   f. Hypersensitivity reactions
   g. Headaches, aseptic meningitis syndrome

F. Splenectomized children
   1. Splenectomized children are susceptible to overwhelming infections with encapsulated bacteria.
   2. Penicillin, amoxicillin, or erythromycin may be used for antibiotics prophylaxis. Dosage recommendations are as follows:
      a. Penicillin
         >14 years: 250–500 mg b.i.d.
         5–14 years: 250 mg b.i.d.
         1–5 years: 125 mg b.i.d.
      b. Amoxicillin
         >14 years: 250–500 mg daily

> 5–14 years: 125–250 mg daily
> 1–5 years: 10 mg/kg/day

   c. Erythromycin (base)
> >8 years: 250–500 mg daily
> 2–8 years: 150 mg daily
> 1–2 years: 125 mg daily

3. Immunization (see Chapter 2, section IA)
   a. Polyvalent pneumococcal vaccine: (See Chapter 2, section IIID)
   b. *Hemophilus* type b conjugate vaccine: 0.5 mL IM for children ≥2 months old
      See the manufacturer's recommendations for the number of injections required
   c. Quadrivalent meningococcal polysaccharide vaccine

IV. PROPHYLAXIS AGAINST FUNGI

Fungal infections are a significant cause of morbidity and mortality in immune-suppressed patients undergoing prolonged periods of antibiotics therapy for fever/neutropenia. The most common fungal infections in patients receiving intensive chemotherapy include Candida and Aspergillus species; however, one should consider mucormycosis, fusarium, coccidiomycosis, and others based on clinical findings and epidemiologic considerations.

A. Candidiasis
   1. Candidiasis is the most common fungal infection in children receiving anticancer therapy.
   2. For prevention of oral or esophageal candidiasis during treatment with steroids or with intensive chemotherapy, use one of the following regimens:
      a. Nystatin oral swish and swallow
         i. Infants: 200,000 units (2 ml) b.i.d.
         ii. Children/adults: 500,000 units (5 ml) b.i.d.
      b. Clotrimazole troche: 1 (10 mg) b.i.d., suck for 10–20 min
      c. Fluconazole oral: 2 mg/kg/d; maximum 200 mg/d

B. Aspergillosis
   1. Aspergillus is primarily an airborne organism. Sinopulmonary colonization is thought to precede infection.

2. Aspergillus infection may be avoided as follows:
   a. Efforts to prevent aspergillus infection should include respiratory isolation, use of laminar flow rooms, and use of high-efficiency particulate air filters.
   b. If the patient is hospitalized at an institution where aspergillus infections are common, consider eliminating plants from the patient's room, monitoring and controlling nasal microbial flora, and scrutinizing construction work (which may be a source of airborne aspergillus spores).
   c. Low-dose amphotericin B (0.1–0.25 mg/kg/day IV) may reduce the incidence of invasive aspergillosis. The inhalant form of amphotericin B, itraconazole, and other agents need to be further evaluated.

V. **PROPHYLAXIS AGAINST INFECTIOUS COMPLICATIONS IN PATIENTS WITH CENTRAL CATHETERS**

A. Background
   Indwelling central catheters are common in children receiving chemotherapy. When these children have surgery or other invasive procedures, they are at risk for colonization of the catheter during episodes of transient bacteremia.

B. Recommendations
   All patients with indwelling central catheters (of either the external catheter type or the subcutaneous reservoir type) should receive standard prophylaxis against subacute bacterial endocarditis, as recommended by the American Heart Association, during invasive procedures including operations on the gastrointestinal or genitourinary tract, endotracheal intubation, and dental manipulation.
   1. Standard regimen
      Amoxicillin 50 mg/kg (maximum 2 g) PO 1 hour before the procedure *or* Ampicillin 50 mg/kg (maximum 2 g) IV, 30 minutes before the procedure.
   2. Regimen for patients allergic to penicillin
      Clindamycin 20 mg/kg (maximum 600 mg) PO 1 hour before the procedure *or* 20 mg/kg (maximum 600 mg) IV within 30 minutes before the procedure.

VI. PROPHYLAXIS AGAINST VIRUSES

Common viral infections that are known to have increased virulence in immune-compromised children include varicella zoster virus (VZV), herpes simplex virus (HSV), cytomegalo-virus (CMV), Epstein-Barr virus (EBV), hepatitis types A and B, respiratory syncytial virus (RSV), and rubeola (measles). Infection with these viruses has resulted in prolonged virus excretion, increased morbidity, and death.

A. General pre-exposure measures
   1. At the time of diagnosis of malignancy
      a. Obtain a history of immunization and previous infection with VZV, HSV, EBV, RSV, measles, and hepatitis A and B.
      b. Obtain viral titers against VZV (preferably using immunofluorescence antibody or a similarly sensitive technique), HSV, CMV, EBV, and, for infants <2 years old, RSV.
   2. Decrease exposure
      a. Siblings should receive their immunizations as recommended in the AAP Red Book.
      b. Notify appropriate teachers, caregivers, and friends of the risk to these children of infection with measles and VZV.
      c. Prevent in-hospital exposure by preadmission screening of other hospitalized children.
      d. Have immune-suppressed patients avoid contact with caregivers and others with active viral infections.

B. Prophylaxis against varicella zoster virus
   1. Indications for, and use of, varicella zoster immune globulin are discussed in Chapter 2, section IIID.
   2. The decision to hold chemotherapy during the incubation period for the development of varicella should be based on the intensity of exposure, the general condition of the patient, and the intensity of the chemotherapy.
   3. If varicella develops, stop chemotherapeutic agents and start acyclovir (1,500 mg/m^2/day IV divided q8h) with adequate hydration.

C. Prophylaxis against herpes simplex virus
1. Patients with recurrent HSV infections are at increased risk of developing significant HSV infections while receiving chemotherapy or during and after bone marrow transplantation. The administration of acyclovir prophylactically may prevent or decrease the severity of recurrent HSV infection. Its use is recommended.
2. Acyclovir
a. Dosage
80 mg/kg/day PO divided into 3–5 doses or 250 mg/m^2 IV q8h during periods of marked leukopenia (maximum dose 1,000 mg/day).
b. Preparations
i.   Vial: 500 mg for IV use
ii. Capsule: 200 mg
c. Acyclovir may be infused in 5% dextrose, 5% dextrose/0.9% saline, Ringer's lactate, or 0.9% saline. Ensure adequate hydration.
d. Acyclovir should not be added to or infused in the same line with blood products, protein hydrolysates or amino acids, or fat emulsions.
e. The clearance of acyclovir is markedly decreased in neonates. The clearance in infants aged 3–12 months is unknown; that of infants >1 year old is the same as that for adults. Adjust the dosage if the patient has renal insufficiency (the drug is excreted by the kidneys). Table 1.1 shows the dosage adjustment for patients with renal impairment.

D. Prophylaxis against cytomegalovirus (CMV)
1. CMV-seronegative patients who are candidates for a bone marrow transplant should receive leukocyte-depleted blood products using third- or fourth-generation filters.
2. Filtering of blood products is more effectively done at the site of collection or dispensing.

E. Prophylaxis against Epstein-Barr virus (EBV)
1. The significance of EBV infection in patients with malignancies is unknown, although children in leukemic remission have died after a hemophagocytic infection associated with EBV.

Table 1.1.
Dosage Adjustment of Acyclovir for Patients with Renal Impairment

Creatinine Clearance Rate (mL/min/1.73 m^2)	% Usual Individual Dose	Dosing Interval
>50	100	q8h
25–50	100	q12h
10–25	100	q12h
<10	50	q24h

2. α-Interferon (αIF) can prevent EBV infections in patients who have undergone renal transplantation.
3. EBV proliferation can be associated with a post-transplant lymphoproliferative disorder. In these cases, the use of Rituximab might be helpful.
4. The routine use of αIF for the prevention of EBV infections in patients receiving chemotherapy is not practical.

F. Prophylaxis against infectious hepatitis types A and B (see Chapter 2, sections IIIB and C)

G. Prophylaxis against respiratory syncytial virus (RSV)
    The risk of nosocomial infection with RSV can be significantly reduced with rapid laboratory diagnosis combined with cohort nursing and the wearing of gowns and gloves for all contacts with RSV-infected children.

H. Prophylaxis against rubeola (measles) (see Chapter 2, section IIIA)

Bibliography

Advisory Committee on Immunization Practices. Preventing pneumococcal disease among infants and young children. *MMWR* 49 (No. RR-9), 2000.

American Academy of Pediatrics. In Pickering, LK, ed., 2000 *Red Book: Report of the Committee on Infectious Diseases,* 25th ed. Elk Grove, Ill.: American Academy of Pediatrics, 2000.

Dajani AS, Tauber KA, Wilson W, et al. Prevention of bacterial endocarditis: Recommendations by the American Heart Association. *Circulation* 96:358–66, 1997.

Hathorn JW. Critical appraisal of antimicrobials for prevention of infections in immunocompromised hosts. *Hematol Oncol Clin North Am* 7:1051–99, 1993.

Hughes WT. Recent advances in the prevention of *pneumocytis carinii* pneumonia. *Adv Pediatr Infect Dis* 11:163–80, 1996.

Madge P, Paton JY, McColl JH, Mackie PL. Prospective controlled study of four infection control procedures to prevent nosocomial infection with respiratory syncytial virus. *Lancet* 340:1079–83, 1992.

Working Party of the British Committee for Standards in Hematology. Clinical Hematology Task Force: Guidelines for the prevention and treatment of infections in patients with an absent or dysfunctional spleen. *Br Med J* 312:430, 1996.

2

Immunization

Caroline Hastings, M.D.

The aggressive therapies that children with cancer receive result in profound immune suppression. Experience with vaccine administration in immune-compromised children is limited, though there are considerable data on HIV-infected infants. These data provide reassurance about the low risk of adverse events following immunization. Though a number of studies in children with cancer demonstrate reduced immunogenicity, many of these children may benefit from routine immunizations. The ability to mount an adequate response depends on the timing of the immune suppression, the underlying disease, and the intensity of the therapy. Killed or inactivated vaccines can be administered to all immune-compromised patients, but live virus vaccines should never be given during periods of active immune suppression. Immunization during chemotherapy or radiation therapy should be avoided, as the immunologic response is blunted; however, protective antibody titers may develop if given during breaks in therapy (between cycles) or during periods of less aggressive therapy. When all immunosuppressive therapy is discontinued, an adequate response to immunization usually occurs between 3–12 months later.

Children immunized before or during therapy may lose or never have attained protective antibody titers. Specific serum titers should be determined at diagnosis, postimmunization, and off therapy to assess the immune response and guide management of future exposures and further immunizations. The recommendations that follow are based on a review of the literature of immunization in immune-compromised hosts, a number of clinical trials of immunization in children with cancer, and guidelines for immunization of immune-suppressed children from the Centers for Disease Control Immunization Practices Advisory Committee (ACIP) and the American Academy of Pediatrics (AAP).

Table 2.1.

Active Immunization of the Child with Cancer on Chemotherapy

Vaccine	Recommendation
DTaP	Per routine childhood schedule (routine boosters can be deferred)
Polio	IPV only, per routine childhood schedule
MMR	Contraindicated
Pneumococcus	PCV, 23PS vaccines per routine childhood schedule
Meningococcus	Should be given to asplenic children
Hib	Per routine childhood schedule
HBV	Per routine childhood schedule; recommended in previously unimmunized children likely to receive blood products
Influenza	Seasonally
Varicella	Consider in children with ALL in remission 1 year

Note: DTaP, Diphtheria tetanus, acellular pertussis; IPV, inactivated killed polio vaccine; MMR, measles, mumps, rubella; PCV, pneumoccal conjugate vaccine; 23PS, 23 valent polysaccharide; Hib, Hemophilus influenzae type B; HBV, hepatitis B virus.

I. **ACTIVE IMMUNIZATION OF CHILDREN ON CHEMOTHERAPY (Table 2.1)**

    A. Immunization against bacterial infection

        1. DTaP (Diphtheria, tetanus, acellular pertussis)

            a. Few infections with these organisms are seen, probably due to some protection from earlier immunizations and herd immunity. Several studies report adequate responses to primary and booster DTaP immunizations given during chemotherapy. Children receiving more aggressive therapies may be less likely to respond as well as those receiving standard therapies.

            b. Recommendation

               Children on maintenance therapy should receive DTaP immunizations at scheduled times. If therapy is short in duration or to be discontinued shortly after the DTaP is due, delay the immunization until the patient is off therapy. DTaP titers may fall during active therapy; therefore, a booster dose of DTaP (dT for children over 7 years of age) is recommended at 3–12 months after completion of therapy.

        2. Polysaccharide vaccines: PCV (Pneumococcal conjugate vaccine) and 23PS (23 valent polysaccharide

pneumococcal vaccine), Hib (*Hemophilus influenzae* type B), meningococcal vaccine

a. Children who are receiving chemotherapy or are asplenic (surgical or radiation induced) are at increased risk of infection with polysaccharide encapsulated pathogens, especially during the first 4 years of life. An increased incidence of *Streptococcus pneumoniae* and *Hemophilus influenzae* is seen in children with acute lymphocytic leukemia (ALL) and in splenectomized patients with Hodgkin disease. Though less frequent, meningococcal disease has been reported in such patients.

b. Several studies have documented an adequate response to the pneumococcal polysaccharide and *H. influenza* vaccines in patients with acute leukemia, Hodgkin disease, and solid tumors. The new pneumococcal vaccine, PCV, has not been formally tested in this population. Approximately 50% to 85% of children with leukemia and 45% of children with solid tumors have a significant antibody response after receiving Hib PRP-D. The response is greatest in children immunized in the first 12 months of therapy for leukemia with antibody levels declining during continued therapy. In Hodgkin disease, the antibody response is only minimally impaired if the vaccine is given before initiation of therapy, yet dramatically impaired if chemotherapy is begun within 10 days of immunization. Responses to polysaccharide vaccines may not be normal for as long as 4 years after treatment in children with Hodgkin disease.

c. Recommendation
   Immunization with the pneumococcal, meningococcal, and Hib conjugate vaccines is recommended by the ACIP and AAP for all immune-compromised patients. However, there is a paucity of data to support immunization against meningococcus in children with cancer receiving chemotherapy. Unimmunized children with ALL or solid tumors should receive Hib and PCV during maintenance therapy per the routine childhood schedule. Immunization with PCV is followed by at

least 1 dose of 23PS (23 valent polysaccharide) vaccine as per the AAP guidelines. If possible, patients with Hodgkin disease should be immunized at least 7–10 days before the initiation of therapy and be given boosters of pneumococcal and Hib vaccines at 3–5 years after completion of chemotherapy. Patients with surgical or functional asplenia (due to radiation) also should be given the meningococcal vaccine in the pretreatment period with a booster 2–3 years later. After completion of therapy, boosters for pneumococcus and meningococcus should be given every 5–6 years, as recommended for high-risk adults. For children with ALL or solid tumors who receive Hib during therapy, a booster should be given 1 year after completion of therapy.

B. Immunization against viral infection
   1. Measles, Mumps, Rubella (MMR)
      a. The safety of the MMR vaccine in immune-compromised hosts has been a concern since the death of a patient who received it while on therapy more than 30 years ago! A further attenuated measles vaccine has been studied in a small group of children with leukemia. Though safe, the patients had a suboptimal and short lasting antibody response.
      b. Recommendation
         MMR is contraindicated for any child with cancer currently undergoing therapy. Primary immunization or re-immunization is recommended at 1 year after completion of therapy, then once every 10 years. Children who have received less aggressive therapies may receive this vaccine as soon as 3 months after completion of therapy.
   2. Polio (IPV, OPV)
      a. Inactivated killed polio vaccine (IPV) may be safely given during therapy and is reasonably immunogenic. The oral polio vaccine (OPV) is contraindicated in immune-compromised hosts due to the increased frequency of vaccine-associated poliomyelitis in these patients.

    b. Recommendation

       IPV can be safely given at appropriate times for patients receiving the primary series. Partially or unimmunized children can receive IPV or OPV at 1 year off therapy. Household contacts should not receive OPV.

3. Hepatitis B (HBV)

    a. Pediatric oncology patients are at risk for blood-borne infections due to numerous invasive procedures including venous access and frequent transfusion of blood products. Additionally, children with cancer have an increased risk of becoming chronic HBsAg carriers. Children with cancer have an impaired, yet adequate, serologic response to HBV. The protective titer of antibody after 3 doses of vaccine is reached in 67–75% of children receiving chemotherapy for solid tumors and hematologic malignancies. Seroconversion rates are even higher after 4 doses of HBV and may be dosage dependent.

    b. Recommendation

       The administration of HBV at 0-, 1-, and 6-month intervals is recommended for previously unimmunized children on therapy. Titers should be obtained after immunization to ascertain the adequacy of response, the possible need for a fourth dose, and provide information in case of exposure with regards to passive immunization.

4. Hepatitis A (HAV)

    a. HAV has not been formally studied in children with cancer. In the United States, infection with hepatitis A in this population is not problematic. The HAV vaccine can be given safely to immune-compromised patients, though the response may be sub optimal and should be assessed by titer.

    b. Recommendation

       HAV vaccine is not routinely recommended unless the patient is felt to be at risk (endemic area, travel).

5. Influenza vaccine

    a. The safety of inactivated influenza vaccine in cancer patients is well established, yet efficacy data are minimal and controversial. Studies of immunization in children and adults with cancer on therapy found significant impairment of antibody response. However, several reports in children who received the vaccine while on chemotherapy demonstrated a protective antibody level and lower attack rate.

b. Recommendation

Influenza vaccine is recommended by ACIP for all children during periods of active immune suppression (on therapy and up to 1 year off therapy) before each flu season. It is recognized that this is not general practice due to incomplete data. It can be given safely to immune-compromised patients over the age of 6 months. For optimal immunogenicity, 2 doses should be given, 4 weeks apart, irrespective of age. Annual immunization is recommended because of declining immunity and potential for antigen change in the vaccine strain. The optimal time to immunize children is between cycles of chemotherapy and when the absolute neutrophil and lymphocyte counts are above 1,000 cells/mL.

6. Varicella vaccine

a. The use of the varicella vaccine in children with ALL in remission should be considered because the risk of natural varicella outweighs the risk from the attenuated vaccine virus. Though shown to be safe and effective in this population, the varicella vaccine has not been licensed for use in children with malignancies. It may be used on a compassionate basis for children with ALL in remission. Studies show that 85% of children with ALL in maintenance therapy have serologic evidence of an immune response after receiving 1 dose and over 90% after 2 doses, independent of whether chemotherapy is withheld. In children in which chemotherapy was withheld for 1–2 weeks before and after immunization, no effect was seen on rate of relapse.

b. Immune-compromised children have a higher incidence of vaccine associated varicella than healthy children ($\leq$40% versus <5%); however, the attack rate is much lower than with exposure to wild type varicella. Additionally, the vaccine-associated illness is usually an extremely mild, often subclinical course. Overall, the vaccine is felt to be more than 80% effective in preventing clinical varicella in children with ALL and is effective in preventing severe varicella in this high-risk population. There are no published data on its use in children with nonhematologic malignancies, though studies are ongoing. Current data indicate that this immunity does not wane over time. An added benefit is that the vaccine provides a protective effect against zoster and, with a booster, reduces the risk from 15% to 3%.

c. Recommendation

i. Varicella vaccine is recommended for all susceptible children with ALL in maintenance, 12 months after documented remission. A first dose confers immunity and a second dose, given 3 months later, boosts the immunity and gives added protection against zoster. Varicella titers should be checked several months after the second dose to determine if seroconversion has occurred and what steps may be necessary if an exposure should occur.

ii. Chemotherapy should be interrupted for 1 week before and 1 week after receiving the first dose of the vaccine and timed such that it is not given within 1 week of the steroid pulse. It is not necessary to interrupt therapy for the second injection. The absolute lymphocyte count should be at least 700 cells/mL at the time of immunization.

iii. Due to the possibility of rash-associated transmission of the virus to other immune-compromised children, care should be taken to not have children in the oncology clinic at 4–5 weeks after the vaccine. Children who develop vaccine-induced varicella tend to have mild clinical courses (<100 lesions, no systemic symptoms). These children typically are treated with oral acyclovir and watched closely. The attenuated vaccine virus

is sensitive to acyclovir, but acyclovir does not
appear to interfere with the development of
an appropriate immune response. If systemic
symptoms appear or the child develops >100
lesions, the child should be hospitalized and
receive intravenous acyclovir.
iv. There are currently no recommendations for
the varicella vaccine in children with solid
tumors.

II. ACTIVE IMMUNIZATION OF CHILDREN OFF CHEMOTHERAPY

The duration and severity of immune dysfunction following
cessation of chemotherapy is not known. Preliminary studies suggest that immune recovery, both humoral and cellular, recover
slowly and at variable rates dependent on the disease, type of
therapy, and timing from the end of therapy. Abnormalities in children with ALL and Hodgkin disease may be more pronounced and
last longer than in children with solid tumors. Some recovery is
evident in the majority of children 3–12 months from the end of
therapy.

A. Recommendation
DTaP, IPV, MMR, Hib, PCV (and 23PS), meningococcal,
HBV, and varicella vaccines require boosters. These killed
vaccines (or boosters) may be resumed per schedule
3–12 months after completion of therapy. Live virus vaccines (MMR) may be given 3–12 months after cessation of
therapy. Titers may need to be checked to guide which vaccines are needed.

III. PASSIVE IMMUNIZATION (Table 2.2)

The use of passive immunization is well established for certain pathogens including measles, hepatitis A, hepatitis B, varicella,
and tuberculosis. Due to possible loss of immunity while receiving
chemotherapy and the potential for exposure, it is worthwhile to
check yearly titers. The recommendations that follow are per the
guidelines of the AAP.

A. Measles
1. Immune-compromised patients who are exposed to
measles should receive immune globulin prophylaxis,

Table 2.2.
Passive Immunization and Chemoprophylaxis of the Child with
Cancer on Chemotherapy

Vaccine	Recommendation
Hepatitis A	Immune globulin 0.02 mL/kg IM (maximum dose 2 mL), within 14 days of exposure. Good personal hygiene and hand washing.
Hepatitis B	Previously unvaccinated children: HBIG 0.06 mL/kg IM (maximum dose 5 mL). Start first of 3 doses of HBV vaccine series.
	Previously vaccinated children (known nonresponder or unknown status): HBIG 0.06 mL/kg IM and HBV vaccine.
	HBIG should be given within 24 hours of exposure and vaccine series initiated within 7 days.
	Previously vaccinated children with positive titer: No prophylaxis
Measles	Immune globulin 0.5 mL/kg IM (maximum 15 mL) within 6 days of exposure, regardless of prior immunization status.
Varicella	VZIG 1 vial/10 kg IM (maximum 5 vials) within 48 hours of exposure for maximal effect up to 96 hours post exposure.
Tuberculosis	Isoniazid (INH) 10 mg/kg/day orally (maximum 300 mg/day) for 12 months. For noncompliance, INH by DOT 20–30 mg/kg/day, twice weekly (maximum 900 mg/day) preferably after 1 month of daily therapy.

Note: HBIG, hepatitis B immune globulin; HBV, hepatitis B virus; VZIG, varicella zoster immune globulin; DOT, directly observed therapy.

even if previously immunized. The efficacy of immune globulin within 6 days of exposure in preventing serious complications in patients with cancer is not clear but is likely to be beneficial.

2. Recommendation

Immune globulin 0.5 mL/kg IM (maximum dose 15 mL) should be given within 6 days of exposure to measles. (Note that this dose is higher than that recommended for immune competent individuals.) Combined prophylaxis with a live virus vaccine is contraindicated in immune compromised children, but recommended in immune-competent contacts that may have been exposed (siblings, household, or school contacts).

B. Hepatitis B

1. Administration of hepatitis B immune globulin (HBIG) effectively prevents hepatitis B for patients with a percutaneous or mucosal exposure or for a household contact with a chronic HBsAg carrier. Postexposure vaccination is highly effective when combined with passive immunization in the prevention of disease,

especially if the vaccine begins within 7 days of exposure. HBsAg titers should be checked yearly to determine the patient's risk and need for combined prophylaxis.

2. Recommendation
    Combined prophylaxis with HBIG and HBV is recommended in the unvaccinated child, or in the child with a documented negative titer despite previous vaccination. For unvaccinated children, the dose of HBIG is 0.06 mL/kg IM, maximum dose 5 mL, to be given within 24 hours of exposure. In vaccinated children with either unknown or negative titers, HBIG should be given (0.06 mL/kg). In the child with a documented positive titer, HBIG is not indicated.

C. Hepatitis A
    1. Hepatitis A immune globulin can prevent clinical disease resulting from HAV in exposed susceptible individuals when given within 14 days of exposure. If ongoing exposure to HAV is likely, the inactivated hepatitis A vaccine is indicated for combined prophylaxis in children over age 2 years. However, the expected immune response may not be obtained.
    2. Recommendation
        The dose of hepatitis A immune globulin is 0.02 mL/kg IM (maximum dose 2 mL) as soon as possible after the exposure and within 14 days. Combined prophylaxis with the hepatitis A vaccine may be indicated for high-risk individuals with ongoing exposure.

D. Varicella
    1. Exposure to varicella is defined as a continuing household exposure to someone with active varicella, or having been in the same room with an individual for at least 1 hour who is in the contagious state 1–2 days before eruption and 5 days after the eruption of vesicles. Varicella Zoster immune globulin (VZIG) is highly effective in preventing primary varicella. The incubation period is prolonged by 7 days when VZIG is administered; thereby, extending the isolation period from day 10 to day 28 after exposure. No data are available on the possible role of acyclovir in the prevention of varicella after exposure.

2. Recommendation
Immune-compromised children with an exposure to varicella and who have unknown or documented negative titers should receive VZIG 1 vial/10 kg IM (maximum dose 5 vials) within 96 hours of exposure. Children who have been previously vaccinated and have documented positive titers do not need to receive VZIG with exposures. Postexposure prophylaxis is recommended only for siblings and household contacts.

E. Tuberculosis
1. Children who are exposed to a potentially infectious case of tuberculosis should undergo tuberculosis skin testing (PPD with appropriate controls) and have a chest roentgenogram. However, children who are immune suppressed may be anergic and negative skin tests do not indicate lack of disease.
2. Recommendation
Prophylactic Isoniazid (INH) 10 mg/kg/day orally (maximum dose 300 mg/day) should be given for 12 months to immune-compromised patients with a significant exposure to tuberculosis, irrespective of skin test findings.

IV. IMMUNIZATION OF SIBLINGS OF CHILDREN WITH CANCER

In general, siblings should continue to receive all their immunizations as per the guidelines of the AAP.

The inactivated poliovirus vaccine (IPV) is now recommended in lieu of OPV for all children to eliminate the risk of vaccine-associated paralytic poliomyelitis. This new recommendation also decreases the risk of exposure to this live virus vaccine for immune-compromised individuals. If OPV is inadvertently given to a sibling or household contact, close contact between the patient and vaccine recipient should be avoided for 4–6 weeks. Specifically, frequent hand washing should be practiced.

Varicella vaccine is recommended for siblings over the age of 12 months. Transmission of vaccine type varicella from healthy children to immune-compromised siblings has not been documented. Additionally, transmission of the virus has only been known to occur when the vaccinee develops a rash (incubation time 1 month), which occurs in less than 5% of immune-competent children. The vaccine type infection is not spread via respiratory secretions but by direct contact with skin lesions. The transmission rate is less than one-fourth that of the wild type virus.

Influenza vaccine is recommended for family members to reduce possible exposure to the immune-compromised child.

Bibliography

Ambrosino DM, Molrine DC. Critical appraisal of immunization strategies for prevention of infection in the compromised host. In: The immunocompromised host II. *Hematol Clin N Am* 7(5):1027–51, 1993.

American Academy of Pediatrics. *Red Book, 2000.* Report of the Committee on Infectious Diseases, 25th edition.

Bernini JC, Mustafa MM, Winick NJ, et al. Evaluation of attenuated live virus measles vaccine in children with cancer. [Abstr] Proceedings of ASCO 13:438, 1994.

Gershon AA, LaRussa P, Steinberg S, et al. The protective effect of immunologic boosting against zoster: An analysis in leukemic children who were vaccinated against chickenpox. *J Infect Dis* 173:450–53, 1996.

Gross PA, Gould AL, Brown AE. Effect of cancer chemotherapy on the immune response to influenza virus vaccine. Review of published studies. *Rev Infect Dis* 7:613–18, 1985.

Hovi L, Valle M, Siimes M, et al. Impaired response to hepatitis B vaccine in children receiving anticancer chemotherapy. *Pediatr Infect Dis J* 14:931–35, 1995.

LaRussa P, Steinberg S, Gershon AA. Varicella vaccine for immunocompromised children: Results of collaborative studies in the United States and Canada. *J Infect Dis* 174 (Suppl. 3):S320–23, 1996.

McFarland E. Immunizations for the immunocompromised children. *Pediatr Ann* Aug; 28(8):487–96, 1999.

Meral A, Sevihir B, Gunay U. Efficacy of immunization against hepatitis B virus infection in children with cancer. *Med Pediatr Oncol* 35:47–51, 2000.

Shenep JL, Feldman S, Gigliotti F, et al. Response of immunocompromised children with solid tumors to a conjugate vaccine for *Haemophilus influenza* type b. *J Pediatr* 125:581–84, 1994.

3

The Management of Fever and Neutropenia

Lawrence J. Wolff, M.D., Arnold J. Altman, M.D., Roger L. Berkow, M.D., and F. Leonard Johnson, M.D.

In the neutropenic child with cancer, the usual signs and symptoms of infection are sometimes absent. A temperature of 38.3°C (101°F) or 38°C (100.4°F) sustained for at least 1 hour indicates infection until proven otherwise. A careful physical examination is important because untreated infection will spread rapidly. Start antibiotic therapy promptly, and consider all organisms potentially pathogenic. Choose antibiotics by the microbial prevalence and institutional antibiotic sensitivity patterns with consideration of the presence or absence of a central venous line (CVL) and symptoms and signs demonstrated by the patient.

I. DEFINITIONS

A. Fever

Fever is one of the most common and obvious signs suggestive of infection. Fever is defined as a single *oral* temperature (or its axillary or tympanic equivalent) >38.3°C (101°F) or ≥38.0°C (100.4°F) taken on two occasions at least 1 hour apart. Do not take rectal temperatures in patients with neutropenia.

B. Neutropenia

Severe neutropenia is defined as an absolute neutrophil count (ANC) <200/μL [total leukocyte count x (% neutrophils + % band cells)]; moderate neutropenia is 200–500/μL; mild neutropenia is 500–1000/μL. The risk for a serious infection in a child being treated for cancer is directly related to the degree and duration of neutropenia. The risk for bacteremia/septicemia escalates when the ANC is <200/μL, while that for serious infections (including pneumonitis, cellulitis, and abscess) begins to increase when the ANC falls below 500/μL. Those patients whose course of neutropenia is brief (ANC ≥500/μL, within 7 days after fever) have a better clinical response than those who remain neutropenic (ANC ≤500/μL) more than 7 days.

C. Indicators of marrow recovery
An increase in circulating monocytes, an increase in platelet count, and the presence of young myeloid precursors, toxic granules, and Döhle bodies imply marrow recovery.

II. EVALUATION OF THE FEBRILE NEUTROPENIC CHILD WITH CANCER

A. History and physical examination
The evaluation of the febrile child with cancer should be thorough but expeditious. If the patient is neutropenic, the usual signs of the inflammatory process may be absent or subdued. Findings such as minimal discharge, faint tenderness, or redness should be regarded as significant. Pay special attention to the skin, nose, pharynx, and perineal and perirectal areas. Palpate over sinuses and evaluate the range of motion in all joints. The identification of an infection in specific areas such as the perirectum, skin, or mouth narrows the spectrum of likely infecting microorganisms.

B. Laboratory evaluation
Laboratory evaluation should include a complete blood count, urinalysis, and generous amounts of blood drawn from all venous access catheter ports and one or two peripheral sites for culture. A catheter site that is inflamed or draining should be cultured. Any suspicious skin lesion, watery blister, or prominent erythema should be aspirated, stained, and cultured for bacteria, fungi, or viruses as appropriate. If periodontal infection is suspected, the patient should be examined by a pediatric dentist and appropriate radiographs and tissue samples obtained. Patients with tenderness over a sinus(es) should have diagnostic imaging studies. A febrile, neutropenic child with cancer who demonstrates mental confusion or central nervous system dysfunction should have a lumbar puncture.

Examine diarrheal stools for bacterial, protozoal, and viral agents as well as *Clostridium difficile* toxin. Culture the urine if there are signs of urinary tract infection, the urinalysis is abnormal, or a urinary catheter is in place. Chest radiographs are indicated if there are clinical symptoms or signs including chest pain, tachypnea, or decreased pulse oximetry suggesting pulmonary disease.

C. Other studies
  1. Acute phase reactants
     Although available to some only as research tools, C-reactive protein and interleukin-6 may give a rapid indication of bacterial or fungal infection.
  2. Imaging
     With prolonged fever, CT scan and/or MRI of the sinuses, chest, abdomen, or pelvis may be useful to locate sites of infection.
  3. Special studies
     The polymerase chain reaction (PCR) and enzyme-linked immunosorbent assay (ELISA) may be helpful in the early diagnosis of invasive bacterial or fungal disease. *Candida* enolase antigenemia can also detect invasive fungal disease.

D. Follow-up monitoring
   Re-examine and re-evaluate patients carefully at least once a day. Obtain blood cultures at least daily while the patient is febrile. Repeat urine, stool, and tissue cultures, obtain diagnostic imaging, and consultation as clinically indicated.

III. MANAGEMENT OF FEVER WITH SEVERE NEUTROPENIA

A. At onset with unknown pathogen
   After diagnostic evaluation, commence empiric broad-spectrum antibiotic coverage promptly (see section IVB). If a central venous catheter is in place, rotate antibiotics infusions to include all ports and lumens. Consider modification of a "standard" selected regimen as follows:
  1. If a patient has a history of penicillin allergy, avoid semisynthetic penicillins and use cephalosporins, an aminoglycoside, or a carbapenem.
  2. If the patient has recently received high-dose cytarabine and has mucositis, *Viridans streptococcus* is highly suspect and vancomycin should be started.

3. If perianal tenderness is present, add anaerobic therapy (e.g., Metronidazole or clindamycin).
4. If peritonitis or typhlitis is suspected, begin vancomycin to cover *Clostridia species*.
5. If a central venous catheter (CVC) is suspected as the source of infection, begin vancomycin, but discontinue its use after 72 hours if cultures are negative for *Staphylococcus epidermidis* and methicillin-resistant *S. aureus* (MRSA).
6. If a pulmonary infiltrate is present and persists after 48 hours with a continued fever, consider the merits of empiric therapy versus bronchial brushings or bronchoalveolar lavage (BAL). If this is not diagnostic, then consider needle or open lung biopsy.
   a. Begin empiric therapy for *Pneumocystis* with trimethoprim-sulfamethoxazole and for *Legionella* or Mycoplasma with erythromycin.
   b. If there is disease progression after 2 days of empiric therapy, then brushings, BAL, needle, or open lung biopsy is strongly indicated. If this is not possible, add empiric antifungal therapy.

B. When a specific pathogen is not identified on culture
   1. Continue antibiotic coverage until the patient is afebrile for 24 hours, and there is evidence of marrow recovery (increase in absolute phagocyte or neutrophil count for 1 or more days).
   2. If fever and granulocytopenia persist for about 3 or more days, and all diagnostic procedures remain negative
      a. Continue broad-spectrum antibiotics and add antifungal therapy if not already included.
      b. Continue daily blood cultures, thorough physical examinations, and repeated histories for clues.
      c. Consider brain, perineal, perianal, and pelvic abscess, as well as pseudomembranous colitis, viral infection. Do not overlook the possibility of recurrent malignancy; use diagnostic imaging as indicated.
      d. Stop antibiotics after 14 days and repeat cultures daily and monitor the patient several times daily.

3. Recurrence of fever demands prompt rehospitalization, complete diagnostic evaluation, and aggressive antimicrobial therapy (bacterial, fungal).

C. When a specific pathogen is identified on culture
1. Staphylococci and streptococci (including *Viridans streptococcus*) are the most frequent pathogens.
2. Organisms seen less frequently in immunocompromised patients are: *Pseudomonas aeruginosa, Escherichia coli, Klebsiella* species, *Hemophilus influenzae, Neisseria* species, *Enterococcus faecalis, Corynebacterium* species, *Bacillus* species, *Listeria monocytogenes,* as well as anaerobic cocci and bacilli. Fungal isolates include *candida, aspergillus,* and *fusarium.*
3. Make certain that the optimal agent or agents are being used for the isolated organism(s) when cultures and sensitivity are known, but continue empiric broad-spectrum coverage until the patient is afebrile and there is evidence of marrow recovery (increases in absolute monocyte, absolute neutrophil, and platelet counts for 2 consecutive days). Then antibiotics may be tailored to the specific infectious agent.
4. Continue antibiotic therapy for a minimum of 10 days total (14 days if an indwelling catheter is present).

D. When a fungal infection is suspected or documented
1. Presume fungal infection when fever and neutropenia persist after 3–7 days of empiric broad-spectrum antibiotics.
2. Predisposing factors leading to fungal infections include prolonged hospitalization, prolonged granulocytopenia, prolonged use of broad-spectrum antibiotics, use of indwelling catheters, damaged mucosal barriers, and hyperalimentation.
3. The most common pathogens are *candida* species and *aspergillus; fusarium, trichosporon,* and *Mucor* are becoming more common.
4. Antifungal agents and doses are shown in Table 3.1.

E. When a viral infection is suspected or documented
1. For documented infection with herpes simplex, treat with acyclovir 750 mg/m^2/day divided q8h intravenous (IV).

Table 3.1.

Antifungal Agents and Doses

Drug	Route	Dose
Amphotericin B (Fungizone)	IV	Test dose 0.1 mg/kg to a maximum dose of 1 mg over 1 hr; if tolerated, may use 0.4 mg/kg and increase to 1 mg/kg/d
Amphotericin B lipid complex (Abelcet)	IV	5 mg/kg/d
Amphotericin B liposomal (Ambisone)	IV	3–5 mg/kg/d
Amphotericin B colloidal dispersion (Amphotec)	IV	3–5 mg/kg/d
Flucytosine	PO	50–150 mg/kg/d divided every 6 hr
Fluconazole	IV, PO	3–12 mg/kg/d (maximum dose 600 mg/d)
Itraconazole	IV, PO	3–10 mg/kg/d, has been used, but dose yet to be established
Voriconazole	IV, PO	6 mg/kg q 12h, IV for 1st 24h and then 4 mg/kg q 12h. Oral dose: >40 kg, 200 mg b.i.d., may increase to 300 mg b.i.d., <40 kg 100 mg b.i.d., may increase to 150 mg b.i.d.
Caspofungin	IV	35–70 mg/d. IV. Not adequately studied in patients <18 years old

2. For documented infection with varicella zoster, treat with acyclovir 1,500 mg/m^2/day divided q8h IV until no new lesions appear. Ensure adequate hydration.

3. For documented infection with cytomegalovirus (CMV), treat with ganciclovir 10 mg/kg/day divided q12h IV plus CMV immune globulin.

F. For documented or suspected infection with *Pneumocystis carinii*

1. Treat with trimethoprim-sulfamethoxazole (TMP/SMX): TMP 15–20 mg/kg/day and SMX 75–100 mg/kg/day divided q8–12h for at least 14 days PO or IV.

2. If TMP/SMX is not tolerated, treat with pentamidine 4 mg/kg/day IV for at least 14 days or TMP 5 mg/kg PO q6h plus dapsone 100 mg/day PO for 21 days.

G. For documented toxoplasmosis

Treat with pyrimethamine loading dose 1 mg/kg/twice daily po for 1–3 days, then 1 mg/kg/day for 4 weeks plus either sulfadiazine or trisulfapyrimidines 100 mg/kg/day PO in 3–4 divided doses for 4 weeks.

IV. ANTIBIOTICS

A. The choice of antibiotics (antimicrobials) to be used at an institution should be determined by the needs of the patient and the local patterns of infection and resistance to antibiotics. The underlying disease, the chemotherapy being used, the prophylactic antimicrobials taken, and the prevalent microorganisms in the hospital, community, and geographical area are factors that affect the empirical choice of initial antimicrobials. The presence of a central venous access device, recent invasive procedures (e.g., bone marrow aspirate/biopsy, lumbar puncture, endoscopy), drug allergy, renal or hepatic dysfunction, and other drugs that may affect hearing and kidney or liver function will influence the choice of antimicrobial.

B. Many combinations of antimicrobials are effective. Prevailing community microorganisms and their antibiotic sensitivity will direct the choices and combinations of antibiotics. The patient with severe mucositis or with a recently diagnosed neoplasm of the gastrointestinal or genitourinary tract should receive coverage for anaerobic bacteria. Various combinations that are used are listed below. For help in making a selection, remember that drug resistance is a major problem and refrain from using vancomycin initially unless the clinical situation suggests its use. (See Table 3.2.)

   1. Aminoglycoside plus an antipseudomonal β-lactam drug
      a. Advantages
         i.   Good gram-negative coverage
         ii. Synergism against some gram-negative bacilli
         iii. Minimal emergence of resistance
         iv. Some anaerobic activity
      b. Disadvantages
         i.   Lack of activity against some gram-positive bacteria
         ii. Nephrotoxicity and ototoxicity
         iii. Hypokalemia
         iv. Anaerobic coverage not optimal

Table 3.2.
Frequently Used Antibiotics for Fever and Neutropenia

Drug	Dose	Route	Schedule
Aminoglycosides			
Amikacin	15 mg/kg/day	IV	Divided q8h
Gentamicin	6.0–7.5 mg/kg/day	IV	Divided q8h
Tobramycin	6.0–7.5 mg/kg/day	IV	Divided q8h
β-Lactam drugs			
Antipseudomonal, semisynthetic penicillins			
Azlocillin	300 mg/kg/day (maximum 24 g/day)	IV	Divided q4–6h
Mezlocillin	300 mg/kg/day (maximum 24 g/day)	IV	Divided q4–6h
Piperacillin	300 mg/kg/day (maximum 24 g/day)	IV	Divided q4–6h
Piperacillin/Tazobactan	300 mg/kg/d of Piperacillin component	IV	Divided q6h
Ticarcillin	300 mg/kg/d (maximum 24 g/day)	IV	Divided q4–6h
Carbenicillin	500 mg/kg/day	IV	Divided q4–6h
Cephalosporins			
Ceftazidime	100–150 mg/kg/day	IV	Divided q8h
Cefazolin	50–100 mg/kg/day (maximum 6 g/day)	IV	Divided q8h
Cefepime	50 mg/kg per dose (maximum 2 g)	IV	q8h
Carbapenem			
Imipenem/Cilastatin	50 mg/kg/day (maximum 4 g/day)	IV	Divided q6–8h
Meropenem	60–120 mg/kg/day (maximum dose 6 g/day)	IV	Divided q8h
Penicillinase-resistant penicillin			
Nafcillin	100–200 mg/kg/day	IV	Divided q4–8h
Other			
Vancomycin	40 mg/kg/day (maximum 2 g/day)	IV	Divided q6–8h
Anaerobic coverage			
Clindamycin	40 mg/kg/day	IV	Divided q6–8h
Metronidazole	30 mg/kg/day (loading dose initially 15 mg/kg)	IV	Divided q6h

    v. Necessity of monitoring serum aminoglycoside
        levels
2. Combination of two β-lactam drugs
    a. Advantages
        i.   Good gram-negative coverage
        ii. Synergism against some gram-negative bac-
             teria
        iii. Low toxicity without need to monitor drug
             levels
    b. Disadvantages
        i.   Possible antagonism with some combinations
        ii. Anaerobic coverage not optimal
        iii. Lack of activity against some gram-positive
             bacteria
        iv. High cost
3. Penicillinase-resistant penicillin or vancomycin plus
    aminoglycoside and β-lactam drug
    a. Advantages
        i.   Broad gram-positive effectiveness
        ii. Good gram-negative coverage
        iii. Synergism against gram-negative bacteria
        iv. Minimal emergence of resistance
        v.   Some anaerobic activity
    b. Disadvantages
        i.   Combination without vancomycin has subop-
             timal effectiveness against *S. epidermidis.*
        ii. Nephrotoxicity and ototoxicity, especially in
             conjunction with vancomycin
        iii. Hypokalemia
        iv. Anaerobic coverage not optimal
        v.   Necessity of monitoring serum aminoglycoside
             and vancomycin levels.
        vi. High cost, especially with vancomycin
4. Monotherapy with third- or fourth-generation cephalo-
    sporin or carbapenem
    a. Advantages
        i.   Less toxic than other combinations
        ii. Fairly good broad-spectrum activity against
             gram-positive, gram-negative, and anaerobic
             bacteria (carbapenems)

   b. Disadvantages
       i.   Insufficient gram-positive and anaerobic effec-
            tiveness (ceftazidime)
       ii. Potential for β-lactam resistance
       iii. Lack of synergistic activity
       iv. Anaerobic coverage not optimal
5. Third-generation cephalosporin plus penicillinase-
    resistant penicillin or vancomycin
    a. Advantage
        Wide antibacterial coverage, including gram-
        positive organisms
    b. Disadvantages
        i.   Combination without vancomycin has subop-
             timal effectiveness against *S. epidermidis*
        ii. Lack of synergism against gram-negative bac-
             teria
        iii. Necessity of monitoring vancomycin levels
        iv. Nephrotoxic and ototoxic with vancomycin
        v.   Expensive

V. MONITORING FOR TOXICITY TO ANTI-INFECTIVE AGENTS

A. Available monitors
    1. Complete blood count (CBC) with differential for
        hematopoietic effect
    2. Serum chemistries for specific effects (e.g., electrolyte
        depletion, hepatic, and renal toxicity)
    3. Serum levels for specific antibiotics
    4. Audiologic testing
    5. Urinalysis for glycosuria, albuminuria, and hematuria
    6. Quantitative urine samples for sodium and potassium
    7. Nucleotide glomerular filtration rate or creatinine
        clearance

B. Specific monitoring
    1. Gentamicin and tobramycin
        a. Check serum creatinine, blood urea nitrogen
            (BUN), and electrolytes every other day to monitor
            renal function. When creatinine rises over baseline,
            monitor renal function daily.
        b. Check peak and trough serum levels of antibiotic
            after 24 hours at a fixed dose.

Table 3.3.
Guidelines for the Desired Serum Concentrations of
Gentamicin and Tobramycin

Concentration	Gentamicin (μg/mL)	Tobramycin (μg/mL)
Peak		
Serious infection	6–8	6–8
Life-threatening infection*	8–10	8–10
Trough		
Serious infection	<1	<1
Life-threatening infection*	1–2	1–2

*Higher peak and trough values have also been suggested.

    c. Modify the dosage or dosage interval according to the guidelines in Table 3.3.
    d. See guidelines for desired serum concentrations in Table 3.3.
  2. Amphotericin B
    a. Monitor serum creatinine, BUN, serum electrolytes, particularly serum sodium, potassium, and magnesium (supplemental K+ almost always necessary), at 1- to 3-day intervals.
    b. With significant persistent abnormality, adjust the frequency of administration to every other day or less frequently.
    c. Infusion of saline for several hours before amphotericin may protect renal function.
    d. Check creatinine clearance or nucleotide glomerular filtration rate as indicated.
  3. Vancomycin
    Monitor serum antibiotic levels. Aim for a peak level of 20–24 μg/mL, and a trough level of 5–10 μg/mL.
  4. Nafcillin
    Monitor liver transaminases.

VI. MANAGEMENT OF FEVER WITHOUT NEUTROPENIA

  A. Evaluation
    1. Detailed history and physical examination
    2. Bacterial cultures

        a.   Obtain blood cultures from a venipuncture site and, for patients with a central venous catheter, from each port of the catheter.

        b.   Obtain cultures of urine and other potential sites of infection as indicated by history and physical examination (e.g., aspiration of cellulitis site or cerebrospinal fluid if meningitis is suspected).

   3.   Imaging studies as indicated by history and physical examination

B.   Therapeutic measures

   1.   When a central venous catheter is not present

        a.   If a specific infection is not documented, continue to examine daily and monitor clinically with daily blood cultures and other relevant laboratory studies but do not start antibiotics. However, if the patient's ANC has increased 2–3 fold above the baseline and there are increased bands or early myeloid precursors, many clinicians would begin IV antibiotics.

        b.   If a specific pathogen is isolated, treat with appropriate antibiotics.

   2.   When a central venous catheter is present

        a.   If only an exit-site infection is suspected, obtain blood cultures from all ports of the catheter, one venipuncture site (if practical), and the exit-site.

            i.   Begin antibiotic therapy with dicloxacillin, 25 mg/kg/day PO divided q6h, or Cephalexin, or amoxicillin/clavulanic acid or start IV antibiotics (see section IV).

           ii.   Re-examine at 24–48 hours.

           iii.   If improved, finish 10-day course of antibiotic therapy

           iv.   If not improved after 48 hours of oral antibiotics, commence therapy with vancomycin 40 mg/kg/day IV divided q8h (maximum 2 g/day) and tobramycin or gentamicin 6–7.5 mg/kg/day IV divided q8h.

           v.   If not improved after 72 hours of parenteral therapy, change antibiotics and consider removing the catheter.

   b. If there is no evidence of local infection, obtain blood cultures from all catheter ports and one venipuncture site. Many physicians would choose to commence parenteral therapy with ceftriaxone 75 mg/kg IV q24h (maximum 2 g/day).

   c. If the cultures are negative and the fever resolves, stop antibiotic therapy after 48 hours.

   d. If the cultures are positive, adjust antibiotic therapy appropriate to sensitivity of the organisms. If cultures remain positive despite 48 hours of appropriate antibiotic therapy, strongly consider removing the central venous line.

   e. If the cultures become negative, complete a 10- to 14-day course of antibiotics and do not remove the catheter.

VII. MANAGEMENT OF FEVER WITH MODERATE NEUTROPENIA

A. Studies show that more than 80% of febrile children with cancer and moderate neutropenia who are carefully chosen as defined below may be managed successfully either as outpatients or hospitalized briefly (12–48 hours) and then followed as outpatients. They should be evaluated carefully as detailed in management of fever without neutropenia (see section VIA1–3) and meet the following criteria:

   1. Be older than 1 year of age.

   2. Have no obvious source of infection (e.g., perirectal abscess, central line tunnel, cellulitis).

   3. Have ANC $\geq 200/\mu L$ and anticipation that it will increase.

   4. Be normotensive.

   5. Have a remission status of their cancer.

   6. Not be a bone marrow transplant recipient.

   7. Have no history of recent surgery.

   8. Have no moderate or severe mucositis.

   9. Have telephone access and transportation and be within approximately 30–40 minutes of a center with expertise in immunocompromised patients.

B. Such patients can receive monotherapy such as ceftazidime, ceftriaxone, cefepime, or one of these agents combined with an aminoglycoside. However, they must be examined and evaluated daily by a physician experienced in caring for immunocompromised children.

Bibliography

Bash RO, Katz JA, Cash JV. Safety and cost effectiveness of early hospital discharge of lower risk children with cancer admitted for fever and neutropenia. *Cancer* 74:189–96, 1994.

Cohen KL, Leamer K, Odom L, et al. Cessation of antibiotics regardless of ANC is safe in children with febrile neutropenia. *J Pediatr Hematol Oncol* 17:325–30, 1995.

Freifeld AG, Pizzo PA. The outpatient management of febrile neutropenia in cancer patients. *Oncology* 10:599–612, 1996.

Hughes WT, Armstrong D, Bodey GP, et al. 2002 guidelines for the use of antimicrobial agents in neutropenic patients with cancer. *Clinical Infectious Diseases* 34:730–51, 2002.

Mustafa MM, Aquino VM, Pappe A, et al. A pilot study of outpatient management of febrile neutropenic children with cancer at low risk of bacteremia. *J Pediatr* 128:847–49, 1996.

Yu LC, Shanneyfelt T, Warrier R, Ode D. The efficacy of ticarcillin-clavulanate and gentamycin as empiric treatment for febrile neutropenic pediatric patients with cancer. *Pediatr Hematol Oncol* 11:181–87, 1994.

4

Blood Component Therapy

Dorothy R. Barnard, M.D., and Zora R. Rogers, M.D.

I. **GENERAL RECOMMENDATIONS FOR BLOOD COMPONENT TRANSFUSION**

A. General risks of transfusions (see Table 4.1)
  1. Hemolytic reactions
     a. Acute, immune: Usually related to mistaken transfusion of ABO-incompatible blood, resulting in acute intravascular hemolysis, shock, chills, fever, dyspnea, chest pain, back pain, headache, disseminated intravascular coagulation, renal failure;
     b. Acute, nonimmune: Related to bacterial contamination of the unit, mechanical damage, heat damage, or administration with a hypotonic solution;
     c. Delayed, immune: Related to antibodies undetectable at time of pretransfusion screening resulting in progressive, otherwise unexplained, fall in hemoglobin 4–14 days after transfusion; may be accompanied by fever, hemoglobinuria, hyperbilirubinemia.
  2. Nonhemolytic reactions
     a. Febrile transfusion reactions: Symptoms related to release of endogenous pyrogens; repeated episodes may require premedication with acetaminophen; antihistamines only effective if associated with hives/allergy; meperidine effective for shaking chills.
     b. Acquired infections
        i. Viral: Cytomegalovirus (CMV), human immunodeficiency virus (HIV), Epstein-Barr virus (EBV), West Nile virus, hepatitis
        ii. Nonviral: Toxoplasmosis, bacteria

Table 4.1.
Complications of Blood Transfusions

Complication	Frequency
Acute hemolytic transfusion reaction	1 per 25,000 RBC units transfused
Delayed hemolytic transfusion reaction	1 per 2,500–9,000 RBC units transfused
RBC alloimmunization	8% of patients transfused with RBC
Febrile reaction	1 per 100 RBC units, higher with platelets
Anaphylaxis	1 per 20,000–50,000 units
Urticaria	1 per 100–300 units
Circulatory overload	1% of transfusions
Death due to transfusion error	1 per 600,000 units

c. Hypotension: ACE inhibitor-related associated with the use of bedside leucopoor filters; anaphylaxis.

d. Iron overload can be found in most patients receiving red cell concentrates during their cancer treatment. The short- and long-term implications of iron overload for children receiving red cell transfusion during cancer treatment are as yet undefined.

e. Immune modulation: Alloimmunization; transfusion-associated immunomodulation-immune suppression, anergy; ameliorated by leucodepletion of transfusion products.

f. Metabolic disturbances: Hyperkalemia, hypernatremia, acidosis, citrate toxicity.

g. Miscellaneous: Allergic reactions, fluid overload, hypothermia, air embolism, post-transfusion purpura, red-eye syndrome.

h. Transfusion-related acute lung injury presents as noncardiogenic pulmonary edema with rapid onset of dyspnea, tachypnea, cyanosis, fever, and hypotension within 4–6 hours of transfusion, usually in already seriously ill patients. Chest x-ray shows bilateral patchy infiltrates without cardiac enlargement. Estimated occurrence is about 1 per 2,000–5,000 transfusions. It is postulated to be induced by immune-mediated reaction of HLA antibodies or other granulocyte leukoagglutins found in donor plasma.

i. Transfusion-associated graft versus host disease (TA-GVHD)

    i. Symptoms are the result of T cell activation (in the transfused product) and include maculopapular rash, fever, diarrhea, hepatitis, and bone marrow hypoplasia. TA-GVHD becomes clinically apparent within 4–30 days after transfusion (median 8 days).

    ii. The diagnosis may be confirmed by demonstration of chimerism of lymphocytes using PCR technology.

    iii. TA-GVHD is resistant to treatment and has a mortality rate of 75–90%.

    iv. This complication can be prevented by irradiation of blood products (see section ID).

B. Precautions to ensure that the correct product is given to the correct patient

1. It is essential that the blood sample taken from a patient for type and screen/cross-match be labeled clearly, checked with the patient's identification, and signed by the phlebotomist as required by health center policy.

2. Before administering blood or blood product, check the physician order, the patient identification, and blood product number and tags.

3. Clerical error and misidentification of patient remain significant transfusion risks potentially leading to hemolytic transfusion reactions. The frequency of deaths related to patients receiving the incorrect blood component is estimated to be at least 30 times greater than the risk of transfusion acquired HIV infection and accounted for 52% of serious transfusion incidents in the SHOT study.

C. Preparation of and indications for leucodepleted products. (See Table 4.2).

1. Definition of leucocyte-depleted product: Total white cell count $<5 \times 10^6$ per transfusion "dose."

2. Leucodepletion decreases recovery of red cell and platelet concentrates but does not affect the function of erythrocytes or platelets.

Table 4.2.
Potential Indications for the Use of Leucodepleted Products

Reduction of risk for/prevention of:*
  Alloimmunization
  CMV (+ other human herpes virus) infection
  Febrile transfusion reactions
  HTLV-1, HTLV-2 infection
  Immunomodulation effect
  Latent virus reactivation
  Postoperative infection
  Post-transfusion thrombocytopenic purpura
  Post-operative infection (controversial)
  Prion disorders (controversial)
  Red cell transfusion associated Yersinia
  Reperfusion injury after cardiac surgery
  Transfusion-associated GVHD**
  Transfusion-related lung injury***

*White cells in transfusion products felt to be responsible for or contributory to disorders listed.
**Not sufficient alone to prevent TA-GVHD.
***Usually secondary to anti-HLA or antigranulocyte antibodies in the donor plasma.

3. Complications related to use of leucodepletion filters: Rarely hypotensive reactions with bedside use of leucodepletion filters, especially in patients receiving angiotensin converting enzyme (ACE) inhibitors, secondary to delay in bradykinin metabolism; not associated with prestorage filtration.

4. Risk of CMV infection decreased to 0.5% with leucofiltration compared with 0.8% with serologic testing of donors and 18% with unscreened, unfiltered products.

5. Prestorage leucocyte-depletion has been adopted by British Transfusion Services and Canadian Blood Services because of the potential advantages including inventory and quality control and greater total reduction in transfusion reactions. The cost-effectiveness of this approach remains unknown.

6. *Not* to be used with granulocyte concentrate transfusions

7. Generally felt not necessary for acellular products such as cryoprecipitate and fresh frozen plasma (will be leucofiltered where prestorage leucofiltration is used).

8. Allergic reactions to platelet transfusion are not decreased by leucofiltration. These may be secondary

to a cytokine known as RANTES (regulated on activation, normal T-cell expressed and secreted) produced by platelets during storage.

9. Indications for CMV "safe" products: (see Table 4.3)

D. Indications for radiation of blood products and effects of radiation on blood products. (See Table 4.4).

1. The dose of viable T cells needed to induce TA-GVHD is approximately 10^4/kg in an immunocompromised host.

2. Irradiation of cellular blood products is currently the only validated method of preventing TA-GVHD. Radiation with a dose of 2,500cGy to the central midplane of the unit with a minimum of 1,500 cGy elsewhere is recommended (1,500 cGy reduces lymphocyte PHA blast transformation by 90%). No lymphocyte response to PHA has been demonstrated in the lymphocytes found in fresh frozen plasma (FFP); therefore, radiation of FFP, cryoprecipitate, or cell free fractionated plasma

Table 4.3.

Indications for CMV "Safe" Products: CMV Seronegative Blood/Leucocyte-reduced

CMV + Patients	CMV − Patients
Receiving chemotherapy or stem cell/marrow transplantation	Receiving aggressive chemotherapy
Leucocyte-reduced products may reduce reactivation	Receiving stem cell/marrow transplant
	Preterm infants
	HIV-infected patients; immunodeficient

Table 4.4.

Potential Indications for the Use of Irradiated Blood Products

Directed donation from a biological relative
Granulocyte transfusions
Donations from HLA-matched donors
Stem cell/marrow transplant
Hodgkin disease and other hematologic malignancies
Immunosuppression from cancer treatment*
Intrauterine transfusion
Exchange transfusion
Congenital cell-mediated immunodeficiency
Extracorporeal membrane oxygenation*

*Controversial

components such as albumin is not indicated. Irradiation of plasma stored unfrozen may be indicated for high-risk patients.

3. The use of third-generation leucopoor filters, whereas not validated to prevent TA-GVHD, may decrease the risk of TA-GVHD by decreasing the number of viable T lymphocytes infused.

4. Photochemical treatment may be effective in decreasing the risk of TA-GVHD, but cannot be used for red cell concentrates.

5. Irradiation does not significantly affect the survival or function of white cells or platelets. Red cell viability may be decreased modestly and levels of plasma potassium are increased in irradiated packed red cell concentrates (PRBC). Storage of PRBC is recommended not to exceed 28 days after radiation.

6. Irradiated blood components are indicated for children under the following circumstances:
    a. Receiving transfusions with shared haplotypes (HLA selected platelet donations, transfusions from first and second degree relatives);
    b. Severe immunodeficiency (congenital);
    c. Acquired T cell defects secondary to disease or treatment (bone marrow/stem cell transplantation: Allogeneic or autologous); single case reports suggest that children receiving markedly immunosuppressive therapy should receive irradiated blood components;
    d. Beginning at least 7 days before harvesting of autologous stem cells and for blood products given from the initiation of the conditioning regime for marrow/stem cell transplantation;
    e. Many institutions transfuse all children with cancer with irradiated blood components for administrative and inventory flexibility.

II. RED CELL TRANSFUSIONS

A. Assessment of anemia
    1. Red blood cell mass should be adequate to maintain oxygen carrying capacity and tissue oxygen delivery—usually hemoglobin >7 g/dl is adequate.

2. Individual variation in tolerance for fatigue, concomitant thrombocytopenia with attendant risk of prolonged bleeding, other health problems (particularly cardiac or pulmonary comorbidities), and patient preference may guide transfusion triggers.

3. Small adult trials suggest that maintaining a higher hemoglobin concentration during chemotherapy results in a better quality of life.

B. Therapeutic approaches to anemia
   1. Transfusion is the simplest and fastest method to correct anemia.
   2. Erythropoietin, 100–300 units/kg/dose via thrice-weekly SC injection will raise hemoglobin by 1–2 g/dl in patients receiving moderately intensive chemotherapy.
   3. Darbepoetin, an analogue of erythropoietin with a longer plasma half-life, 1.5 to 4.5 mcg/kg/dose at 2–4-week intervals may produce the same effect.

C. Red cell transfusion products available
   1. Packed red blood cells unit parameters depend on preservative
      a. CPDA (citrate-phosphate-dextrose-adenine) 250 ml per unit with hematocrit of 65–80%; stored for up to 35 days.
      b. AS (adsol) units have a volume of 350 ml with a hematocrit of 55–60%; stored for up to 42 days.
   2. Double red cell units obtained by pheresis, not usually used in pediatric patients.
   3. Whole blood is rarely available and offers no advantage over packed red cells.
   4. Red cell substitutes, including cell-free hemoglobin solutions, are in advanced clinical trials. All have a short duration of action, 12–24 hours, of limited value to the average pediatric oncology patient.

D. Indications for red cell transfusion
   1. Hemoglobin below 6–7 g/dl with symptoms of anemia such as lassitude, malaise, deceased activity, or irritability transfusion should be considered. Comorbidities must be considered.

   2. Transfusion need not be given routinely if recovery from chemotherapy-induced aplasia is imminent and symptoms are mild.
   3. If invasive procedures are planned, a hemoglobin of 9–10g/dl may minimize perioperative bleeding.
   4. If the patient is concomitantly thrombocytopenic, a hemoglobin of 10 g/dl may minimize the need for platelet transfusion support while prophylaxing against the risk of hemorrhage.

E. Usual transfusion volumes and expected count increment
   1. Transfusion volume should be ordered in mL/kg of recipient weight.
   2. Standard transfusion volume is 10 mL/kg (adult dose 2 units).
      a. CPDA cells should raise hemoglobin by 2.5 g/dl or hematocrit by 8–9%.
      b. AS cells will raise hemoglobin by 2 g/dl or hematocrit by 6–7%.
   3. Maximum transfusion volume generally 15–17 mL/kg over 4 hours.
   4. Hemoglobin <5 g/dl, particularly with congestive heart failure or hypertension, requires small repeated transfusion accompanied by a diuretic.
      a. Safe initial transfusion volume: mL/kg equal to the hemoglobin value given over 4 hours.
      b. The blood bank can use sterile technique to divide a single unit of red cells into smaller aliquots and provide several transfusions from one unit, and thus one donor exposure.
      c. Partial exchange transfusion, either manual or automated, can also isovolemically raise the hemoglobin.

III. PLATELET TRANSFUSIONS

A. Assessment of thrombocytopenia
   1. Platelet transfusion is always indicated for a bleeding patient with thrombocytopenia.
   2. Prophylactic use of platelet products is more controversial. Some indications include:
      a. Platelet count alone is a poor indicator of bleeding risk.

Table 4.5.
Platelet Transfusion Triggers in Children with Cancer

Clinical Status	Platelet Count per mm^3	Intervention
Well	>5,000–7,000	Observe for bleeding
Febrile, stable	<10,000	Transfusion
Mucosal bleeding or febrile, unstable	<20,000	Transfusion
Extensive mucosal or internal bleeding	<50,000	Transfusion
Invasive procedure		
Surgery	<50,000	Transfusion
Lumbar puncture	<20,000	Transfusion
Bone marrow	<5,000	Transfusion

Source: Rogers, Aquino, and Buchanan, 2002, Table 40-2, p. 1208.

    b. Suggested platelet counts for transfusion are shown in Table 4.5.

    c. At any given platelet count, a patient will bleed less with a hemoglobin of at least 10 g/dl.

  3. Thrombopoietic agents such as IL1, IL3, IL6, IL11, or thrombopoietin have all been tried in pediatric cancer patients with no definitive success in maintaining platelet counts.

B. Therapeutic approaches to thrombocytopenia

  1. Avoidance of bleeding precipitants may decrease the need for platelet transfusions.

    a. Invasive procedures such as urinary catheters, NG tubes, or IM injections should be minimized.

    b. Pressure for 5–15 minutes after venipuncture or injections.

    c. Caution against use of antiplatelet agents such as ibuprofen, naproxen, or aspirin.

  2. Nonspecific treatments for bleeding

    a. Topical agents such as gelfoam or topical thrombin promote local hemostasis and are useful for cutaneous bleeding.

    b. Antifibrinolytics such as epsilon amino caproic acid (Amicar) or tranexamic acid may help maintain a clot in mucosal hemorrhage (contraindicated in urinary tract bleeding).

    c. Prednisone may improve capillary stability and decrease bleeding.

       d. Desmopressin (DDAVP) enhances platelet adhesion to vascular endothelium and shortens bleeding time. It is of unclear value with platelet counts below 50,000/mm^3.

       e. Estrogen, alone or in oral contraceptives, is useful for menometrorrhagia.

C. Platelet transfusion products

   1. Random donor platelet concentrates

       a. Platelets separated from whole blood by centrifugation.

       b. Stored for up to 5 days with continuous agitation.

       c. 5.5–10 × 10^{10} platelets in 40–70 mL of plasma and anticoagulant.

       d. Pooled if multiple units needed, can be volume reduced with loss of 10–20% of platelets.

   2. Apheresis platelets

       a. Platelets from donors with good veins in 90-minute procedure.

       b. 3–6 × 10^{11} platelets in 200–300 mL of plasma and anticoagulant.

       c. Apheresis unit equivalent to 6–10 random donor platelet units.

       d. Theoretically preferred due to decreased donor exposure, but with leukofiltration there are no data that apheresis platelets decrease alloimmunization or platelet refractoriness.

D. Risks of platelet transfusion

   1. General risks of transfusion as discussed above.

   2. Bacterial contamination much more common since platelets are stored at room temperature.

E. Indications for platelet transfusion

   1. Any platelet count below 50,000/mm^3 and clinical bleeding.

   2. No benefit to prophylactic platelet transfusion with platelet count >10,000/mm^3 in absence of bleeding or procedure.

   3. Specific recommendations in Table 4.5.

F. Usual transfusion volumes and expected count increment

   1. Random donor units: Transfusion volume 10 mL/kg or 1 unit/10 kg (adult dose 5 units)

2. Apheresis units (equivalent to 6–10 random donor units): Estimate $\frac{1}{4}$, $\frac{1}{2}$ unit or order by mL/kg.
3. Expected increment 50–100,000/uL in previously untransfused patients, or 1 unit per m^2 will raise count by 10–12,000/uL.

G. Options for platelet transfusion-refractory patients
  1. Poor numerical increment with transfused platelets common in multiply transfused patients.
     a. Obtain post-transfusion platelet count, 1 and 8–24 hours later.
     b. Consumption: 1-hour count will show the expected response, second count will be at or below baseline value.
     c. Sensitization: Both count more than 50% below expected values.
     d. Sensitized patient is deemed refractory to platelets and should be transfused only for bleeding.
  2. Patients refractory to platelets should be encouraged to meticulously use the nonspecific strategies for prevention and management of bleeding above.
     a. Management of platelet sensitization or refractoriness
        i. HLA A- and B-matched platelets.
        ii. Platelet cross-matching.
        iii. Transfuse only for bleeding.
        iv. Better to prevent the problem by leukofiltration and judicious use of platelets than to try to manage it once it occurs.

IV. GRANULOCYTE TRANSFUSIONS

A. Assessment of need for granulocyte transfusion
  1. Neutropenia (absolute neutrophil count [ANC] below 500/mm^3) may predispose to bacterial and fungal infection and may delay recovery from infection once it occurs.
  2. If there is an expected delay in neutrophil recovery for more than 5–7 days in a patient with a documented infection that either does not, or would not be expected to, respond promptly to available antibiotics, then granulocyte transfusions should be considered.

3. Granulocyte transfusions require extensive preparation and are not usually available for 48 hours or more, and need to be given for 3 or more days for greatest efficacy.

B. Therapeutic approaches to granulocytopenia
1. Widespread use of G- and GM-CSF has decreased the depth and duration of the neutrophil nadir following chemotherapy.
2. Increase in the dose (from 5 to 10 mcg/kg/day), frequency of dosing (from 1 to 2 times daily), and route of administration (SC to IV) of G-CSF may result in a faster response.
3. Studies to evaluate the efficacy of GCSF-stimulated granulocytes in the prevention of infection in neutropenic cancer patients are in progress.

C. Granulocyte transfusion product
1. Collected by apheresis for a specific patient, not stored.
2. Unstimulated donors yield $0.5-1.0 \times 10^{10}$ cells per liter of donor blood processed.
3. Donor can be mobilized with GCSF or corticosteroid to increase yield.
4. Historically commitment for 3 or more daily infusions required to begin therapy.

D. Specific risks of granulocyte transfusion
1. Transfusion to patients alloimmunized to HLA or neutrophil specific antigens may result in fever and acute pulmonary symptoms including chills, dyspnea, check tightness, hypoxia, and pulmonary infiltrates.
2. Concurrent administration of amphotericin B and granulocyte concentrates should be separated by at least 4 hours to minimize risk of a particularly severe pulmonary syndrome.
3. Premedication with acetaminophen, diphenhydramine, and possibly corticosteroids should be considered before granulocytes are administered.

E. Indications for granulocyte transfusion
1. Persistent bacterial or fungal infections in profoundly neutropenic patients (ANC $<500/\text{mm}^3$) despite appropriate antibiotics or antifungal agents and no evidence of marrow recovery.

2. Once granulocyte transfusion has been initiated, the usual course of treatment is at least 5 days.
3. Clearance of the infection and recovery of endogenous neutrophils obviate the need for further transfusion.

V. ALBUMIN TRANSFUSIONS

A. Assessment of hypoalbuminemia
   1. Acute phase reactant: Albumin is a negative acute phase reactant; mRNA for albumin is decreased in response to stress.
   2. Serum albumin level: Albumin normally binds lipophilic substances, hormones, drugs, cations, and metals. Albumin binding is unlikely of clinical importance except for drugs >80% bound. It contributes up to 80% of normal colloidal oncotic pressure and responsible for 50% of normal anion gap. Synthesis is regulated by oncotic pressure near hepatocytes. Serum level is a poor indicator of total body albumin stores.
   3. Etiology of hypoalbuminemia: Stress, poor nutrition, increased loss.
   4. Signs and symptoms of hypoalbuminemia include peripheral edema, pulmonary edema, edematous bowel wall producing diarrhea, and, perhaps, delayed wound healing.

B. Therapeutic approaches to hypoalbuminemia
   1. An infusion of 25 grams of 25% albumin increases plasma volume by ~400 mL at 2 hours after infusion.
   2. 5% albumin increases plasma volume equal to the volume infused.
   3. Infused albumin disperses into the extracellular fluid at a rate of 5–10% per hour; therefore, the longer the infusion time, the longer the albumin remains in the intravascular space. Infused albumin has a plasma half-life of 24 hours.
   4. For resuscitation, 1 volume of 5% albumin achieves a plasma volume expansion equivalent to that of 4 volumes of crystalloid.

C. Albumin transfusion products available
   1. 25% albumin in 50 mL, 100 mL bottles;
   2. 5% albumin in 50 mL, 250 mL, 500 mL bottles.

Table 4.6.
Indications for Albumin Transfusion

Accepted Indications	Possible Indications
Fluid replacement in plasma exchange	Fluid resuscitation in shock/sepsis
Nephrosis resistant to diuretics	Stabilization of intravascular volume
Following large-volume paracentesis	

D. Specific risks of albumin transfusion
1. If used during sepsis, may aggravate pulmonary capillary leakage.
2. Volume overload.
3. Hypertension if infused rapidly.
4. The assessment of the risks of albumin infusion as reviewed by the Cochrane Injuries Group Albumin Reviewers remains controversial. The article concludes, "Because this review was based on relatively small trials in which there were only a small number of deaths, the results must be interpreted with caution."

E. Indications for albumin transfusion (the following are the least contentious indications/nonindications). (See Table 4.6).
1. Not indicated for nutritional support.
2. Indicated for volume maintenance during plasmapheresis as replacement fluid.

F. Dose for albumin transfusion
1. One gram per kilogram (25%), given as slowly as possible when used for severe hypoalbuminemia to achieve intravascular stability; may be given in TPN solution if added under hood to ensure sterility;
2. 10–20 mL/Kg for resuscitation with 5% solution.

G. Administration of albumin through transfusion does not require a leucopoor filter but does require meticulous handling to ensure sterility and the use of a micropore filter.

VI. FACTOR CONCENTRATE TRANSFUSIONS

See Chapter 5 on hemorrhagic and thrombotic complications in children with cancer.

VII. CRYOPRECIPITATE TRANSFUSIONS

See Chapter 5 on hemorrhagic and thrombotic complications in children with cancer.

A. Cold precipitated protein fraction prepared from fresh-frozen plasma; suspended in a minimum volume of plasma (~9–16 mL/unit); contains >80 IU of FVIII:C, FVIII:vWF activity; fibrinogen 100–350 mg; FXIII 40–60 IU;

B. Stored frozen at −18°C;

C. Fibrinogen half-life of 3–5 days, recovery approximately 50%;

D. Indicated to replace fibrinogen <0.6–1.0/L, especially when associated with clinical bleeding or contemplated surgery;

E. Dose about 1 unit per 5 kg body weight will increase plasma fibrinogen content by 1.0 gm/L;

F. Administered through a "platelet administration" filter.

VIII. PLASMA TRANSFUSIONS

A. Plasma transfusion products available
   1. Fresh-frozen plasma (FFP) obtained from a single unit donation (~160–250 mL), frozen within 8 hours of donation contains approximately 1 unit/mL of each blood coagulation factor;
   2. Cryoprecipitate depleted FFP is FFP frozen after cryoprecipitate removal and should not be used for patients with von Willebrand disease, or factor V, VIII, XIII, or fibrinogen deficiency;
   3. Single-donor, apheresed fresh-frozen plasma, volume ~400–600 mL;
   4. Solvent-detergent treated plasma obtained from pooled plasma donations contains decreased amounts of most coagulation factors (15–50%) and is more costly than FFP. The solvent processing does not prevent all transfusion-transmitted infections, specifically viruses not enveloped by a lipid membrane.

B. Specific risks of plasma transfusion
   1. Allergic, anaphylactic reactions. Diphenhydramine and epinephrine should be readily available;
   2. Volume overload.
   3. Transmission of infectious agent.

C. Indications for plasma transfusion (See also Chapter 5 on Hemorrhagic and Thrombotic Complications in Children with Cancer).
   1. Documented single and/or combined clinically significant coagulation protein deficiencies (II, V, X, XI; ATIII, protein C, protein S) for which specific factor concentrates are not readily available;
   2. Patients receiving warfarin with clinically concerning bleeding or who require emergency surgery;
   3. PT and/or PTT>1.5 times normal in a nonbleeding patient scheduled for surgery or invasive procedure or as a result of massive transfusion or in disseminated intravascular coagulation. However, elevation of PT and/or PTT in these circumstances does not necessarily correlate with bleeding risk. INR values are comparable only from lab to lab in patients with coagulation factor deficiencies related to warfarin therapy and not from other causes.
   4. Thrombotic thrombocytopenic purpura.

D. Dose for plasma transfusion: Usual dose 10–15 mL/Kg given over 1–2 hours or as tolerated. This is expected to increase plasma concentration of coagulation factors by 15–20% after transfusion.

E. Administration of plasma transfusion
   1. Administered through a millipore or 120 micron filter
   2. Must be ABO compatible.

IX. ALTERNATIVES TO PLASMA TRANSFUSIONS

A. Single coagulation factor concentrates;
B. Synthetic colloids for volume expansion in resuscitation;
C. Albumin solutions for volume replacement in plasmapheresis;
D. Pentastarch for volume expansion or blood product sparing during surgery; contraindicated in children less than 4 years of age, with underlying disorders predisposing to hemorrhage or thrombosis, congestive heart failure, anuria, renal failure, or allergy to hydroxyethyl starch;
E. Pharmacologic agents such as DDVAP, aminocaproic acid, tranexamic acid, aprotinin;

F. Fibrin glue: Purified, virally inactivated fibrin sealant may be useful for some surgical bleeding. Fibrin glue may rarely be followed by the development of factor inhibitors most commonly to factor V.

G. Recombinant Factor VII a (NovoSeven®)—see Chapter 5: Bleeding Complications in Children with Cancer, section IC4.

X. INTRAVENOUS GAMMA GLOBULIN TRANSFUSIONS

A. Approximately 95% IgG, remaining 5% other plasma proteins;

B. Specific products available: Intravenous immune globulin, Rho (D) immune globulin, cytomegalovirus immune globulin, RSV immune globulin;

C. Rho (D) immune globulin is indicated for Rh-negative girls receiving platelet units not typed for Rh status; dose 300 mcg for every 35 units of platelets transfused (or 120 mcg for every 12 units transfused); repeat every 4 weeks if platelet transfusion given; 1 dose of anti-D effective for 28 days;

D. IV IgG supplied as a 5%, 6%, or 10% solution in 2.5 gm, 5 gm, 10 gm, and 20 gm vials; anti-D supplied as 50, 120, or 300 mcg vials;

E. Adverse effects include headache, fluid retention, complement activation, allergic/anaphylactic reactions, nausea, aseptic meningitis, flushing, hypotension, chest tightness, hemolysis, dermatitis, edema, infusion site pain, renal dysfunction, hepatitis;

F. Adverse reactions decreased by premedication with acetaminophen and midinfusion furosemide (0.5 mg/Kg);

G. Intravenous gamma globulin not effective in improving poor platelet transfusion response;

H. Intravenous gamma globulin may be indicated in severe hypogammaglobulinemia associated with chemotherapy; indicated in hypogammaglobulinemia after BMT;

I. Renal dysfunction or failure is related to rapid infusion of hyperosmolar concentrates (high-sucrose products in particular). Patients should be adequately hydrated before receiving the IgG infusion. Patients with pre-existing renal dysfunction, diabetes, volume depletion, sepsis, or receiving concomitant nephrotoxic drugs. The recommended maximum infusion rate for each product should not be exceeded;

J. Administration of intravenous gamma globulin should carefully follow the recommendations of the appropriate hospital policy and/or the instructions provided with the gamma globulin concentrate.

Bibliography

Boldt J, Knothe C, Schindler E, et al. Volume replacement with hydroxyethyl starch solution in children. *Brit J Anaesth* 70:661–65, 1993.

British Committee for Standards in Haematology, Blood Transfusion Task Force. The administration of blood and blood components and the management of transfused patients. *Transfusion Med* 9:227–38, 1999.

British Committee for Standards in Haematology, Blood Transfusion Task Force. Guidelines on the clinical use of leucocyte-depleted blood components. *Transfusion Med* 8:59–71, 1998.

British Committee for Standards in Haematology, Blood Transfusion Task Force. Guidelines on gamma irradiation of blood components for the prevention of transfusion-associated graft-versus-host disease. *Transfusion Med* 6:261–71, 1996.

Cochrane Injuries Group Albumin Reviewers. Human albumin administration in critically ill patients: Systemic review of randomised controlled trials. *Brit Med J* 317:235–340, 1998.

Consensus Working Group. Present and future uses of IVIG: A Canadian multidisciplinary consensus-building initiative. *Can J Allergy Clin Immunol* 2:176–208, 1997.

Doweiko JP, Nompleggi DJ. Role of albumin in human physiology and pathophysiology. Review. *J Parent Enteral Nutr* 15:207–11, 1991.

Goodnough LT. Universal leukoreduction of cellular blood components in 2001? - No. *Am J Clin Pathol* 115:674–77, 2001.

Guidelines for red blood cell and plasma transfusion for adults and children. Report of the Expert Working Group. Supplement to Can Med Assoc J 156:s1–23, 1997.

Hiruma K, Okuyama Y. Effect of leucocyte reduction on the potential alloimmunogenicity of leucocytes in fresh-frozen plasma products. *Vox Sang* 80:51–56, 2001.

Kluter H, Bubel S, Kirchner H, Wilhelm D. Febrile and allergic transfusion reactions after the transfusion of white cell-poor platelet preparations. *Transfus* 39:1179–84, 1999.

Letters to editor. *Brit Med J* 317:882–86, 1998.

McCelland DBL, McMenamin JJ, Moores HM, Barbara JAJ. Reducing risks in blood transfusion: Process and outcome. *Transfusion Med* 6:1–10, 1996.

Moroff G, Luban NLC. The irradiation of blood and blood components to prevent graft-versus-host disease: Technical issues and guidelines. *Transfusion Med Reviews* 11:15–26, 1997.

Pereira A. Cost-effectiveness of transfusing virus-inactivated plasma instead of standard plasma. *Transfusion* 39:479–87, 1999.

Perrotta PL, Snyder EL. Non-infectious complications of transfusion therapy. *Blood Reviews* 15:69–83, 2001.

Przepiorka D, LeParc GF, Werch J, Lichtiger B. Prevention of transfusion-associated cytomegalovirus infection, practice parameter. *Amer J Clin Pathol* 106:163–69, 1996.

Rogers A, Aquino V, Buchanan GR. Hematologic supportive care and hematopoietic cytokines. In Pizzo PA, Poplack DG, ed., *Principles and Practice of Pediatric Oncology*, 4th ed. Philadelphia: Lippincott Williams & Wilkins, 2002.

Schuh A, Atoyebi W, Littlewood T, Hatton C, Bradburn M, Murphy MF. Prevention of worsening of severe thrombocytopenia after red cell transfusion by the use of leucocyte-depleted blood. *Brit J Haematol* 108:455–57, 2000.

Sharma AD, Sreeram G, Erb T, Grocott HP. Solvent-treated fresh frozen plasma: A superior alternative to standard fresh frozen plasma? *J Cardio Vasc Anesth* 14:712–17, 2000.

Sweeney JD. Universal leukoreduction of cellular blood components in 2001?—Yes. *Am J Clin Pathol* 115:666–73, 2001.

Vamvakas EC, Blajchman MA. Deleterious clinical effects of transfusion-associated immunomodulation: Fact or fiction? *Blood* 97:1180–95, 2001.

Williamson LM, Warwick RM. Transfusion-associated graft-versus-host disease and its prevention. *Blood Reviews* 9:251–61, 1995.

Williamson LM, Lowe S, Love EM, Cohen H, Soldan K, McCelland DBL, Skacel P, Barbara JAJ. Serious hazards of transfusion [SHOT] initiative: Analysis of the first two annual reports. *Brit Med J* 319:16–19, 1999.

5

Hemorrhagic and Thrombotic Complications

J. Nathan Hagstrom, M.D., and Paul T. Monagle, M.B.B.S.

Evaluating Hemostasis in Children with Cancer

I. HEMOSTASIS AND CANCER

When there is vascular injury, multiple pathways are activated, which interact through complex positive and negative feedback loops to cease blood loss while maintaining tissue perfusion. The critical step is thrombin generation, which produces fibrin deposition and activates platelets at the site of injury. Thrombin generation is regulated by the inhibition of activated procoagulants and thrombus formation is contained by fibrinolysis. With injury, tissue factor is exposed initiating coagulation. In addition, injury exposes subendothelial collagen resulting in platelet adhesion, which is mediated in part by von Willebrand factor. In malignancy, *intravascular* initiation of hemostasis may occur from abnormal expression of tissue factor by tumor cells or by injured or activated endothelium.

When treating children with cancer, one must consider that the hemostatic system in neonates and children has significant developmental differences from that of adults. These differences must be considered physiologic.

    A. Primary hemostasis
        1. Platelets: Thrombocytopenia is often present in children with cancer. In addition, certain medications including nonsteroidal anti-inflammatory drugs, complementary or alternative medicines, and selective serotonin reuptake inhibitors may affect platelet function (see Table 5.1).

Table 5.1.
Factors That Adversely Affect Platelet Function

Medication (partial list)	Herbal Medicine (partial list)	Condition
Clinically significant	Herbs, spices, and foods	Uremia
Aspirin	Garlic	Cholestasis
Ibuprofen	Ginger	Malnutrition
Ketorolac	Cumin	Inherited defects
Other NSAIDS*	Clove	
Minimal effect	Black tree fungus	
Antihistamines	Turmeric	
High-dose penicillin and	Ethanol	
cephalosporins		
Guiafenesin		
Specific serotonin reuptake		
inhibitors (e.g., Prozac)		

*NSAIDS, nonsteroidal anti-inflammatory drugs.

2. Von Willebrand factor: Increased levels of von Willebrand factor during times of stress or endothelial damage may help to offset the decreased platelet capacity.

3. Vascular constriction is an important first event when there is vascular injury. Endothelium normally promotes an antithrombotic luminal surface. However, activated endothelial cells can express various adhesion molecules and prothrombotic proteins. Bacteremia, chemotherapeutics, and invading tumor cells can lead to endothelial activation.

B. Procoagulant system

1. Tissue factor pathway: Because malignant cells may express tissue factor, a localized low-grade consumption may occur, depleting the system of procoagulants such as factor VII, and anticoagulants such as tissue factor pathway inhibitor (TFPI).

2. Vitamin K-dependent procoagulants (prothrombin, factors VII, IX, and X): Levels of these factors are normally lower in neonates compared to children, and children have slightly lower levels compared to adults. The functional levels of these proteins are reduced by warfarin therapy and are especially sensitive to mild liver dysfunction or dietary vitamin K deficiency.

3. Cofactors (factors VIII and V): Levels of these two proteins in children are similar to those in adults. Factor VIII is an acute phase reactant that is often elevated in malignancy. Persistently elevated levels of factor VIII have been associated with thromboembolic disease.
4. Contact factors (factors XI and XII, high molecular weight kininogen and prekalikrein): Levels are lower in neonates compared to children and adults.

C. Anticoagulant system
1. Antithrombin (formerly known as antithrombin III): Levels in children are comparable to adults except in early infancy. It circulates in an alpha (fully glycosylated) and a beta form; the beta form binds to heparan sulfate on the surface of endothelium with more avidity and; therefore, may be more important physiologically. Antithrombin levels are often decreased with L-asparaginase therapy.
2. Protein C pathway: Proteins C and S are both vitamin K-dependent proteins. Levels of proteins C and S are lower in children than adults and are lowest during early infancy. Acquired protein S and/or protein C deficiency can be associated with severe infections in children.
3. Alpha-2-macroglobulin is a major inhibitor of thrombin throughout childhood.
4. Tissue factor pathway inhibitor (TFPI): TFPI, in the presence of factor Xa, can bind to, and thereby inhibit, the factor VIIa-tissue factor complex.

D. Fibrinolytic system: Hyperfibrinolysis is associated with certain disease states and treatments and may lead to an increased risk of bleeding. Hypofibrinolysis is associated with thrombosis.
1. Profibrinolytics: Plasminogen, tissue plasminogen activator.
2. Antifibrinolytics: Plasminogen activator inhibitor-1, thrombin-activated fibrinolysis inhibitor (TAFI). TAFI is a major "link" protein decreasing fibrinolysis as thrombin formation increases.

II. LABORATORY EVALUATION

A. Primary hemostasis
1. Platelet count and morphology: A peripheral smear should always be reviewed to confirm thrombocytopenia.
2. Bleeding time: The bleeding time lacks sensitivity and specificity for predicting risk of bleeding. It has limited practical use in children with cancer.
3. PFA-100: A method for measuring an in vitro "bleeding time" on a small volume of whole blood. As blood is passed through an aperture lined with collagen/ADP or collagen/epinephrine, a platelet plug forms obstructing blood flow, which results in a closure time. The hematocrit and leukocyte count are inversely correlated with the closure time. PFA-100 is very sensitive to even mild thrombocytopenia. Therefore, its use in oncology patients may be limited.
4. Von Willebrand factor assays: Von Willebrand disease is common and; therefore, may be present in a child with cancer. Acquired von Willebrand factor deficiency has been described in patients with Wilms tumor.
5. Vascular integrity: Currently there is no specific clinical assay for evaluating vascular integrity. A vitamin C level can be done to rule out scurvy. Tissue biopsies are the most specific and sensitive method for diagnosing vasculitis.

B. Coagulation
1. Prothrombin time (PT): The PT is performed by adding an excess of tissue factor and calcium and does not reflect normal physiology; nonetheless, it can be useful in assessing hemostasis. The prothrombin time is especially sensitive to deficiencies in factors VII and II. It may also be elevated in combined mild factor deficiencies involving factors II, VII, and X, which might be seen in mild liver dysfunction, mild vitamin K deficiency, or early disseminated intravascular coagulation (DIC). The PT is less sensitive to heparin and to the presence of a lupus anticoagulant compared to the aPTT, but the PT can be prolonged when these two substances are present in high concentrations.

2. Activated partial thromboplastin time (aPTT): The aPTT is performed by activating the contact system, which is not essential for maintaining hemostasis in vivo and; therefore, does not reflect true physiology. Despite this, the PTT remains useful for detecting deficiencies in factors VIII, IX and XI, and vWF. With the PT, the aPTT assists in evaluating the common pathway (factors II, V, X, and fibrinogen). Elevations in the PTT may be related to heparin, the presence of a lupus anticoagulant, a factor deficiency, or factor inhibitor.

3. Thrombin time (TT): The TT is elevated in hypofibrinogenemia and is very sensitive to the presence of heparin; therefore, it is a rapid way to screen for heparin contamination in samples drawn from a central venous catheter.

4. Factor assays are performed by adding diluted plasma to factor deficient plasma then performing a PT- or PTT-based clotting assay. The results are compared to a standard curve. Performing factor assays are helpful when evaluating an elevated PT and/or PTT.

C. Plasma samples drawn from an indwelling catheter may contain heparin and, therefore, give erroneous results for clotting-based tests. It is recommended that samples drawn from catheters be drawn using a validated discard volume protocol before sampling or be treated with hepzyme. Samples drawn for the purposes of monitoring heparin therapy or for measuring heparin levels may need to be drawn peripherally.

D. Regulatory pathways
1. Antithrombin should be measured using a functional assay whenever possible; heparin contamination of the sample should be avoided.

2. Protein C pathway
a. Protein C can be measured using a clotting-based, chromogenic, or immunologic assay. Chromogenic assays (which reflect function) are most readily available, although clotting-based assays probably provide a more physiologic measurement.

b. Protein S is a cofactor for protein C and circulates as free (active) form and bound to C4b-binding protein (inactive). A functional assay for protein S is sufficient as a screen for protein S deficiency. Total and free protein S may be helpful follow-up tests in someone found to be deficient.

   c. Activated protein C resistance (APCR) is measured by a clotting-based assay. Newer methods that dilute the test sample in factor V deficient plasma only test for APCR due to defects in factor V. However, resistance of factor VIIIa to APC cleavage could also result in APCR. In the majority of cases, APC resistance can be explained by an inherited defect in the factor V protein (factor V Leiden) that renders it less readily inactivated by APC. The factor V Leiden mutation can be detected using PCR followed by restriction enzyme digestion.

  3. Fibrinolytic system

   a. D-dimers reflect the breakdown of cross-linked fibrin, whereas fibrin degradation products (FDPs) may reflect fibrinogen or fibrin degradation. Elevated fibrin/fibrinogen split products may be indicative of hyperfibrinolysis.

   b. Elevated PAI-1 and lipoprotein (a) levels, as well as hypoplasminogenemia, create a hypofibrinolytic state.

E. Endothelium/vascular system

  1. Surrogate markers for endothelial damage (e.g., soluble thrombomodulin) can be measured, but their clinical utility is marginal.

  2. Disorders of nitric oxide production and metabolism may play a role in thrombotic and bleeding complications; however, useful clinical assays are not available.

III. ASSESSING THE RISK FOR HEMORRHAGIC AND THROMBOTIC COMPLICATIONS

Many tests are available for evaluating hemostasis. However, there is no one test that can accurately characterize one's risk of bleeding or thrombosis (see Section II). A history of bleeding or thrombotic problems in the patient or their family, the patient's underlying disease and treatment, the presence of comorbid conditions, physical examination findings, and laboratory results must all be considered when assessing a patient's risk.

  A. Risk assessment for bleeding
    1. History and physical: A personal history of bleeding symptoms or complications is suggestive of an underlying bleeding problem more so than a comprehensive laboratory evaluation. In particular, a history of previous dental or surgical procedures should be obtained. In children, family history is especially relevant as many patients themselves have not had previous surgical or dental challenge. Careful inspection of the skin and mucous membranes of the oral and nasal cavity should be performed. The pattern of any bruises, petechiae, or mucosal bleeding may provide clues to the likely bleeding abnormality.
    2. Disease specific: Certain cancers are more associated with abnormalities in hemostasis (see Table 5.2). Tumor invasion of medium and large vessels may result in severe localized hemorrhage. Hemorrhage into a friable, vascular solid tumor can result in significant blood loss (especially neuroblastoma). Hemorrhage into an intracranial tumor can result in permanent neurologic sequelae and may precipitate clinical presentation. Acute promyelocytic leukemia (APML) and other subtypes of AML, especially acute monoblastic leukemia, are associated with a consumptive coagulopathy secondary to hypercoagulable and hyperfibrinolytic states.
    3. Comorbid conditions: Liver dysfunction, malnutrition, renal insufficiency, and cholestasis can be associated with bleeding complications (see Table 5.2). Certain fungal and bacterial infections can be associated with severe bleeding secondary to invasion of blood vessels (e.g., aspergillosis, pseudomonas). Fever and sepsis increase the likelihood of bleeding associated with thrombocytopenia.
    4. Treatment specific: L-asparaginase, especially when given with prednisone, is associated with hypofibrinogenemia. Platinum drugs are associated with more severe and prolonged thrombocytopenia. Surgery,

Table 5.2.

Clinical Disorders Associated with Abnormalities in Hemostasis, and Their Treatment

Clinical Disorder	Hemostatic Tests	Treatment
Infiltration of bone marrow (e.g., leukemia, neuroblastoma)	↓platelet count	Platelet transfusion. If no response, consider using aminocaproic acid, desmopressin, or NovoSeven® (rFVIIa)
Liver dysfunction due to metastatic disease or chemotherapy	↑PT, ± ↑PTT, ↓factors II, V, VII, IX, and X	FFP NovoSeven® Platelet transfusions
Acute promyelocytic leukemia	↑PT, ↑PTT, ↑TT, ↑d-dimers, ↓factors V, VII, VIII, fibrinogen	ATRA Heparin Platelet transfusions
Vitamin K deficiency due to antibiotic therapy, chronic diarrhea, poor nutrition (also applies to warfarin overdose)	↑PT, ± ↑PTT, ↓factors II, VII, IX, and X	Vitamin K PCC FFP
DIC	↑PT, ↑PTT, ↑TT, ↑d-dimers, ↓factors II, V, VII, VIII, IX, and X, fibrinogen	FFP Platelet transfusion Cryoprecipitate NovoSeven® Heparin Antithrombin APC
L-asparaginase therapy (±prednisone)	↓fibrinogen ↓antithrombin	Cryoprecipitate FFP Antithrombin
Wilms tumor	↓von Willebrand factor	DDAVP Humate-P®

especially neurosurgery, can be associated with a hypercoagulable state or, if sufficient consumption occurs, a hypocoagulable state.

5.   Laboratory evaluation: Initially a platelet count, PT, PTT, and fibrinogen are performed. Clinically abnormal bleeding in the setting of these first line tests being normal suggest the possibility of vWD, platelet function defect, Factor XIII deficiency, fibrinolytic or endothelial cell dysfunction, or alternatively local vascular factors.

6. Thrombocytopenia is the most common reason for bleeding in children with cancer. The platelet count is useful in predicting bleeding in a patient. However, when considering a threshold for prophylactic platelet transfusions, the clinician should consider the clinical condition of each individual patient and perform a full risk assessment (see Chapter 4 Section III and Table 4.5). Multiple conditions and medications can decrease platelet function (see Table 5.1).

B. Risk assessment for thrombosis
1. History: The presence of a central venous access device (CVAD) is the most important risk factor for thromboembolic complications. A previous history of a thrombotic event is a strong risk factor for developing new thrombosis. A strong family history is also important.
2. Disease specific: Tumors, which lead to compression of a vascular structure, can result in thrombosis. Direct invasion into a vessel can also result in thrombosis. APML is often associated with a hypercoagulable state. Hyperleukocytosis may be associated with thrombosis.
3. Treatment specific: DVT secondary to CVAD are reported to occur in up to 60% of adults with malignancy receiving TPN. Studies in children with cancer report DVT incidences of 1–74% depending on the diagnostic technique used. L-asparaginase is associated with thrombotic events including stroke, dural sinus thrombosis, and deep venous thrombosis, which is often associated with an acquired antithrombin deficiency. Hormonal therapies are associated with thrombosis. The use of oral contraceptives can increase the risk of thrombosis. Megestrol acetate (Megace) at high doses has been associated with thrombosis. Post-CNS radiation vasculitis may be associated with stroke.
4. Laboratory evaluation: The d-dimer has been used as a screening test for the presence of active venous thrombosis in adults. However, its usefulness has not been tested in children with cancer. Measurement of the F1.2 fragment, a marker for thrombin generation, has been used as a screening test for hypercoagulability. However, its clinical utility is questionable.

Bleeding Complications in Children with Cancer

I. **APPROACH TO ABNORMAL BLEEDING IN A CHILD WITH CANCER**

   A. Assess clinical status and stabilize as appropriate.
      1. Determine source of bleeding and estimate blood loss.
      2. Inspect for other bleeding manifestations to assist in determining if bleeding is a localized or systemic phenomenon.
      3. Administer colloid and PRBCs as appropriate to maintain intravascular volume and oxygen delivery.

   B. Rapid assessment of hemostasis
      1. CBC, PT, PTT, fibrinogen, d-dimer.
      2. Individual factor assays as appropriate.
         a. Factors V and VIII to differentiate between DIC and liver dysfunction.
         b. Factors II and VII to explore vitamin K-dependent procoagulants.

   C. Choose initial therapy based on severity of bleeding and the clinical and laboratory data (see therapeutic armamentarium).
      1. Platelets at a dose of 0.1–0.2 U per kg if thrombocytopenic.
      2. Plasma (FFP) at a dose of 10–20 cc per kg if PT (INR > 2.0) and/or PTT (> 1.5 times normal) are elevated.
      3. Cryoprecipitate at a dose of 1 bag per 10 kg if fibrinogen less than 100 mg/dl and patient still bleeding after plasma.
      4. NovoSeven® (rFVIIa) should be administered at a dose of 30–90 mcg/kg if the bleeding is severe and there has been no response to other measures.

   D. Further evaluation
      1. Thrombocytopenia is usually related to decreased platelet production following cytotoxic therapy. However, other possible causes should be investigated, especially when the thrombocytopenia is not fully explained by therapy-related bone marrow aplasia. Infection, severe mucositis, veno-occlusive disease, large venous thrombosis, hypersplenism, DIC, immune-mediated

Table 5.3.
Medical Therapies Used to Treat Bleeding

	Dose According to Severity of Bleeding		
	Mild	Moderate	Severe
Platelets	0.1 U/kg	0.2 U/kg	Continuous infusion
Plasma (FFP)	10–20 cc/kg x1	10–20 cc/kg q6hr	Continuous infusion
Cryoprecipitate	1 bag per 10 kg	2 bags per 10 kg	
Aminocaproic acid	100 mg/kg IV/PO	100 mg/kg q6hr	Continuous infusion
Desmopressin	0.3 mcg/kg		
NovoSeven		10–60 mcg/kg	60–90 mcg/kg q2hr (higher doses have been used)
Prothrombin complex concentrates (PCCs)			50 U/kg
Vitamin K1	2.5–5 mg po qd	2–5 mg SC (0.1 mg/kg)	2–5 mg IV (0.1 mg/kg)
Protamine		1 mg for every 100U of heparin	
Aprotinin			4 mg/kg

thrombocytopenia, heparin-induced thrombocytopenia, hemophagocytosis, drug-induced and microangiopathic disease (e.g., BMT-associated HUS/TTP) are among the various potential causes of thrombocytopenia in children with cancer. Rarely, tumor associated consumption of platelets may occur (e.g., disseminated osteogenic sarcoma).

2. It is always important to assess a patient's response to therapy. This should be done with both follow-up clinical assessment and laboratory data.

II. THERAPEUTIC ARMAMENTARIUM (See Table 5.3)

A. Platelets contain factors V and XI, fibrinogen, fibronectin, and von Willebrand factor. Platelet function can be adversely affected by multiple factors. Therefore, even in a patient with mild thrombocytopenia, if bleeding is present, the patient may benefit from a platelet transfusion.

B. Fresh-frozen plasma contains variable amounts of all the clotting factors because factor levels can vary significantly from one donor to another. Only pooled plasma from multiple donors would have a final concentration of a specific factor equal to 1 U/ml. Furthermore, the concentration of a specific factor needed to achieve hemostasis differs from factor to factor. For example, only small amounts of factor V are needed to achieve hemostasis, whereas a higher concentration of prothrombin is needed.

C. Cryoprecipitate contains fibrinogen, factor VIII, von Willebrand factor, fibronectin, and factor XIII.

D. Red cells not only will replace lost RBCs and volume, but also will improve hemostasis by improving blood viscosity.

E. Aminocaproic acid has been used to treat bleeding associated with thrombocytopenia and factor deficiencies such as von Willebrand disease and hemophilia.

F. Desmopressin has been used also, in bleeding associated with uremia, von Willebrand disease, factor VIII deficiency, and platelet dysfunction.

G. Recombinant factor VIIa (NovoSeven) has been used to treat bleeding associated with thrombocytopenia, DIC, and liver failure. It is also used in hemophilia patients with inhibitors as well as in people with factor VII deficiency.

H. Prothrombin complex concentrates contain factors II, VII, IX, and X, as well as protein C and S.

I. Local measures
    1. Nasal packing is used for persistent epistaxis in cases where medical intervention has failed.
    2. Interventional radiology can sometimes be used to embolize arteries that are supplying blood to an area that is hemorrhaging despite less invasive therapeutic maneuvers.
    3. Surgical intervention is sometimes necessary to control severe localized bleeding by ligating vessels, packing specific sites, or removing a bleeding tumor or organ.

III. PRIMARY PROPHYLAXIS

A. Severe thrombocytopenia
    Platelet transfusion (See Table 4.5)
B. Hypofibrinogenemia
    FFP or cryoprecipitate has been used to prevent bleeding in patients with ALL receiving steroids and L-asparaginase who develop severe hypofirinogenemia. However, there are

no data to suggest that this approach is either necessary or helpful. We do not recommend checking fibrinogen levels unless the patient has bleeding not explained by thrombocytopenia alone.

C. Menstrual bleeding can be severe in patients with thrombocytopenia or other bleeding disorders. Therefore, it may be advisable to take measures to decrease menstrual bleeding. Oral contraceptives can decrease menstrual bleeding when used for the conventional 21 days on, 7 days off schedule. However, when oral contraceptives are continued daily, amenorrhea often can be achieved. Another option is to use daily progestin therapy. Medroxyprogesterone acetate (DEPO-PROVERA) is also an option. Gonadotropin-releasing hormone analogs are an option, but may take 1–2 months before halting the menstrual cycle.

IV. MINOR BLEEDING COMPLICATIONS

A. Definition: No evidence for hypovolemia and a drop in hgb of less than 2 g/dl.

B. Specific therapeutic considerations
   1. Epistaxis, oral bleeding, gastrointestinal bleeding will usually respond to a platelet transfusion in patients with thrombocytopenia.
   2. Hematuria should be treated with aggressive hydration.
   3. Menstrual bleeding can be stopped by taking a combination monophasic oral contraceptive every 6 hours for 4–7 days.

V. MAJOR BLEEDING COMPLICATIONS

A. Definition: Signs of hypovolemia or Hgb dropped 2 g/dL or more.

B. Specific therapeutic considerations
   1. Epistaxis that is severe and refractory to medical intervention may require anterior packing either with Vaseline gauze or gelfoam. Consult ENT.
   2. Gastrointestinal bleeding that is severe may require octreotide to decrease splanchnic blood flow. Consult a GI specialist.

3. Hematuria and hemorrhagic cystitis can be severe enough to threaten the integrity of the renal system and result in significant blood loss. Initial management includes overhydration and correction of any hemostatic abnormalities. Bladder instillation of various substances, including formalin and prostaglandin E2, has been used. NovoSeven has been used to treat life-threatening hemorrhagic cystitis with success.

4. Severe menstrual bleeding can be treated with intravenous conjugated estrogen, 40 mg every 6 hours, or oral estrogen, 2.5 mg every 6 hours, in addition to treating underlying abnormalities of hemostasis.

5. Pulmonary hemorrhage including diffuse alveolar hemorrhage is a rare but serious and life-threatening complication of high-dose chemotherapy. Often a multi-faceted therapeutic approach is needed to stabilize the patient including positive pressure ventilation with a high-frequency oscillator, multiple transfusions of various blood products, vascular and surgical interventions, and steroids. Both Amicar and NovoSeven have been used to treat severe pulmonary hemorrhage with a positive response.

6. DIC
   a. FFP, cryoprecipitate, and platelets are most commonly used to treat bleeding associated with DIC. However, factor VIIa (NovoSeven) has also been used in DIC.
   b. Recombinant activated protein C has been proven beneficial in adults with sepsis and multiorgan dysfunction.
   c. Heparin may be helpful when the predominant feature of the DIC is microvascular thrombosis, not bleeding.
   d. Antithrombin concentrate may be useful in patients with DIC and thrombotic complications who are not responsive to heparin.
   e. Eradicating the underlying cause is critical to the management of DIC.

7. Liver dysfunction
   a. FFP is used frequently to treat the coagulopathy associated with liver disease. However, in severe liver failure, plasmapheresis is often needed to adequately reverse the coagulopathy.

      b. NovoSeven (rFVIIa) can be used to treat bleeding associated with liver dysfunction.

    8. Vitamin K deficiency

      a. Vitamin K1 will take 4–6 hours to have a significant effect on hemostasis.

      b. Prothrombin complex concentrate is often easier to administer and may be obtained faster than FFP.

      c. FFP is usually effective in treating bleeding associated with the factor deficiencies caused by vitamin K deficiency; however, FFP also contains factors that are not vitamin K dependent.

    9. L-asparaginase-induced coagulopathy—bleeding FFP and cryoprecipitate

Thrombotic Complications in Children with Cancer

I. RISK FACTORS

A. Acquired: A central venous access device (CVAD) is the most important risk factor for thrombosis in children with cancer. CVAD-related DVT accounts for more than 60% of all thrombosis seen in childhood. Younger age probably increases the risk of CVAD-related DVT. This risk factor explains the predominance of childhood thrombosis in the upper venous system. The presence of antiphospholipid antibodies and lupus anticoagulants are important acquired risk factors for thrombosis.

B. Inherited: Protein C, S, and antithrombin deficiencies have long been recognized as inherited risk factors. However, the factor V Leiden and prothrombin 20210A mutations are the most common inherited risk factors for thrombosis. The methylenetetrahydrofolate reductase thermolabile variant, elevated factor VIII activity, and excess lipoprotein (a) are also common risk factors. There are conflicting data regarding the association of these factors to the thrombotic complications encountered in children with cancer. Primary screening for these conditions in children with cancer cannot be advocated at this time.

C. Malignancy related: Active malignancy is a thrombotic risk factor, presumably through expression of procoagulant molecules. Hyperleukocytosis, local vascular compression, and vascular invasion are other potential risk factors. Dehydration secondary to vomiting or fluid loss may increase the risk of sinovenous thrombosis.

D. Treatment related: Chemotherapy, in particular L-asparaginase, is associated with increased risk of thrombosis. Infusion of TPN likely increases the risk of thrombosis associated with CVADs.

II. DIAGNOSIS

A. Clinical symptoms and signs: Clinical presentation of thrombosis is variable and is often subtle in children. Sinovenous thrombosis may be present with non-specific headache or neurologic signs that are difficult to distinguish from (for example) methotrexate toxicity. Upper system DVT associated with CVADs may be present with CVAD dysfunction, increasing superficial collaterals on the chest wall, or the classic SVC syndrome. Pulmonary embolus is frequently diagnosed only at autopsy and may be the cause of nonspecific cardiorespiratory deterioration in critically ill children.

B. Ultrasound is sensitive and specific for venous thrombosis when compression of the vein is possible, such as jugular veins or femoral veins. Comparative studies show ultrasound fails to detect up to 80% of major vessel thrombosis in the central veins (subclavian/brachiocephalic/SVC).

C. Venograms: Bilateral upper limb venography remains the gold standard for the detection of upper system thrombosis.

D. CT scan with IV contrast may be used for the diagnosis of CVAD-related DVT, but its use has not been validated by comparative studies in children. Studies do show that CT is insensitive for detecting sinovenous thrombosis especially in small children when compared to magnetic resonance venography (MRV).

E. MRI (MRV) is the first line investigation for sinovenous thrombosis. While anecdotally MRV is promising for CVAD-related DVT, comparative studies with venography have not been reported.

F. Ventilation perfusion scans: V/Q scans remain the first line investigation for pulmonary embolus, although interpretation may be difficult in children with other pulmonary lesions.

G. Spiral CT scan with rapid administration of IV contrast is rapidly replacing VQ scans as the image of choice to rule out pulmonary embolism. This imaging modality has not been thoroughly tested in children. It is likely better than VQ scans but may not equal the sensitivity of pulmonary angiogram.

III. THERAPEUTIC ARMAMENTARIUM

Objectively proven DVT usually require anticoagulation therapy, even in the absence of major clinical symptoms, because of the risk of extension and embolization. However, routine surveillance for asymptomatic catheter-related DVT is not done, nor is it recommended. Data from long-term, prospective observation studies, specifically looking at poor outcomes related to asymptomatic catheter-related DVT, are not available. Much of the treatment guidelines are extrapolated from adult data and guidelines; however, there are emerging data about the use of anticoagulant therapy in children.

A. Antithrombotic agents
1. Unfractionated heparin (UFH): UFH is rapidly being replaced by low molecular weight heparin as the agent of choice for the acute management of thromboembolic disease. However, in some centers UFH remains the anticoagulant recommended for short-term rapid anticoagulant therapy. Usually given intravenously, it has variable pharmacokinetics. Response may be diminished if antithrombin levels are reduced. The half-life is prolonged in renal failure. Therapeutic doses are those required to maintain an aPTT 2–2.5 times baseline. The usual doses required vary with age, being increased in infants (See Table 5.4). Nomograms for monitoring and dosing UFH in children have been established. Potential adverse effects include bleeding, heparin-induced thrombocytopenia, and osteoporosis (usually seen with longer-term treatment).
2. Warfarin: Oral anticoagulation using coumadin derivatives remains the mainstay of longer-term anticoagulation. Warfarin is monitored using the INR, and the usual target of DVT management is 2.5. Warfarin is particularly problematic in children with cancer due to

Table 5.4.
Use of Standard Unfractionated Heparin in Children

Initiating heparin:
- Loading dose:
  For children <15 years old: 75 U/kg IV over 10 minutes
  For adolescents ≥15 years old: 50 U/kg IV over 10 minutes
- Initial maintenance infusion dose:
  For infants <12 months old: 28 U/kg/hour
  For children 1–15 years old: 20 U/kg/hour
  For adolescents ≥16 years old: 17 U/kg/hour
- Check aPTT 4 hours after initiating heparin therapy and adjust dose according to below.
- Check CBC daily.

Dose adjustments:

APTT	Heparin Bolus	Hold Infusion	Infusion Rate Change	Repeat aPTT
<32	50 U/kg	0	+20%	4 hours
32–42	0	0	+10%	4–6 hours
42–65	0	0	0	12–24 hours
66–80	0	0	−10%	4–6 hours
81–90	0	30 min	−10%	4 hours
>90	0	60 min	−15%	4 hours

Reversal of heparin therapy in the event of significant bleeding:
- Discontinue heparin infusion (for minor bleeding this may be all that is needed)
- Check PTT and CBC
- Protamine at a dose of 1 mg for every 100 U of heparin received in the last 2 hours (max = 50 mg).

If heparin has already been discontinued:

Time since Last Heparin	Dose of Protamine per 100U Heparin
<30 min	1 mg
30–60 min	0.5–0.75 mg
60–120 min	0.375–0.5 mg
>120 min	0.25–0.375 mg

the variable gut absorption, variable liver metabolism affected by chemotherapy and antibiotics, the additive bleeding risk from chemotherapy-induced thrombocytopenia, and the long lag time to stop and restart therapy around procedures such as lumbar punctures. Guidelines for warfarin monitoring and management in children have been published. (See Table 5.5).

Table 5.5.
Use of Warfarin in Children

Initiating Warfarin Therapy:
   If a patient has not reached the therapeutic range within 5 days of initiating OAT[†],
   adjustments will need to be made on an individual basis in consultation with
   hematology.
   Warfarin is given daily at the same time each day, preferably in the evening.
Warfarin Loading Dose: 0.2 mg/kg/day (maximum dose 10 mg po qd)
   For patients with liver dysfunction, history of Fontan procedure, a baseline INR
   >1.2, or who are not receiving heparin, use a initial dose of 0.1 mg/kg/day with
   a maximum of 5 mg po qd.
Monitoring:
• For those patients receiving heparin, daily PT/INRs are required.
• For those initiated on a maintenance dose, PT/INR should be checked every
   2–3 days for the first two weeks.
Dose Adjustments:
   For patients currently receiving a parenteral anticoagulant, adjustments to the
   loading dose are made based on the results of the INR as follows:

INR	Warfarin Adjustment
1.1–1.39	repeat initial loading dose
1.4–3.09	50% of initial loading dose
3.1–3.5	25% of initial loading dose
>3.5	hold until INR <3.5 then restart at 50% less than previous dose

• When the INR is therapeutic two days in a row, discontinue the heparin.
   For patients initiated on a maintenance dose, adjustments to the dose are made
   based on the results of the INR as follows:

INR	Warfarin Adjustment
1.1–1.49	increase dose by 10%
1.5–1.99	increase dose by 10% if > day 5, otherwise no change
2.0–3.09	no change
3.1–3.5	decrease dose by 10% (if < day 5 then recheck in 24 hours)
>3.5	hold until INR <3.5, then restart at 20% less than previous dose (check INR qod)

Maintenance Warfarin Therapy:
• The INR should be checked twice weekly for 1–2 weeks after therapeutic INR
   achieved following the initiation of warfarin therapy (see below for initiation of
   warfarin therapy).
• The INR is then checked weekly for 3–4 weeks, then if stable every 2 weeks for
   4 weeks, then every 3 weeks for 6 weeks, then every 4 weeks thereafter.
• 5–7 days after the start of any new medications, the INR should be checked, then
   follow above sequence starting with weekly INRs.
• After a dose adjustment of the warfarin, the INR should be checked in 5–7 days,
   then the above sequence is followed starting with weekly INRs.

cont.

Table 5.5.
continued

INR	Warfarin Adjustment
1.1–1.49	increase dose by 20%
1.5–1.99	increase dose by 10%
2.0–3.09	no change
3.1–3.5	decrease dose by 10%
>3.5	hold until INR <3.5, then restart at 20% less than previous dose (check INR qod)

†OAT, oral anticoagulant therapy.

3. Low molecular weight heparin (LMWH) (see Table 5.6): Numerous LMWH are in clinical use in adults, and there are subtle variations in their efficacy in different clinical circumstances. Enoxaparin (Lovenox) is the most commonly used LMWH in children, and dose finding studies in children have been performed. Twice daily subcutaneous therapy is the most common dose schedule, although IV use in neonates has been reported. The advantages over UFH are more predictable pharmacokinetics and less bleeding risk. However, LMWH is not completely reversible with protamine. Before any procedure, especially lumber puncture, at least 2 doses of LMWH should be excluded.

4. Organan is a glycosaminoglycan with high anti-Xa activity. In adults, it is used for surgical thromboprophylaxis and management of heparin-induced thrombocytopenia (HIT). In children, organan is the most common agent used for HIT.

5. Argatroban: There are insufficient published data on the use of argatroban in children to make worthwhile comment.

6. Hirudin: There are case reports of hirudin being used for HIT in children.

7. Drotrecogin alfa (activated protein C) is used in severe sepsis for its antithrombotic, anti-inflammatory, and profibrinolytic properties. There are not sufficient data in children to guide its use in this population.

8. Fibrinolytic agents. The actions of thrombolytic agents are mediated by converting endogenous plasminogen into plasmin. Newborns have plasminogen levels

Table 5.6.
Protocol for Monitoring Enoxaparin for Treating Thrombosis

Dose:
  <2 months old: 1.5 mg/kg/dose SC q12h
  >2 months old: 1.0 mg/kg/dose SC q12h
Check antifactor Xa level 4–6 hours after first or second dose.

Antifactor Xa Level (U/ml)	Dose Change	Hold Dose?	Repeat Antifactor Xa Level
<0.35	Increase by 25%	No	4–6 hrs after next dose
0.35–0.49	Increase by 10%	No	4–6 hrs after next dose, or after 2nd new dose
0.5–1.0	No	No	1–4 days later, then weekly. May increase interval to every 2–4 weeks if stable.
1.1–1.5	Decrease by 20%	No	4–6 hrs after next dose, or after 2nd new dose.
1.6–2.0	Decrease by 30%	3 hours	Before dose and 4–6 hrs after next dose
>2.0	Decrease by 40%	Until antifactor Xa <0.5 U/ml	Follow antifactor Xa q12h until <0.5 U/ml, then 4–6 hrs after next dose.

Monitoring of Low Molecular Weight Heparin
1. Draw blood from fresh venipuncture. There must be no contamination from standard heparin.
2. On day 1 and/or day 2, a blood sample should be drawn 4 hours after the SQ administration of Enoxaparin. If therapeutic, a weekly check on the antifactor Xa level is sufficient while the patient is an inpatient, then every two weeks if level has been stable.
3. The therapeutic anti-Xa level for treatment dose therapy is 0.5–1 units/mL.
4. For patients on long-term Enoxaparin therapy (>3 months), consider bone densitometry studies at baseline and then every 6 months to assess for possible osteoporosis.

Enoxaparin Antidote

If anticoagulation with Enoxaparin needs to be discontinued, termination of the SC injection will usually suffice. If an immediate effect is required, protamine sulfate has been shown in experimental animal models to decrease microvascular bleeding produced by very high concentrations of Enoxaparin. If protamine is given within 3–4 hours of the Enoxaparin, then a maximal neutralizing dose is: 1 mg of protamine sulfate per 1 mg of Enoxaparin given in last dose. The protamine should be administered IV and over 10–20 minutes. Protamine sulfate should be given only after consultation with hematology.

cont.

Table 5.6.
continued

Low Molecular Weight Heparin Dilution Procedure
For doses less than 5 mg only:

Ingredient	Quantity
Enoxaparin syringe 30 mg/0.3 ml	1 syringe
Water for injection	qs to 1.5 ml
Enoxaparin injection 20 mg/ml	0.1 ml = 2 mg

Procedure:
- Withdraw water for injection into 3 ml syringe, almost to 1.5 ml
- Inject contents of the enoxaparin syringe directly into the water for injection and fill to a total volume of 1.5 ml. Inject into a sterile vial.
- Fill dose syringe to volume required plus 0.05 ml overfill (for needle) from this vial
- Cap and label syringe.

Storage: Refrigerate.
Expiration: 24 hours.

reduced to 50% of adult values. Many children with thrombosis may have acquired plasminogen deficiency. Supplementation with plasma before thrombolysis increases the thrombolytic effect and reduces the bleeding risk. Tissue plasminogen activator (tPA) is the most commonly used thrombolytic agent in children. The indications for thrombolysis in children are limited; however, most commonly acute arterial thrombosis is secondary to intravascular access. Acute central vein CVAD thrombosis, especially when there is an ongoing need for central venous access, may benefit from thrombolysis. There are very few data on the use of thrombolysis in stroke or sinovenous thrombosis in children. Local, low-dose thrombolysis is used frequently to restore patency to dysfunctional CVAD. (See Table 5.7).

B. Interventional strategies
1. IVC filters placed by interventional radiologic techniques are useful in patients with recurrent pulmonary embolism who are not responding to or cannot tolerate medical therapy.

Table 5.7.
Guidelines for Local Instillation of Tissue Plasminogen Activator

Weight	Single-Lumen CVL	Double-Lumen CVL	SC Port
<30 kg	110% of estimated internal lumen volume of 1 mg/ml conc. or 1ml of a 0.5 mg/ml conc. diluted with 0.9% NaCl	Treat one lumen at a time with 1mg/ml conc. or use 0.5 mg/ml conc. to treat both lumens simultaneously.	110% of estimated internal lumen vol. + reservoir vol. of 1 mg/ml conc. or 3 ml of a 0.5 mg/ml conc. 0.5 mg diluted with 0.9% NaCl
≥30 kg	2 ml of a 1mg/mL conc. (0.5 mg/ml conc. has also been used).	Treat one lumen at a time with 2 ml of a 1mg/ml conc. or use 2 ml of a 0.5 mg/ml conc. to treat both lumens simultaneously.	2 ml of a 1 mg/ml conc. (may need to dilute 2 mg to 3 ml with 0.9% NaCl for some larger patients)

Note: CVL, central venous line; SC, subcutaneous port; TPA, tissue plasminogen activator; kg, kilograms; mg, milligrams; NaCl, sodium chloride; mL, milliliters.

    2.   Stents are being used with increasing frequency to treat persistent or severe postphlebitic syndrome.

    3.   Intrathrombus delivery of thrombolytic therapy has been used successfully in both adults and children. However, evidence-based guidelines for the use of catheter directed thrombolytic therapy do not exist for children.

IV. PRIMARY PROPHYLAXIS

    A.   L-asparaginase-induced hypercoagulable state
        1.   FFP contains all the procoagulant and anticoagulant proteins but only at a concentration of 1 u/ml, limiting its usefulness for replacing anticoagulant proteins, which require higher levels to restore physiologic function. There are insufficient data supporting the use of FFP for asymptomatic AT deficiency in patients receiving L-asparaginase.
        2.   Antithrombin concentrate can be used to treat the acquired AT deficiency associated with L-asparaginase. However, there are insufficient data supporting its use for prophylaxis.

3. Low molecular weight heparin is used in adults for pro-
    phylaxis in high-risk situations. The risk/benefit ratio
    cannot be accurately evaluated for children due to a
    lack of data.

B. Central venous catheter-related thrombosis
    1. Low molecular weight heparin is being studied, but at
        this time, no specific recommendations can be made.
    2. Warfarin at a low dose of 1 mg has been used in adults
        with some studies showing a benefit with minimal ad-
        verse effects. However, no study in children with cancer
        has been performed.

C. Short-term prophylactic anticoagulation in high-risk situ-
    ations such as immobility, significant surgery, or trauma
    is an option for children with known congenital prothrom-
    botic disorders. However, there are no published data on
    which to base a formal recommendation.

D. Veno-occlusive disease (VOD)—see also Section VG
    1. Antithrombin concentrate can be used in BMT patients
        with acquired AT deficiency who are at risk for VOD.
    2. Low molecular weight heparin has been used to pre-
        vent VOD and has been shown to be beneficial in
        some studies. However, data for its use in children are
        lacking.

V. MANAGEMENT OF SPECIFIC THROMBOTIC COMPLICATIONS

A. Deep venous thrombosis
    1. First thromboembolic event (TE): Children (over
        2 months of age) with an initial TE should be acutely
        treated with IV heparin sufficient to prolong the APTT
        to a range that corresponds to an antifactor Xa level
        of 0.3 to 0.7 units/ml; or LMWH sufficient to achieve an
        antifactor Xa level of 0.5 to 1.0 units/ml,4 hours after
        an injection. This recommendation is based on current
        recommendations for adults and cohort studies in chil-
        dren.
        a. Initial treatment with heparin or LMWH should be
            continued for 5–10 days. For patients in whom sub-
            sequent oral anticoagulant therapy will be used, it

can be started as early as day 1 and heparin/LMWH discontinued on day 6 if the INR is therapeutic on 2 consecutive days. For massive PE or extensive DVT, a longer period of heparin or LMWH therapy should be considered. This recommendation is based on recommendations for adults and two cohort studies in children.

b. Anticoagulant therapy should be continued for at least 3 months using oral anticoagulants to prolong the PT to a target INR of 2.5, range 2.0 to 3.0, or alternatively LMWH, to maintain an antifactor Xa level of 0.5 to 1.0 units/ml. This recommendation is based on recommendations for adults, two cohort, and six case series in children.

c. For children with an idiopathic TE, treatment should be continued for at least 6 months with either oral anticoagulants or LMWH. This recommendation is based on recommendations for adults.

d. After the initial 3 months of therapy, for children with a first CVL-related DVT, prophylactic doses of oral anticoagulants (INR 1.5 to 1.8) or LMWH (antifactor Xa levels of 0.1 to 0.3) are an option until the CVL is removed. However, there are no published data on which to base a formal recommendation.

2. Recurrent thromboembolic event. Recurrent TEs should be treated longer and a more extensive search for underlying prothrombotic states should be carried out.

a. For recurrent non-CVL-related TEs, following the initial 3 months of therapy, indefinite therapy with either therapeutic or prophylactic doses of oral anticoagulants or LMWH should be used. This recommendation is based on recommendations for adults.

b. For recurrent CVL-related TEs, following the initial 3 months of therapy, prophylactic doses of oral anticoagulants (INR 1.5 to 1.8) or LMWH (*antifactor* Xa levels of 0.1–0.3) should be continued until removal of the CVL. If the recurrence occurs while on prophylactic therapy, therapeutic doses should be continued until the CVL is removed or for a minimum of 12 months.

B. Sinovenous thrombosis (dural sinus thrombosis): Treatment with low molecular weight, heparin has been used in children and adults with DST. However, in children with cancer, the risk of intracranial hemorrhage is higher and; therefore, anticoagulant therapy should be used only if there is extensive and/or progressive thrombosis.

C. Stroke: The use of antithrombotic therapy in children with cancer who experience stroke cannot be recommended given the risk of hemorrhagic transformation. Management should focus on treating the underlying cause(s).

D. DIC can occur in children with cancer from a number of different causes. Treating the underlying cause is critical. Activated protein C is available, but its use in children with cancer has not been adequately studied.

E. Atrial thrombosis is often associated with CVLs, and the risk of PE is unclear. Therefore, treatment should be decided on an individual basis. Evaluation for occult PE is advised.

F. Endocarditis: There is no clear role for antithrombotic therapy in the management of endocarditis. If a TE has occurred, consider antithrombotic therapy.

G. Veno-occlusive disease
   1. Antithrombin concentrate (Thrombate III) has been used to treat and prevent VOD because of the association of antithrombin deficiency with VOD.
   2. Alteplase (TPA) has been used to treat life-threatening VOD, but the risk of serious bleeding is very high in these patients.
   3. Heparin, including low molecular weight heparin, has been used to prevent and treat VOD.
   4. Defibrotide has been shown to be beneficial in some patients with VOD but is not yet available in the United States.

H. Purpura fulminans is rare in children with cancer. It is usually associated with severe protein C or S deficiency.

Treatment with protein C concentrate or FFP is advised. Antithrombotic therapy can also be used.

VI. MANAGEMENT OF CANCER PATIENTS ON ANTITHROMBOTIC THERAPY

Multiple factors can increase the risk of bleeding in patients with cancer who are also being treated with antithrombotic therapy; thrombocytopenia, liver dysfunction, consumptive coagulopathies, invasive procedures, local tissue disruption from infections, or neoplasm are among a few.

Those patients being treated with antithrombotic therapy should have the platelet count kept above 20,000 in low-risk situations, 30,000 in moderate-risk situation, and 50,000 in high-risk situation (see below).

Before undergoing a lumbar puncture, patients on warfarin should have an INR of 1.5 or less, and those on LMWH should have 2 doses held.

In summary, bleeding and clotting are potentially important complications in children with cancer and are often multifactorial in origin. Careful history, examination, and routine coagulation tests are critical to appropriate assessment. An increasing number of therapeutic agents can be used to treat clotting or bleeding complications; however, the evidence for the benefit of many of these treatments remains low, especially in children. Considerably more research is required into coagulation abnormalities in children with cancer and multicenter trials of primary prophylaxis and treatment will be necessary to optimize care.

Bibliography

Andrew M, Monagle P, Brooker L. *Thromboembolic Complications during Infancy and Childhood*. Hamilton, Ont.: B. C. Decker, Inc., 2000.

Monagle P, Michelson AD, Bovill E, Andrew M. Antithrombotic therapy in children. *Chest* Jan. 119 (1 Suppl.):344–70S, 2001.

6

Hematopoietic Growth Factors

Jeffrey D. Hord, M.D., and Julia Cartwright, R.Ph.

Several recombinant human (rh) hematopoietic growth factors are approved and in clinical use. Granulocyte-colony stimulating factor (rhG-CSF, filgrastim) and granulocyte-macrophage-colony-stimulating factor (rhGM-CSF, sargramostim) stimulate the proliferation, maturation, and function of granulocytes. Interleukin-11 (rhIL-11, oprelvekin) stimulates the proliferation of megakaryocyte progenitor cells and the maturation of megakaryocytes resulting in increased platelet production. Erythropoietin (rhEPO, epoetin alfa) stimulates the proliferation and differentiation of committed erythroid progenitors, including burst-forming unit-erythroid cells and colony-forming unit-erythroid cells.

Even though hematopoietic growth factors are approved for use in children, both the indications and doses for children are largely unsettled. Although the severity of neutropenia after myelo-suppressive chemotherapy may be unaffected by the administration of filgrastim or sargramostim, the duration of neutropenia is typically shortened. While there is some evidence that the prophylactic administration of filgrastim reduces the incidence of febrile episodes with neutropenia, there has been no documented impact on survival. The intensification of some chemotherapeutic regimens might not be feasible without the administration of filgrastim or sargramostim to accelerate granulocyte recovery. Information about the use of epoetin alfa and oprelvekin in children with cancer is very limited. The available data suggest that many children with cancer will have higher hemoglobin levels and require fewer transfusions with the administration of epoetin alfa. Similarly, the administration of oprelvekin in a small number of children following myelosuppressive chemotherapy shortened the duration of thrombocytopenia and led to fewer platelet transfusions.

Most recently, both filgrastim and epoetin alfa have been modified (pegylation of filgrastim and addition of 2 N-glycosylation sites to epoetin alfa) to lengthen the half-life of these growth factors and decrease the frequency of administration. At this time, there is no experience with the administration of these specific agents in children.

Consider the following guidelines as a general framework that will be refined as additional data become available. When no specific recommendations for the use of hematopoietic growth factors exist within a study protocol or the patient is not enrolled in a study, the following guidelines may prove useful.

Recombinant Human Granulocyte-Colony-Stimulating Factor (rhG-CSF, filgrastim, Neupogen manufactured by Amgen)

I. **INDICATIONS AND CONTRAINDICATIONS**

A. Proven indications
1. To accelerate granulocyte recovery after dose-intensive myelosuppressive chemotherapy for high-risk malignancies such as AML, B cell non-Hodgkin lymphoma, neuroblastoma, soft-tissue sarcoma, and osteosarcoma.
2. To accelerate granulocyte recovery in patients who have undergone bone marrow transplantation for non-myeloid malignancies.
3. To mobilize peripheral blood stem cells before leukapheresis in stem cell donors.

B. Controversial indications
1. To accelerate granulocyte recovery, when an ANC of <500 cells/mcL for ≥7 days is anticipated, secondary to noncytotoxic myelosuppressive agents (e.g., ganciclovir, zidovudine).
2. To accelerate granulocyte recovery in patients with febrile neutropenia or neutropenia and sepsis when filgrastim was not administered empirically.

C. Contraindications
1. History of hypersensitivity to filgrastim or *E. coli*–derived proteins.
2. Sickle cell anemia

II. ADMINISTRATION

A. Dosage
   1. Starting dose is 5 mcg/kg/d SC or IV over 15–30 minutes once daily.
   2. No studies in children have demonstrated a significant difference in neutrophil response with higher doses (>5 mcg/kg/d).
   3. In patients preparing for stem cell collection, the usual dose is 10 mcg/kg/d SC or IV for at least 4 days before leukapheresis and to continue until collection is complete.

B. Duration
   In cancer patients following myelosuppressive chemotherapy, start filgrastim 24 hours after the last chemotherapeutic agent and continuing until the ANC is 5,000–10,000 cells/mcL after the expected chemotherapy-induced nadir. The ANC will often increase transiently 2 days after the initiation of filgrastim. Avoid premature discontinuation before the expected ANC nadir. Do not administer filgrastim within 24 hours of the administration of chemotherapy.

C. Monitoring
   Monitor complete blood, differential, and platelet counts before starting filgrastim, and 1–2 times weekly, past the neutrophil nadir until target ANC reached. More frequent monitoring of WBC might be needed to avoid excessive leukocytosis.

D. Formulation and preparation
   1. Filgrastim (rh G-CSF, Neupogen®) is supplied as single-dose, preservative-free vials containing 300 mcg or 480 mcg both at a concentration of 300 mcg/mL and in single-use syringes of 300 mcg/0.5 ml and 480 mcg/0.8 ml.
   2. Each vial or syringe contains 300 mcg of filgrastim in a solution containing 10 mM sodium acetate buffer at pH 4.0, with 5% sorbitol and 0.004% Tween 80 and 0.035 mg sodium in 1 mL or 0.5 ml, respectively, of water for injection, USP.
   3. Vials and syringes are single-dose and should not be re-entered or reused for later administration, since filgrastim is supplied as a preservative-free solution.

E. Dilution
    1. Dilute filgrastim only in dextrose 5% in water (D5W). Avoid shaking. Do not dilute in saline.
    2. If the concentration of the diluted filgrastim is 5–15 mcg/mL, add albumin to the D5W to make an albumin concentration of 2 mg/ml before adding the filgrastim. Dilutions of less than 5 mcg/mL are not recommended.

F. Storage
    1. Store filgrastim at 2–8°C. Do not freeze. Vials are stable for a maximum of 24 hours at room temperature.
    2. After dilution in D5W, the solution is stable in the refrigerator or room temperature for 7 days. Since the solution is preservative-free, practice caution to maintain sterility.

III. ADVERSE EFFECTS

A. Common: Mild to moderate bone pain, elevation of uric acid, lactate dehydrogenase (LDH), and alkaline phosphatase.
B. Occasional: Fever, nausea and vomiting, rash, diarrhea, splenomegaly, exacerbation of psoriasis, hypotension, and erythema at the injection site.
C. Rare: Allergic reactions, acute respiratory distress syndrome, splenic rupture.

PEGylated Recombinant Human Granulocyte-Colony Stimulating Factor (PEG-rhG-CSF, pegfilgrastim, Neulasta manufactured by Amgen)

I. INDICATIONS AND CONTRAINDICATIONS

A. Proven indications
    1. There is no experience with pegfilgrastim in pediatrics.
    2. To decrease the incidence of infection, as manifested by febrile neutropenia, in patients weighing ≥45 kilograms with non-myeloid malignancies receiving myelosuppressive chemotherapy.

B. Contraindications
    1. Weight less than <45 kilograms

2. Scheduled to receive chemotherapy within the next 14 days
3. History of hypersensitivity to filgrastim or *E. coli*–derived proteins
4. Sickle cell anemia

II. ADMINISTRATION

A. Dosage
There is one standard dose of 6 mg SC for all those weighing ≥45 kilograms and should be administered only once per chemotherapy cycle, no sooner than 24 hours after the last dose of chemotherapy.

B. Formulation and preparation
Pegfilgrastim is supplied as 0.6 mL prefilled syringes containing 6 mg pegfilgrastim in a sterile, clear, colorless, preservative-free solution containing acetate, sorbitol, polysorbate 20, and sodium in water for injection, USP.

C. Storage
Store pegfilgrastim at 2–8°C. Do not freeze. Do not shake syringe.

III. ADVERSE EFFECTS

The adverse effects observed with pegfilgrastim therapy are similar in type and frequency to those observed with filgrastim therapy.

Recombinant Human Granulocyte-Macrophage-Colony-Stimulating Factor (rhGM-CSF, sargramostim, Leukine manufactured by Immunex)

I. INDICATIONS AND CONTRAINDICATIONS

A. Proven indications
1. To accelerate myeloid recovery after autologous stem cell/ bone marrow transplantation for non-Hodgkin lymphoma, Hodgkin lymphoma, or acute lymphoblastic leukemia.
2. To accelerate myeloid recovery in patients with delayed or failed engraftment after autologous or allogeneic stem cell/ bone marrow transplant.

3. Mobilization of hematopoietic progenitors cells into peripheral blood for collection by leukapheresis.
4. To accelerate myeloid recovery after peripheral blood stem cell transplantation.

B. Controversial indications
1. To accelerate myeloid recovery in patients who have undergone autologous bone marrow transplantation for myeloid malignancy.
2. To shorten the time to neutrophil recovery and to decrease the incidence of life-threatening infections in adults after induction chemotherapy for acute myelogenous leukemia.

C. Contraindications
1. Excessive myeloid blasts ($\geq 10\%$) in bone marrow or peripheral blood
2. Juvenile chronic myeloid leukemia or monosomy 7 syndrome
3. History of hypersensitivity to sargramostim or yeast-derived proteins
4. Concomitant use of chemotherapy or radiation therapy
5. Sickle cell anemia

II. ADMINISTRATION

A. Dosage
Starting dose is 250 mcg/m^2/day SC or IV over 2–24 hours.

B. Duration
1. When given after stem cell or marrow transplantation, the first dose should be given within 24 hours after the stem cell or bone marrow infusion, then once a day until the ANC >1,500 cells/mcL for 3 consecutive days.
2. In case of engraftment delay or failure of bone marrow transplant, 14 days of treatment may be necessary.
3. For mobilization of peripheral stem cells, sargramostim is infused daily, usually starting 5 days before the date of planned collection, and is continued until the collection is complete.

C. Monitoring
1. CBC with differential and platelet counts should be monitored 1–2 times weekly and sargramostim should be discontinued when ANC is 5,000–10,000 cells/mcL.

2. If blasts appear or disease progresses, discontinue sargramostim.
3. Monitor renal and hepatic function twice a week and more often for patients with organ dysfunction.
4. Due to possible fluid retention syndrome, monitor patients for weight gain, respiratory distress, and pleural or pericardial effusions.

D. Formulation and preparation
1. Sterile, white, preservative-free, lyophilized powder in vials containing 250 mcg of sargramostim to be reconstituted with 1 mL of Sterile Water for Injection, USP or 1 mL of Bacteriostatic Water for Injection, USP. Avoid shaking.

    Administer product reconstituted with sterile water within 6 hours of preparation: Product reconstituted with bacteriostatic water may be stored for up to 20 days at 2–8°C.
2. Liquid Leukine is a sterile, preserved (1.1% benzyl alcohol), injectable solution in multiple-dose vials containing 500 mcg of sargramostim with 40 mg of mannitol, 10 mg of sucrose, and 1.2 mg of tromethamine in 1 mL of water. Since this product is preserved, once the vial is entered, the drug may be stored for up to 20 days at 2–8°C. Discard any remaining solution after 20 days.

    Both Leukine liquid and lyophilized Leukine reconstituted with Bacteriostatic Water for Injection, USP contains benzyl alcohol and should *not* be administered to neonates due to fatal gasping syndrome.

E. Dilution
For IV infusion, dilute with 0.9% NaCl. If the concentration of sargramostim is <10 mcg/mL, to prevent absorption to the drug delivery system, add albumin to the saline before adding the sargramostim to make a 0.1% albumin solution.

F. Storage
Store all preparations at 2–8°C. Do not freeze.

III. ADVERSE EFFECTS

A. Common: Bone pain, injection site reactions.
B. Occasional: Fluid retention (peripheral edema, pleural effusion, pericardial effusion), leukocytosis, diarrhea, asthenia,

rash, malaise, headache, fever, chills, arthralgias, chest pain, thrombocytopenia, dyspnea, thrombophlebitis, eosinophilia.

C. Rare: Allergic reactions, dyspnea, respiratory distress syndrome, weight gain, thrombosis of vena cava, hypotension, facial flushing, bundle branch block, supraventricular arrhythmias, and elevation of serum creatinine or bilirubin or hepatic enzymes in those with preexisting renal or hepatic disease.

Recombinant Human Erythropoietin (rhEPO, epoetin alfa, Procrit manufactured by Ortho-Biotech, Epogen manufactured by Amgen)

Three points must be emphasized if the use of epoetin alfa is being considered: (1) disproportionate anemia compared with neutropenia and thrombocytopenia suggests other causes of low hemoglobin/hematocrit (iron deficiency, bleeding, or hemolysis) that will not be resolved with epoetin alfa; (2) not all patients will respond to epoetin alfa, sometimes due to "end-organ" problems (myelodysplastic syndrome and some anemias of chronic disease); and (3) some patients receiving cisplatin-containing regimens (due to renal damage) might respond better to epoetin alfa.

I. INDICATIONS AND CONTRAINDICATIONS

A. Proven indications
There are no proven indications in pediatric oncology.

B. Controversial indications
1. Anemia of chronic disease or secondary to chemotherapy to decrease the need of blood transfusions
2. Anemia associated with radiation therapy
3. Anemia secondary to myelodysplastic syndrome when baseline serum EPO is low
4. Anemia after allogeneic bone marrow transplantation

C. Contraindications
1. Anemia secondary to nutritional deficiencies (iron, folic acid, or vitamin B_{12}), bleeding, or hemolytic anemia
2. Uncontrollable hypertension

3. Hypersensitivity to mammalian cell-derived products
4. Hypersensitivity to human albumin
5. Anemia unresponsive to 6–8 weeks of epoetin alfa with adequate iron stores present

II. ADMINISTRATION

A. Baseline laboratory tests
   1. Before starting epoetin alfa therapy, all patients should have a baseline ferritin measurement and other causes for the anemia should be excluded.
   2. If ferritin is <100 ng/mL, prescribe iron supplementation (ferrous sulfate).
   3. Ferritin should be measured monthly during therapy.

B. Dosage
   1. Starting dose: 150 U/kg/day SC or IV 3 times a week
   2. If there is no response within 4 weeks, the dose can be increased to 300 U/kg/day SC or IV 3 times a week.
   3. If the hematocrit (Hct) reaches ≥36% decrease the dose by 25%, if it reaches 40%, stop the epoetin alfa dose until the Hct is <36%; restart at a 25% dose reduction. Titration might be necessary.
   4. If the Hct increases very rapidly (>4 percentage points in 2 weeks), reduce the epoetin alfa dose by 25%.
   5. Adult data support the use of once per week dosing of epoetin alfa instead of 3 times per week for the treatment of chemotherapy-induced anemia. Adult patients begin with a dose of 40,000 U/week, with an increase to 60,000 U/week if no response is seen in 4 weeks. If an additional 4-week treatment shows no response, the patient is usually considered a nonresponder. Once weekly dosing is being studied in the pediatric oncology population currently.

C. Duration
   1. Continue epoetin alfa until the patient is considered no longer at risk for red blood cell transfusion.
   2. Epoetin alfa can be given concurrently with chemotherapy treatment.

D. Monitoring
   1. Perform a baseline CBC with platelet count and reticulocyte count. Thereafter, monitor the hematocrit and

hemoglobin weekly to monthly until the HCT becomes stable.
2. Monitor blood urea nitrogen, creatinine, and potassium every 2 weeks for the first month and once a month thereafter.
3. Monitor ferritin once a month.

E. Formulation and preparation
1. Single-dose, preservative-free 1 mL vial containing epoetin alfa: 2,000, 3,000, 4,000, 10,000, 20,000, or 40,000 U/ml of injectable solution. Each 1 mL of preservative-free solution contains the above amounts of epoetin alfa with 2.5 mg of albumin (human), 5.8 mg of sodium citrate, 5.8 mg of sodium chloride, and 0.06 mg of citric acid in water.
2. Multiple-dose, preserved 2 mL vial containing epoetin alfa: 10,000 U/mL. Each 1 mL of preserved solution contains 10,000 U of epoetin alfa, 2.5 mg of albumin (human), 1.3 mg of sodium citrate, 8.2 mg of sodium chloride, 0.11 mg of citric acid, and 1% benzyl alcohol as preservative in water.

F. Dilution
Do not dilute epoetin alfa or give with other drugs. However, before subcutaneous injection, it can be mixed in bacteriostatic 0.9% sodium chloride with benzyl alcohol 0.9% at 1:1. The benzyl alcohol acts as an anesthetic.

G. Storage
Store at 2–8°C. Do not freeze or shake.

III. ADVERSE EFFECTS

A. Common: Hypertension, local pain at site of injection, headache, fever, and diarrhea
B. Occasional: Nausea, flulike symptoms, thrombosis of vascular access devices, and seizures

Darbepoetin Alfa (Aranesp, manufactured by Amgen Pharmaceuticals)

I. INDICATIONS AND CONTRAINDICATIONS

A. Proven indications
1. Treatment of anemia associated with chronic renal failure including patients on dialysis.

2. Treatment of chemotherapy-induced anemia.

Note: There are currently no pediatric indications for this agent. A relatively small pharmacokinetic study showed similar pharmacokinetics in pediatric and adult chronic renal failure patients, although children may absorb the drug more rapidly.

B. Contraindications
1. Patients with uncontrolled hypertension.
2. Known hypersensitivity to the active substance or any of the excipients. (Two formulations exist, one containing polysorbate 80 and one containing albumin.)

II. ADMINISTRATION

A. Dosage
1. The estimated starting dose for epoetin alfa treatment-naïve patients is 0.45 mcg/kg SC or IV once per week for chronic renal failure (round dose to nearest vial size for convenience when reasonable). The dose for chemotherapy-induced anemia is the same but given every two weeks rather than weekly (i.e., 100 mcg/week = 200 mcg every 2 weeks). Verify iron stores approximately every month while the patient is on darbepoetin alfa.
2. To convert patients currently on epoetin alfa, the guidelines in Table 6.1 may be useful.

B. Monitoring
1. Doses should be adjusted to achieve and maintain a target hemoglobin ≤ 12 g/dL.
2. Do not increase doses any more frequently than monthly.
3. If the hemoglobin is increasing and approaching 12 g/dL, decrease the dose by 25%.
4. If the hemoglobin continues to rise, hold the dose until it is <12 g/dL and decreasing. Decrease the dose by 25%.
5. If the hemoglobin increases by more than 1 g/dL in a 2-week period, decrease the dose by 25%.
6. If the patient is not responding to darbepoetin alfa (response = hemoglobin increase by at least 1 g/dL in 4 weeks), verify iron stores. If iron stores are adequate, the dose may be increased by 25%.

Table 6.1.
Dosage Adjustments for Conversion from Epoetin
to Darbepoetin

Previous Weekly Epoetin Dose	Weekly Darbepoetin Dose
<2500 units	6.25 mcg
2,500–4,999 units	12.5 mcg
5,000–10,999 units	25 mcg
11,000–17,999 units	40 mcg
18,000–33,999 units	60 mcg
34,000–89,999 units	100 mcg
$\geq 90,000$ units	200 mcg

7. If no response is seen in 6–8 weeks (and adequate iron stores are present), the patient is likely a nonresponder.

C. Formulation and preparation
Darbepoetin alfa is available in 25, 40, 60, 100, and 200 mcg/1mL vials in solutions containing either polysorbate 80 or albumin.

D. Storage
Store darbepoetin alfa at 2–8°C. Do not shake; protect from light.

III. ADVERSE EFFECTS

The adverse effects observed with darbepoetin alfa are similar in type and frequency to those observed with epoetin alfa. *Note*: Much of these data were collected from the chronic renal failure patient population.

A. Common: Hyper- and hypotension, headache, diarrhea, nausea, vomiting, myalgia, infection, upper respiratory infection
B. Occasional: Peripheral edema, abdominal pain, arthralgia, limb/back pain, dizziness, cough, pruritis
C. Rare, serious: Vascular access thrombosis, congestive heart failure, sepsis, cardiac arrhythmia/arrest
D. Rare, other: Injection site reactions, fever, chest pain, fluid overload, constipation, bronchitis

Recombinant Human Interleukin-11 (rhIL-11, Oprelvekin, Neumega, manufactured by Wyeth-Ayerst Pharmaceuticals)

I. INDICATIONS AND CONTRAINDICATIONS

A. Proven indications

Oprelvekin has FDA approval for prevention of severe thrombocytopenia and reducing the need for platelet transfusions after myelosuppressive chemotherapy in patients who have non-myeloid malignancies and are at high-risk of severe thrombocytopenia. Oprelvekin efficacy studies have not been conducted in children.

B. Contraindications
1. Hypersensitivity to the agent
2. Not approved for use in children, especially children younger than 12 years of age
3. Myeloid malignancies
4. Not indicated after myeloablative chemotherapy
5. Use with caution in patients with: Left ventricular dysfunction or congestive heart failure, other conditions in which volume expansion may be detrimental (hypertension, effusions, etc.), history of atrial arrhythmias, thromboembolic disorders, hepatic dysfunction, renal dysfunction, respiratory dysfunction, effusions, hypokalemia, papilledema, CNS tumors

II. ADMINISTRATION

A. Dosage
1. The approved dose in adults in 50 mcg/kg/day SQ beginning 6–24 hours after chemotherapy for 14–21 days.
2. The optimal dose in children has not been determined but may be in the range of 50–75 mcg/kg/day, although this dose is not approved. Dose-limiting papilledema has been reported in children receiving 100 mcg/kg/day of oprelvekin.
3. Pharmacokinetics studies of oprelvekin in renal failure have not been conducted, but the drug is eliminated primarily by the kidneys. Fluid balance should be closely monitored in patients with mild to moderate renal failure.

B. Duration
1. Therapy should not continue for longer than 21 days.
2. Treatment should be discontinued at least 2 days before the next course of chemotherapy.

C. Monitoring
1. Check CBC frequently during therapy (once or twice weekly) until PLT $\geq$50 x 10^9/L.
2. Periodically check heart rate, blood pressure, respiratory rate, temperature, and electrocardiogram.
3. Check for signs and symptoms of peripheral edema, check weight.
4. Observe for signs of toxicity such as dyspnea, arthralgias, fatigue, palpitations, or irregular heart beats.

III. ADVERSE EFFECTS

A. Common: Edema, peripheral edema, palpitations, tachycardia, headache, fatigue, dizziness, anorexia, nausea, conjunctivitis and papilledema in children, dyspnea (probably related to plasma volume expanding effects), skin rashes, arthralgia, myalgia.
B. Occasional: Atrial arrhythmia, thrombosis at indwelling central catheter site.
C. Rare, serious: Cerebral infarction
D. Rare, other: Syncope, weight gain, papilledema

Bibliography

2000 Update of recommendations for the use of hematopoietic colony-stimulating factors: Evidence-based clinical practice guidelines. *J Clin Oncol* 18:3558–85, 2000.

Aranesp, product information. Amgen. Issue date 9/17/2001.

Cairo MS, et al. Prospective randomized trial between two doses of granulocyte colony-stimulating factor after ifosfamide, carboplatin, and etoposide in children with recurrent or refractory solid tumors: A Children's Cancer Group report. *J Pediatr Hematol Oncol* 23:30–38, 2001.

Drugdex Editorial Staff. Darbepoetin Alfa (Drugdex Drug Evaluation). In Hutchison TA, Shahan DR, eds., *Drugdex System*. MicroMedex, Greenwood Village, Colorado (Edition expires 6/2002).

Gabrilove JL, et al. Clinical evaluation of once-weekly dosing of epoetin alfa in chemotherapy patients: Improvements in hemoglobin and quality of life are similar to three-times-weekly dosing. *J Clin Oncol* 19:2875–82, 2001.

Grabenstein, J, Drugdex Editorial Staff. Oprelvekin (Drugdex Drug Evaluation). In Hutchison TA, Shahan DR, eds., *Drugdex System*. MicroMedex, Greenwood Village, Colorado (Edition expires 6/2002).

Kushner BH, et al. Granulocyte-colony stimulating factor and multiple cycles of strongly myelosuppressive alkylator-based combination chemotherapy in children with neuroblastoma. *Cancer* 89:2122–30, 2000.

Lerner GR, et al. The pharmacokinetics of novel erythropoiesis stimulating protein (NESP) in pediatric patients with chronic renal failure (CRF) or end-stage renal disease. American Society of Nephrology 33rd Annual Meeting 2000 – Toronto, Canada. Poster #SU624.

MacMillan ML, et al. Recombinant human erythropoietin in children with cancer. *J Pediatr Hematol Oncol* 20:187–89, 1998.

Porter JC, et al. Recombinant human erythropoietin reduces the need for erythrocyte and platelet transfusions in pediatric patients with sarcoma: A randomized, double-blind, placebo-controlled trial. *J Pediatr* 129:656–60, 1996.

Schaison G, et al. Recommendations on the use of colony-stimulating factors in children: Conclusions of a European panel. *Eur J Pediatr* 157:955–66, 1998.

Tepler I, et al. A randomized placebo-controlled trial of recombinant human interleukin-11 in cancer patients with severe thrombocytopenia due to chemotherapy. *Blood* 87(9); 360 7–14, 1996.

Varan A, et al. Recombinant human erythropoietin treatment for chemotherapy-related anemia in children. *Pediatrics* 103:e16, 1999.

7

Monitoring and Management of Drug Toxicity

Prevention and Treatment of Renal and Urinary Tract Toxicity

Dorothy R. Barnard, M.D.

I. **ASSESSMENT OF RENAL FUNCTION**

    A.   Renal function can be considered under 3 major headings:
        1.   Excretory
            a.   Excretion of nonprotein nitrogenous compounds (amino acids, creatinine, urea, uric acid)
            b.   Excretion of inorganic electrolytes (Na^+, K^+, Cl^-, Ca^{++}, $PO_4^=$, Mg^{++}, $SO_4^=$, HCO_3^-)
            c.   Excretion of foreign chemicals (including heavy metals, drugs, toxins)
        2.   Regulatory
            a.   Water and electrolyte regulations
            b.   Acid-base regulations
        3.   Endocrine
            a.   Erythropoietin production
            b.   Vitamin D metabolism
            c.   Renin and others

    B.   Renal function is typically assessed by:
        1.   Measurement of urine output—oliguria is defined as urine output <0.5 ml/Kg/hr or <300 mL/M^2/hr
        2.   Assessment of glomerular filtration

   a. Measurement of blood urea nitrogen (BUN) and creatinine levels offers a crude assessment of glomerular filtration. The interpretation of these values must take the following confounding factors into account:

     i. BUN level may be elevated because of dehydration

     ii. Serum creatinine may be elevated by factors other than impaired glomerular filtration. These include:

       (1) Agents that interfere with the assay (ketosis, cephalosporins)

       (2) Factors that increase the creatinine pool (vigorous activity, muscle growth, anabolic steroids, meat ingestion)

       (3) Agents that interfere with tubular secretion of creatinine (cimetidine, probenecid, trimethoprim)

     iii. Serum creatinine may be decreased by dietary protein restriction

   b. Glomerular filtration function may be more sensitively assessed by measurement of creatinine clearance or glomerular filtration rate (GFR) scintigraphy study.

     Creatinine clearance may be estimated from plasma creatinine by using the following formula:

$$\text{GFR (mL/min./1.73 m}^2) = k \times L/PCr$$

     $k = 0.55$ for children and adolescent girls; 0.7 for adolescent boys

     L = height (cm.)

     PCr = plasma creatinine (mg/dl)

3. Renal tubular function can be assessed by:

   a. Urinary concentrating and diluting abilities

   b. Fractional excretion of sodium and phosphate

   c. Screening for glucosuria, aminoaciduria, and phosphaturia

   d. Ability to acidify urine

   e. Screening for "tubular" proteinuria (beta-2-microglobulin, retinol-binding protein)

II. SYMPTOMS OF RENAL DAMAGE

A. Symptoms
1. Hypocalcemia: Symptoms associated with hypocalcemia include vomiting, muscle weakness, irritability, tetany, ECG changes (prolonged QT interval), and seizures. Long-term consequences include rachitic changes.
2. Hypokalemia: Symptoms associated with hypokalemia include fatigue, neuromuscular disturbances (weakness, hyporeflexia, paresthesia, cramps, restless legs, rhabdomyolysis, paralysis), gastrointestinal disorders (constipation and ileus), cardiovascular abnormalities (orthostatic hypotension, worsening of hypertension, and arrhythmias), ECG changes (T wave flattening, prominent U waves, and ST segment depression), and renal abnormalities (metabolic alkalosis, polyuria, polydipsia, and glucose intolerance).
3. Hypomagnesemia: Symptoms related to hypomagnesemia include anorexia, nausea, lethargy, confusion, tremor, fasciculations, ataxia, nystagmus, tetany, seizures, and ECG changes (prolonged PR and QT intervals, and arrhythmias). Hypomagnesemia can cause hypokalemia or hypocalcemia.
4. Hyponatremia: Symptoms may occur if hyponatremia develops rapidly. These signs/symptoms can include lethargy, muscle cramps, anorexia, nausea and vomiting, agitation, disorientation, hypothermia, and seizures. The manifestations of hyponatremia depend on whether the hyponatremia results from water overload or sodium deficiency.
5. Hypophosphatemia
   a. Etiology of hypophosphatemia can be related to:
      i. Inadequate input (i.e., starvation, continuous vomiting, or impaired absorption)
      ii. Excessive losses (tubular reabsorptive defect, acidosis, massive diuresis, glycosuria, ketonuria, and catabolic states)
      iii. Acute volume expansion (syndrome of inappropriate antidiuretic hormone)
      iv. Redistribution (respiratory alkalosis, metabolic alkalosis, carbohydrate load, corticosteroids,

and insulin). Hypophosphatemia can be exaggerated by hypomagnesemia.

    b. Symptoms associated with hypophosphatemia result from decreased availability of phosphate for synthesis of adenosine triphosphate and 2,3-diphosphoglycerol. Superimposition of an acute shortage of inorganic phosphate on cells with disturbed energy metabolism may result in clinical symptoms. Hypophosphatemia can lead to osteomalacia, paresthesia, paralysis, irritability, malaise, seizures, coma, myalgias, bone pain, increased oxygen binding by hemoglobin, dysfunctional granulocytes, increased platelet aggregation, hypercalcuria, anorexia, cardiac arrhythmias, metabolic acidosis, and poor diaphragmatic function.

    6. Metabolic acidosis (secondary to urinary bicarbonate losses): Symptoms/signs of metabolic acidosis include tachypnea, hyperventilation, abdominal pain, vomiting, fever, and lethargy.

B. Grading of renal, genitourinary, and other toxicities

Grading of toxicities caused by therapeutic interventions allows an assessment of an individual patient's response and comparison of complications of one treatment program with another (see Table 7.1).

III. RENAL TOXICITY TO BE EXPECTED WITH SPECIFIC CHEMOTHERAPEUTIC AGENTS

A. 5-Azacytidine

5-Azacytidine can produce tubular dysfunction with polyuria, glucosuria, acidosis, hypokalemia, and hypophosphatemia.

B. Aziridinybenzoquinone (AZQ)

AZQ given in high doses commonly leads to proteinuria and renal tubular dysfunction; can lead to renal failure.

C. Carmustine (BCNU)/Lomustine (CCNU)

BCNU/CCNU, along with other nitrosoureas, can cause a progressive chronic nephropathy with uremia and proteinuria (glomerulosclerosis, tubular atrophy, interstitial fibrosis). The renal tubular disease infrequently occurs after the completion of chemotherapy and can be irreversible.

Table 7.1.
Criteria for Toxicity and Complications

Site	Measure	Grade				
		0/WNL	I (Mild)	2 (Moderate)	3 (Severe)	4 (Unacceptable)
Blood	WBC/uL	≥4.0	3.0–3.9	2.0–2.9	1.0–1.9	<1.0
	ANC/uL	≥2.0	1.5–1.9	1.0–1.4	0.5–0.9	<0.5
	PLT/uL	WNL	75.0–normal	50.0–74.9	25.0–49.9	<25.0
	Hgb, g/dl	WNL	10.0–normal	8.0–10.0	6.5–7.9	<6.5
	Lymphocytes/uL	≥2.0	1.5–1.9	1.0–1.4	0.5–0.9	<0.5
Marrow	cellularity	Normal	Mildly hypoplastic 25%↓	Moderate hypoplastic 50%↓	Marked hypoplastic 75%↓ >3 weeks to recovery	Aplastic 3 weeks to recovery
Liver	ALT	WNL	≤2.5×N	2.6–5.0×N	5.1–20.0×N	>20.0×N
	AST	WNL	≤2.5×N	2.6–5.0×N	5.1–20.0×N	>20.0×N
	Alkaline phosphatase	WNL	≤2.5×N	2.6–5.0×N	5.1–20.0×N	>20.0×N
	Total bilirubin	WNL		<1.5×N	1.5–3.0×N	>3.0×N
	Liver-clinical	WNL			Precoma	Hepatic coma
Pancreas	Amylase/creatinine clearance	WNL	<1.5×N	1.5–2.0×N	2.1–5.0×N	>5.0×N
	Amylase	WNL	<1.5×N	1.5–2.0×N	2.1–5.0×N	>5.0×N
	Glucose, mg/dL	WNL	55–64/116–160	40–54/161–250	30–39/251–500	<30/>500/ketoacid
	Ultrasound size and sonolucency	Normal	Increased	Increased localized	Increased generalized	Pseudocyst hemorrhagic
Renal and genitourinary	BUN	<20	20–39	40–59	60–79	≥80
	Creatinine	WNL	<1.5×N	1.5–3.0×N	3.1–6.0×N	>6.0×N
	Creatinine clearance	WNL	75%	50–74%	25–49%	<25%

	Grade 0	Grade 1	Grade 2	Grade 3	Grade 4
Blood pressure					
Systolic	Baseline	±10%	±20%	±30%	±40%
Diastolic	Baseline	±5%	±10%	±15%	±20%
Proteinurla	Negative	1+/or <3 g/l	2-3+/or 3-10 g/L	4+/or >10 g/L	Nephrotic syndrome
Hematuria	Negative	Micro only	Gross, no clots	Gross and clots	Transfusion required
Bladder—frequency and dysuria	None	Slight	Moderate, responds to treatment	Severe, no response to treatment	Incapacitating, with severe hemorrhage
Stomatitis	None	Erythema or Mild soreness	Painful/edema can eat	Cannot eat or drink	Requires parenteral or enteral support
Gastro-intestinal					
Abdominal pain					
Severity	None	Mild	Moderate	Moderate-severe	Severe
Treatment		Not required	Required—helps	Required—no help	Hospitalization, heavy sedation
Constipation	No change	Mild ileus	Moderate ileus	Severe ileus	Ileus >96 hours
Diarrhea	None	↑2-3 stools/day	↑4-6 stools/day or moderate cramps	↑7-9 stools/day or Severe cramps	↑≥10 stools/day, bloody, parenteral support required
Nausea	None	Reasonable intake	Decreased intake	No significant intake	
Vomiting	None	1x/day	2-5x/day	6-10x/day	>10x/day or IV required

cont.

Table 7.1.
continued

Site	Measure	Grade				
		0/WNL	I (Mild)	2 (Moderate)	3 (Severe)	4 (Unacceptable)
Pulmonary	Vital capacity	WNL	10–20%↓	21–35%↓	36–50%↓	>51%
	pAO$_2$	>90	80–89	65–79	50–64	<49
	Functional	Normal	Tachypnea	Dyspnea	O$_2$ required	Assist ventilation
	DLCO	100–75%	74–65%	64–65%	54–40%	<40%
	Clinical	No change	Abnormal PFTs/ asymptomatic	Dyspnea on significant exertion	Dyspnea at normal activity	Dyspnea at rest
Cardiac	Cardiac rhythm	WNL	Asymptomatic/ transient No treatment required	Recurrent/persistent	Requires treatment	Hypotension/ V tach/fibrillation
	Echo %FS	>30	24–30	20–24	<20	
	%STI	<0.35		<0.40	>0.40	
	Ischemia	None	Nonspecific T-wave flattening	Asymptomatic/ECG change suggests ischemia	Angina/without evidence of infarction	Acute myocardial infarction
	Pericardial effusion	None	Asymptomatic effusion; no treatment required	Pericarditis	Drainage required	Tamponade; drainage urgently required
	Cardiac function	WNL	Asymptomatic	Asymptomatic	Mild CHF/responds to treatment	Severe or refractory CHF
	Hypertension	No change	Asymptomatic/ transient ↑20%, no treatment required	Recurrent/ persistent ↑20%, no treatment required	Requires treatment	Hypertensive crisis

	No change	No treatment required	Treatment but no hospitalization	Treatment and hospitalization <48 hours after stop agent	Treatment and hospitalization >48 hours after stop agent
Hypotension	No change				
Nervous system					
Peripheral					
Sensory	No change	Mild paresthesias, loss of tendon reflex	Moderate sensory loss, moderate paresthesias	Interferes with function	
Motor	No change	Subjective weakness/no objective findings	Mild objective weakness/no significant impairment	Objective weakness/impaired function	Paralysis weakness/impaired
Central					
Cerebellar	No change	Slight incoordination/dysdiadokinesis	Intention tremor/dysmetria/slurred speech/nystagmus	Locomotor ataxia	Cerebellar necrosis
CNS					
General	No change	Drowsy/nervous	Confused	Seizures/psychosis	Comatose
Headache	No change	Mild	Transient/moderate/severe	Severe, unrelenting	

cont.

Table 7.1.
continued

Site	Measure		0/WNL	1 (Mild)	2 (Moderate)	3 (Severe)	4 (Unacceptable)
					Grade		
	Cortical		No change	Mild somnolence/agitation	Moderate somnolence/agitation	Severe somnolence/agitation/confusion/hallucination	Coma/seizures/toxic psychosis
Skin	Skin		No change or WNL	Scattered eruption or erythema, asymptomatic	Urticaria/scattered eruption, symptomatic	Generalized eruption, treatment required	Exfoliation/ulcerative dermatitis
	Alopecia		No loss	Mild hair loss	Marked/total hair loss		
Allergy			None	Transient rash	Mild bronchospasm	Moderate bronchospasm, serum sickness	Hypotension, anaphylaxis
Coagulation	Fibrinogen		WNL	$0.99–0.75 \times N$	$0.74–0.50 \times N$	$0.49–0.25 \times N$	$\leq 0.24 \times N$
	PT		WNL	$1.01–1.25 \times N$	$1.26–1.50 \times N$	$1.51–2.00 \times N$	$>2.00 \times N$
	PTT		WNL	$1.01–1.66 \times N$	$1.67–2.33 \times N$	$2.34–3.00 \times N$	$>3.00 \times N$
	Hemorrhage (clinical)		None	Mild/no transfusion	Gross/1–2 transfusions/episode	Gross/3–4 transfusions/episode	Massive/>4 transfusions/episode
Hearing	Objective		No change	20–40 dB loss >4 kHz	>40 dB loss >4 kHz	>40 dB loss 2 kHz	>40 dB loss <2 kHz
	Subjective		No change	Loss on audiometry only	Tinnitus, soft speech	Loss correctable with hearing aid	Deafness not correctable

	0	1	2	3	4
Electrolytes					
Na, mEq/L	WNL	↓130–134/↑146–149	125–129/150–155	116–124/156–164	<115/>165
K, mEq/L	WNL	↓3.1–3.4/↑5.5–5.9	2.6–3.0/6.0–6.4	2.1–2.5/6.5–6.9	<2.0/>7.0
Ca, mg/dL	WNL	8.4–7.8/10.6–11.5	7.7–7.0/11.6–12.5	6.9–6.1/12.6–13.5	≤6.1/≥13.5
Mg, mEq/L	WNL	1.4–1.2	1.1–0.9	0.8–0.6	≤0.5
Infection	None	Mild	Moderate	Severe	Life threatening
Fever	<38°C	38°–40°C	>40°C <24 hours	>40°C >24 hours	
Local	None	Pain	Pain/swelling with inflammation/phlebitis	Ulceration	Plastic surgery indicated
Mood	No change	Mild anxiety or depression	Moderate anxiety or depression	Severe anxiety or depression	Suicidal ideation
Vision	No change			Subtotal vision loss ≥20%	Blindness
Weight change	<5.0%	5.0–9.9%	10–19.9%	≥20%	
Performance (Karnoisky %)	Normal (90–100)	Mild restriction (70–<90)	Ambulatory up to 50% (50–<70)	Bed or wheelchair (30–<50)	No self-care (<30)

Source: Modified from the Children's Cancer Group from the National Cancer Institute Common Toxicity Criteria.

Abbreviations: ANC, absolute neutrophil count; BUN, blood urea nitrogen; CHF, congestive heart failure; CNS, central nervous system; DLCO, diffusion capacity of carbon monoxide; ECG, electrocardiogram; FS, fractional shortening; HgB, hemoglobin; pAO$_2$, partial pressure of arterial oxygen; PFTs, pulmonary function tests; PLT, platelets; PT, prothrombin time; PTT, partial thromboplastin time; AST, aspartate aminotransferase; ALT, alanine aminotransferase; STI, systolic time interval; V tach, ventricular tachycardia; WBC, white blood cell count.

Infusion-related hypotension can lead to a transient increase in creatinine.

D. Busulfan/melphalan
Busulfan and melphalan have been associated with hemorrhagic cystitis and can increase the risk of hemorrhagic cystitis in patients who receive cyclophosphamide.

E. Carboplatin
1. The nephrotoxic potential of carboplatin appears to be less than that of cisplatin; however, dose escalation with stem cell rescue has produced severe nephrotoxicity.
2. Renal tubular damage resulting in hyponatremia secondary to increased urinary loss can occur but is reported rarely; hypomagnesemia occurs more often.
3. Rarely, hematuria can occur.

F. Cisplatin
Proximal and distal renal tubular damage and decreased GFR (acute and chronic) have been associated with cisplatin; rarely, hemolytic uremic syndrome.
1. Hypomagnesemia, hyponatremia, and hypocalcemia due to proximal tubular damage are common.
2. Renal tubular damage is exacerbated by coincident hyperperuricemia, hypoalbuminemia, metoclopramide (perhaps by decreasing renal blood flow), amphotericin B, iodinated intravenous contrast dyes, abdominal radiation, and perhaps, aminoglycoside therapy.
3. Renal toxicity is decreased if the cisplatin is given as a continuous infusion of ≤ 40 mg/m^2/d or if the patient is receiving concomitant phenytoin.
4. Cisplatin can increase nephrotoxicity related to ifosfamide or methotrexate.
5. The extent of GFR or renal tubular damage recovery after the completion of cisplatin is uncertain. In some patients, deterioration of renal function continues after the completion of treatment.

G. Cyclophosphamide
1. Hemorrhagic cystitis (microscopic to gross, life-threatening) is associated with cyclophosphamide therapy.

    a. The cystitis is accompanied by irritative voiding complaints. It can be diminished or prevented with vigorous hydration or Mesna when doses $> 1.2\,g/m^2$ are used.

    b. Radiation to the bladder can increase the risk of hemorrhagic cystitis. Vesicoureteral reflux and hydronephrosis have also been reported.

    c. Symptoms frequently recur, with and without further exposure to cyclophosphamide or related compounds, radiation, or other radiomimetic therapy. The risk of recurrence is higher and the symptoms more severe with additional bladder-toxic treatments.

    d. Bladder fibrosis and bladder cancer are long-term risks.

  2. Transient dilutional hyponatremia and oliguria can occur 8–12 hours after moderate- to high-dose cyclophosphamide treatment due to syndrome of inappropriate antidiuretic hormone.

H. Cyclosporine
  1. Cyclosporine may cause hemolytic uremic syndrome;
  2. Cyclosporine is associated with increased serum creatinine and decreased GFR; these changes are dose dependent and usually reversible;
  3. Rarely associated with interstitial fibrosis.

I. Fludarabine
Fludarabine rarely leads to hemorrhagic cystitis.

J. 5-fluorouracil
5-fluorouracil can lead to renal failure through glomerulus arteriolar damage.

K. Gemcitabine
Gemcitabine can induce hemolytic uremic syndrome.

L. Ifosfamide
  1. Ifosfamide has been associated with proximal renal tubular dysfunction (impaired reabsorption of glucose, amino acids, sodium, calcium, and inorganic phosphate).
  2. Nephrotoxic effects on the proximal tubule appear to be more severe in younger children, particularly the increased urinary excretion of phosphate and glucose.

3. Distal renal tubular dysfunction is less common, and glomerular toxicity has not been reported without associated severe tubular dysfunction.

4. Fanconi syndrome (glucosuria, aminoaciduria, low fractional excretion of phosphate, and elevated fractional excretion of sodium bicarbonate) secondary to proximal tubular damage has been reported. High urinary excretion of sodium in the presence of impaired concentrating ability can lead to significant dehydration.

5. Although the acute effects of each treatment are generally partially to completely reversible between courses of treatment, there is evidence that the capacity to recover from acute tubular damage is increasingly impaired after each course of therapy. Tubular damage, once established, may persist long term. Progression of renal toxicity can continue after the completion of treatment.

6. The incidence of ifosfamide-related nephrotoxicity increases with increasing cumulative doses.

7. The nephrotoxicity of ifosfamide and cisplatin may be additive. Ifosfamide nephrotoxicity is increased after abdominal irradiation or nephrectomy.

8. The onset of laboratory and clinical nephrotoxicity may occur during or years after the completion of treatment.

9. Hematuria resulting from bladder wall damage is common without the use of the uroprotective agent Mesna.
   a. The use of Mesna gives a false-positive result for ketones on urine dipstick measurements.
   b. Mesna does not prevent nephrotoxicity.

10. Rarely, renal toxicity has led to a syndrome resembling that of inappropriate antidiuretic hormone, clinical nephrogenic diabetes insipidus, hypophosphatemic rickets, or renal tubular acidosis.

11. One study found decreased bone mineral density in 20% of children receiving ifosfamide.

M. Interferon
Interferon can induce proteinuria; rarely leads to renal failure secondary to interstitial nephritis, membranoproliferative glomerular sclerosis, focal segmental glomerular

sclerosis, thrombotic microangiopathy, or renal tubular necrosis.

N. Methotrexate
1. High-dose methotrexate can produce renal damage by a variety of mechanisms:
    a. Precipitation of methotrexate in renal tubules or collecting ducts resulting in renal tubular necrosis; this is more likely to occur with acidic urine.
    b. Direct biochemical damage of renal tubules.
    c. Pharmacologic effect on proliferating cells resulting in renal failure.
2. In general, renal failure secondary to methotrexate resolves within 21 days. Proteinuria and enzymuria frequently have resulted from treatment with methotrexate. These laboratory changes are usually clinically insignificant.
3. Systemic complications of methotrexate are increased in the presence of a decreased GFR. Patients with ileal conduits are at increased risk of methotrexate-induced renal complications. Patients receiving both methotrexate and cisplatin are at increased risk of nephrotoxicity.
4. Methotrexate may induce vasoconstriction of the afferent arteriole of the glomerulus.
5. The risk of nephrotoxicity may be increased by concomitant use of nonsteroidal anti-inflammatory drugs or procarbazine.

O. Mitomycin
Mitomycin can lead to renal insufficiency secondary to hemolytic uremic syndrome.

P. Vincristine
Vincristine can lead to urine retention and hyponatremia secondary to inappropriate antidiuretic syndrome.

Q. Interleukin-2
1. High-dose IL-2 is associated with frequent acute renal failure;
2. Usually, this renal failure is rapidly reversible;
3. Probably mediated through vasoconstriction; therefore, it is recommended that IL-2 not be given with nonsteroidal anti-inflammatory drugs;

        4.   Renal toxicity is decreased when IL-2 is given by continuous infusion.

R. Aminoglycosides
1. Aminoglycosides can induce renal tubular dysfunction, decreased GFR, proteinuria, and urinary renal casts.
2. Most patients with aminoglycoside nephrotoxicity develop nonoliguric azotemia.
3. An occasional patient develops Fanconi renal syndrome or electrolyte wasting of calcium, magnesium, and potassium.
4. Aminoglycosides may potentiate the renal damage of other nephrotoxic treatments.
5. Usually, the renal effects of aminoglycosides reverse after the discontinuation of the drug.
6. Gentamicin is associated with the greatest renal toxicity.

S. Amphotericin B
1. Nephrotoxicity occurs to some degree in 50–80% of patients receiving amphotericin B.
2. Amphotericin B decreases GFR through toxic effects on the renal vasculature.
3. Decreases in GFR and renal plasma flow occur almost universally.
   a. These changes may be mediated by sodium status and intrarenal glomerulotubular feedback.
   b. Adequate hydration and sodium loading can decrease nephrotoxicity.
4. Damage to proximal and distal renal tubules by amphotericin B frequently results in excess loss of potassium, magnesium, and protein.
5. Renal tubular acidosis without systemic acidosis can develop.
6. Patients receiving amphotericin B are predisposed to nephrocalcinosis.
7. Alkalinization of the urine can decrease the risk of nephrocalcinosis and permanent renal damage.
8. Hyposthenuria can precede azotemia.
9. Nephrotoxicity is increased in the presence of high cumulative dose of amphotericin B, baseline renal dysfunction, hypovolemia, and the use of diuretics and concomitant nephrotoxic medications.

10. The nephrotoxic effects of amphotericin B usually resolve over several months after the drug is discontinued.
11. The nephrotoxic effects are decreased with lipid soluble formulations or colloidal dispersion compared with conventional amphotericin B.

T. Radiation
1. Modern techniques of delivering abdominal irradiation have decreased the risk of renal damage (primarily by reducing vascular damage).
2. Abdominal radiation in patients receiving cisplatin increases the renal toxicity of cisplatin.
3. Renal interstitial fibrosis has been induced by radiation.
4. Radiation of the bladder can increase the risk of hemorrhagic cystitis.

U. Dacarbazine
Dacarbazine can lead to azotemia without nephrotoxicity

V. L-asparaginase
L-asparaginase can lead to azotemia without nephrotoxicity.

IV. MONITORING STUDIES TO BE PERFORMED

A. Baseline and information to be documented for monitoring of possible renal complications for all patients receiving cancer treatment:
1. Current nephrotoxic medications and medications that alter renal perfusion include diuretics, acetylcholinesterase inhibitors, nonsteroidal anti-inflammatory drugs, β-blockers, steroids, and contrast media.
2. Hydration status during nephrotoxic cancer treatments.
3. Nutritional status, including serum albumin.
4. Urinary tract infections; coincident episodes of sepsis while receiving nephrotoxic treatments.
5. Radiation delivered to the kidney or bladder; presence of a single kidney.
6. Presence of hydronephrosis or obstructive uropathy.

      7. Tumor lysis syndrome, degree of hyperuricemia, and management of tumor lysis or hyperuricemia during remission induction treatment.

B. Laboratory data to consider before each course of chemotherapy: (see section I).

V. SUPPORTIVE CARE MEASURES TO AVOID/AMELIORATE TOXICITY

A. Children with a single kidney or hydronephrosis:
1. Are ineligible to receive ifosfamide in rhabdomyosarcoma protocols. The use of ifosfamide is discouraged for all patients with a single kidney.
2. Have greater nephrotoxicity with cisplatin than those without hydronephrosis, in spite of adjustment of doses for decreased GFR.

B. Primary prevention of nephrotoxicity includes adequate to increased hydration, maintenance of normal intravascular fluid status, and avoidance of intravascular volume depletion.
1. Adequate intravascular hydration and diuresis can be enhanced by the use of 0.45% or 0.9% saline, mannitol, and diuretics.
2. Use mannitol and diuretics to increase diuresis *only* after determining that the child has adequate intravascular hydration.

C. Where possible, avoid:
1. Nephrotoxic antimicrobials and other renal-toxic medications.
2. The use of IV contrast dye for computed tomographic scanning during and after infusion of nephrotoxic chemotherapy.

D. Prevention of bladder toxicity
1. Provide hyperhydration to ensure increased urine output to dilute and decrease the bladder mucosal contact time of toxic oxazaphosphorine metabolites.
2. Strongly encourage ample oral intake for 12–14 hours preceding cyclophosphamide or ifosfamide infusion.
3. Maintain a urine output of >65 mL/m^2/h for at least 18 hours after cyclophosphamide or ifosfamide therapy.
4. Encourage the patient to void at least every 2 hours for the 24 hours after oxazaphosphorine treatment.

E. Specific measures to prevent renal toxicity from renal-toxic drugs
1. Hydration
   a. Before infusion of high-dose methotrexate, moderate- to high-dose cyclophosphamide, cisplatin, or ifosfamide, give hydration at 125 mL/m^2/h (2 x maintenance) for a minimum of 2 hours to increase urine output to >100 mL/m^2/h (>3 mL/kg/h). Hydration appears to decrease the acute, but not chronic, toxicity of cisplatin.
   b. Before the chemotherapy infusion, urine specific gravity should be ≤1.010.
   c. The hydration fluid most frequently used is 5% dextrose/0.45%NaC1 + 10 mEq/L KCl.
   d. During infusion of these agents, in general, maintain hydration at 125 mL/m^2/h and urine output at >90 mL/m^2/h.
   e. After the infusion of nephrotoxic chemotherapy (including high-dose melphalan), maintain urine output at 65–100 mL/m^2/h (depending on agent and protocol) with oral/IV fluids to equal 90–125 mL/m^2/h.
   f. Where needed to maintain isovolemic fluid balance (avoidance of over- and underhydration), diuresis can be forced (in the presence of adequate hydration) through the use of mannitol 6 gm/m^2 (200mg/kg) in at least 25 mL of fluid over 15–60 minutes and/or furosemide 0.5–1 mg/kg push IV.
2. Alkalinization
   a. Before infusion of high-dose methotrexate, urine alkalinization of >pH 6.5 can be achieved with 40–60 mEq NaHC0$_3$/L added to the IV hydration fluid.
   b. Alkalinization of the urine decreases the risk of nephrocalcinosis with amphotericin B.
3. Uroprotectant
   a. Mesna has been used as a uroprotectant with high-dose cyclophosphamide and ifosfamide (oxazaphosphorines). Mesna, which has a half-life of 90 minutes, binds the toxic oxazaphosphorine metabolite acrolein within the urinary collecting system to detoxify it. In adult patients, Mesna may not be more effective in preventing bladder toxicity than vigorous hydration.

    b. The dosage guidelines for Mesna vary. The majority of Children's Oncology Group protocols recommend a total Mesna dose equivalent to the total ifosfamide dose (i.e., 1 mg of Mesna/ 1 mg of ifosfamide) and a total Mesna dose of about 80% of the total cyclophosphamide dose. Oral doses may be used when tolerated (bioavailability of 40–50%).

    c. Studies have shown that lower doses of Mesna may be uroprotective.

4. Hypertonic saline

    a. The effectiveness of prevention of cisplatin nephrotoxicity by infusion in 3% saline is controversial.

    b. Prevention or diminution of nephrotoxicity associated with cisplatin is possible with hydration with normal saline, continuous infusion of cisplatin, and prophylactic supplementation with magnesium.

5. Magnesium

    a. During infusion of cisplatin, add mannitol in a dose of 15 g/m^2 (10–24 g/m^2/L) and MgSO$_4$ in a dose of 20 mEq/L to the hydrating solution to prevent hypomagnesemia.

    b. Continue postchemotherapy hydration with 5% dextrose/0.45%NaCl + 20 mEq/L KCl + 20 mEq/L MgSO$_4$ + mannitol 20 g/L.

    c. When chemotherapy includes cisplatin, routine magnesium supplementation with a minimum of 6 mEq/Kg/day by mouth (PO) is recommended.

6. Continuous versus intermittent infusion

    a. For cisplatin or ifosfamide, preliminary data suggest that continuous infusion reduces nephrotoxicity.

    b. Dosing by pharmacokinetic measurement of area under the curve also can decrease nephrotoxicity. Calvert suggested the formula dose = target-AUC × (GFR +25).

7. Adjust the administered dose of chemotherapeutic agents according to the GFR (Table 7.2).

8. Limited total dose of agent

More than eight courses of ifosfamide (approximately 72 g/m^2) are not recommended, as the incidence of serious nephrotoxic complications increases markedly when this does is exceeded.

Table 7.2.
Suggested Percentage Dose of Chemotherapeutic Agents Adjusted for Glomerular Filtration Rate

>60 mL/min	30–60 mL/min (50–75% baseline)*			10–30 mL/min (25–49% baseline)		<10 mL/min (<25% baseline)	
100% dose	75%	50%	Omit	75%	Omit	50%	Omit
Adrlamycin†	Bleomycin‡	Cisplatin	Nitrosureas	Carboplatin§	Cisplatin	Cyclophosphamide	Cisplatin
Bleomycin		Methotrexate	Bleomycin*	Ifosfamide§	Methotrexate		Methotrexate
Cisplatin			Cisplatin	Nitrosureas	Nitrosureas		
Cyclophosphamide							
Cytarabine†							
5-fluorouracil†							
Ifosfamide							
Melphalan†							
Methotrexate							
Nitrosureas							
Vinblastine†							
Vincristine							

Source: Modified from Patterson (1992).

* Percentage of baseline may not be suitable if high urine output renal dysfunction present.

† No dose modification for decreased glomerular filtration rate.

‡ Recommendations vary per protocol.

§ Reduce by 50%.

9. Amifostine
   a. Amifostine has decreased the nephrotoxicity of cisplatin in adult patients without adversely affecting treatment outcome.
   b. Side effects of amifostine include nausea, vomiting, and hypotension.

F. Measures to treat/limit hematuria
   1. Microscopic hematuria
      a. Transient microscopic hematuria (no more than two abnormal urinalyses on two separate days during a course of therapy); no modification of the oxazaphosphorine or Mesna.
      b. Persistent microscopic hematuria (>2 abnormal urinalyses during a course of therapy)
         i. Do not modify the oxazaphosphorine dose.
         ii. Change the Mesna to a continuous infusion: 360 mg/m^2 during oxazaphosphorine, followed by $120 \text{ mg/m}^2/\text{h}$ for 24 hours.
   2. Gross hematuria
      Evaluate all episodes of gross hematuria by cystoscopy. Also consider further testing such as urine culture, excretory urogram, and voiding cystogram and perform as indicated.
      a. Transient gross hematuria during or after a course of therapy (only one episode, which clears to less than gross hematuria)
         i. Do not modify the oxazaphosphorine dose.
         ii. Change the Mesna to a continuous infusion: 360 mg/m^2 during oxazaphosphorine, followed by $120 \text{ mg/m}^2/\text{h}$ for 24 hours.
      b. Persistent gross hematuria after completion of a course of therapy
         i. Hold subsequent oxazaphosphorine until the urine shows less than gross hematuria.
         ii. Reinstitute oxazaphosphorine at full dose with the Mesna changed to a continuous infusion: 360 mg/m^2 during oxazaphosphorine followed by $120 \text{ mg/m}^2/\text{h}$ for 24 hours after each dose of oxazaphosphorine therapy.
         iii. If gross hematuria does not resolve to microscopic hematuria or less, withhold further oxazaphosphorine therapy.

c. Persistent gross hematuria occurring during a course of oxazaphosphorine
   i. Interrupt the oxazaphosphorine.
   ii. Withhold further oxazaphosphorine until the next course of therapy.
   iii. If the gross hematuria resolves to microscopic hematuria or less, subsequent courses of oxazaphosphorine may be administered at full dose with Mesna changed to a continuous infusion: 360 mg/m^2 during oxazaphosphorine followed by 120 mg/m^2/h for 24 hours.
d. Occurrence of a second episode of gross hematuria or persistence of microscopic hematuria on the continuous infusion regimen.
   i. Continue the oxazaphosphorine when the urine shows less than gross hematuria.
   ii. Double the loading dose of Mesna to 720 mg/m^2 and the subsequent hourly dose to 240 mg/m^2/h.
   iii. Continue to give Mesna by continuous infusion for 48 hours after the last dose of oxazaphosphorine.
e. Persistent gross hematuria in the face of the double dose, continuous infusions regimen. Discontinue oxazaphosphorine.

G. Measures to limit renal tubular dysfunction
   If significant renal Fanconi syndrome (serum phosphate <3.5 ml/dL, potassium <3 mgEq/L; 1 + glycosuria with serum glucose <150 mg/dL, bicarbonate <17 mgEq/L, and ratio of urine protein/urine creatinine <0.2) develops while receiving ifosfamide, consider substituting cyclophosphamide.

H. Measures for methotrexate and renal dysfunction
   Emergency access IV carboxypeptidase-G$_2$ should be considered for markedly delayed excretion of methotrexate secondary to renal dysfunction.

I. Measures for management of syndrome of inappropriate antidiuretic hormone include:
   1. Restriction of fluid intake, particularly free water intake;

2. Aim to increase sodium by 10%/24 hours; more rapid increase is associated with risk of central pontine myelinolysis.
3. In the setting of coma or seizures, treatment with hypertonic saline can be used. Dose of 3% saline = 7–10 mL/kg over 60 minutes to raise the serum sodium to 125 mEq/L.

VI. LONG-TERM FOLLOW-UP/LATE EFFECTS

A. Cyclophosphamide and ifosfamide
Cyclophosphamide and ifosfamide can lead to vesicoureteral reflux, hydronephrosis, or contracted bladder, which may not become symptomatic for months to years after treatment. These complications are usually preceded by acute episodes of hemorrhagic, cystitis and are increased in patients who have received pelvic radiation.

B. Ifosfamide and cisplatin
Both ifosfamide and cisplatin have caused persistent renal Fanconi syndrome, occasionally resulting in hypophosphatemic rickets, growth failure, and/or renal tubular acidosis.
1. The onset of renal tubular dysfunction can occur years after the completion of chemotherapy.
2. Ifosfamide has been associated with persistent nephrogenic diabetes insipidus.

Monitoring for Cardiotoxicity

Debra L. Friedman, M.D.

I. ANTINEOPLASTIC THERAPIES LEADING TO CARDIOTOXICITY

A. Anthracyclines
1. The anthracycline antibiotics include doxorubicin, daunorubicin, idarubicin, epirubicin, and mitoxantrone.
2. Anthracyclines can cause both acute and long-term cumulative cardiotoxicity, and the damage is primarily to the myocytes.

3. Risk factors for cardiotoxicity from anthracyclines include fractional and cumulative dose, age at time of exposure, latency since time of exposure, race, and gender.

   a. Fractional doses higher than 50 mg/m^2 are associated with increased risk. Divided dosing, prolonged versus bolus infusion may be more cardioprotective in adults, but this has not been found in children.

   b. Cumulative doses of greater than 200–300 mg/m^2 increases risk. (See section IA6 about dose equivalence.) Risks increase more sharply with increased doses above 300 mg/m^2.

   c. Younger age at time of exposure is associated with increased risk. Young children under age 5 years, and especially infants are at higher risk, even at lower cumulative doses than 200 mg/m^2.

   d. Risk increases with longer latency time from exposure.

   e. Risk is higher in female patients and African Americans.

   f. Therapy with other cardiotoxic agents (Cyclophosphamide at doses of 100–200 mg/kg, Amascrine, radiotherapy with heart in the radiation field) can increase the toxicity of the anthracyclines.

4. Individual patients may exhibit subclinical toxicity (e.g., decreases in fractional shortening or ejection fraction) at lower doses than those noted above.

5. In considering the maximum allowable dose of anthracyclines, consider the possibility of the future administration of other cardiotoxic therapies such as thoracic radiotherapy or hematopoietic stem cell transplantation where the patient may be exposed to both total body irradiation and high-dose cyclophosphamide.

6. In calculating cumulative doses, consider dose equivalency of anthracyclines.

   a. Most pediatric studies treat daunomycin and doxorubicin as dose equivalent, and thus combined daunomycin and doxorubicin doses should be used to calculate cumulative doses of potential concern.

       b. Epirubicin, rarely used in the United States in pediatric patients, is roughly dose equivalent to doxorubicin.

       c. 12 mg/m^2 of Idarubicin is roughly the equivalent of 45 mg/m^2 of daunomycin.

       d. 1 mg/m^2 of mitoxantrone is roughly equivalent to 5 mg/m^2 of doxorubicin.

B. Radiation therapy

    1. Radiation damages the endothelial cell, altering the fine vasculoconnective stroma of the myocardium.

    2. Late cardiotoxic effects include: Restrictive cardiomyopathy, constrictive pericarditis, coronary artery disease, valvular heart disease, and intracardiac conduction abnormalities.

    3. The effects of thoracic radiotherapy are difficult to separate from those of anthracyclines, as few children are exposed to thoracic radiotherapy in the absence of anthracyclines.

    4. The risks to the heart are related to the amount of radiation delivered to different depths of the heart, the volume and specific areas of the heart irradiated, the total and fractional irradiation dose, and age at exposure

       a. Careful blocking to doses of up to 25 Gy is generally safe, and 40 Gy may be administered to small cardiac regions.

       b. Younger age at exposure increases risk.

       c. Fractionation of dose may decrease risk.

    5. Individual patients may have a lower threshold and develop toxicity at lower doses.

    6. In considering the maximum allowable dose of thoracic radiotherapy, consider the possibility of the future administration of other cardiotoxic therapies such as anthracyclines or hematopoietic stem cell transplantation where the patient may be exposed to both total body irradiation (TBI) and high-dose cyclophosphamide.

II. THE SPECTRUM OF CARDIOTOXICITY EFFECTS

A. Late effects of radiation to the heart include the following potential effects.

1. Delayed pericarditis; pancarditis, which includes pericardial and myocardial fibrosis, with or without endocardial fibroelastosis; myopathy; coronary artery disease and functional valve injury and conduction defects (however, with current techniques of radiotherapy and reduced doses, these effects following treatment for childhood cancer are most unlikely).
2. Arrhythmias can be seen in patients who receive spinal radiation or TBI.
3. The risk of delayed coronary artery disease after lower radiation doses requires additional study of patients followed for longer time intervals to definitively ascertain lifetime risk. Nontherapeutic risk factors for coronary artery disease such as family history, obesity, hypertension, smoking, diabetes, and hypercholesterolemia are likely to impact risk.
4. Late effects of anthracyclines include the following potential effects. The incidence may be potentiated by thoracic radiotherapy.
   a. Cardiomyopathy
   b. Arrhythmia, including prolongation of QTc
5. There are some other modifying risks for cardiomyopathy from anthracyclines.
   a. Isometric exercise may increase risk and anecdotally has been associated with episodes of acute cardiac decompensation and sudden death. This has not been rigorously studied.
   b. Pregnancy, and more specifically labor and delivery, may be associated with increased risk of congestive heart failure.
   c. Febrile illnesses may increase risk of acute events.
   d. Congenital heart disease may increase risk depending on the anatomic anomaly.

III. MONITORING TECHNIQUES

A. Electrocardiogram for rhythm abnormalities
   1. Evaluate rate and rhythm.
   2. Calculate QTc.

B. Two-dimensional or M-mode echocardiography
   1. Follow the fractional shortening (FS), which is normally $\geq 29\%$ or ejection fraction, which is normally $\geq 55\%$.

2. Other parameters that can be followed are end-diastolic internal diameter and volume, systolic time intervals, end-systolic wall stress compared with velocity of circumferential fiber shortening, parameters of diastolic function, and increase of contractility with exercise or chemically induced stress.

C. Radionuclide cardiac cineangiography (RNA, also known as MUGA or RNCA)
    Normal systolic function is defined by a left ventricular ejection fraction (LVEF) $\geq$55%. Normal stress response is defined as an increase in the LVEF by at least 5 percentile points.

D. Cardiopulmonary exercise testing
    1. A number of studies have examined cardiac function after radiation therapy and anthracycline exposure using cardiopulmonary exercise stress tests.
    2. These studies have found abnormalities in exercise endurance, cardiac output, aerobic capacity, echocardiography during exercise testing, and ectopic rhythms.
    3. While these studies are quite useful for assessment of coronary artery disease, they are nonspecific for cardiomyopathy.
    4. The gold standard test for cardiomyopathy is assessment of maximal myocardial oxygen consumption with exercise.

IV. TESTING FOR CARDIOTOXICITY

There are no evidence-based guidelines that have been rigorously evaluated regarding the frequency and type of testing for patients at risk of cardiotoxicity. The following recommendations are extrapolated from the literature and practice of pediatric oncologists with expertise in long-term effects of therapy. These should not be treated as absolute.

A. Before therapy with anthracycline or thoracic radiotherapy:
    1. Any patient with underlying cardiac disease should be evaluated by a cardiologist and obtain clearance for dose and schedule. Any patient with tumor invasion of the heart, or compression of the heart and associated

vasculature, should be evaluated by a cardiologist and obtain clearance for dose and schedule.

2. An ECG and echocardiogram should be performed before anthracycline treatment or thoracic radiotherapy as a baseline. RNA may be substituted for an echocardiogram.

3. If there is an abnormality, obtain consultation from a pediatric cardiologist before starting anthracycline therapy.

B. During therapy:
1. One modality, either echocardiogram or RNA, should be the consistent method of testing at every evaluation, with the other added, if needed, by the consulting cardiologist, when confirmatory testing is required.

2. For a planned cumulative dose of daunomycin/doxorubicin of <300 mg/m^2, testing is generally repeated after one-half of the cumulative dose has been administered.

3. Once a dose of >300 mg/m^2 has been reached, testing is generally repeated before each course of anthracycline.

a. These recommendations should be dose adjusted for idarubicin and mitoxantrone.

b. The most efficient manner is to convert idarubicin and mitoxantrone doses to daunomycin/doxorubicin equivalent for monitoring purposes.

C. After completion of therapy:
1. Patients should be followed off therapy based on risk factors for cardiotoxicity, which include those discussed in sections IA and IB. There is no known lower dose that should be considered risk free, although to date, no adverse effects have generally been reported in patients who have received <100 mg/m^2. However, there is little long-term follow-up for this group of patients. Therefore, long-term monitoring should be considered for all children who have been treated with anthracyclines.

2. Perform a complete history and physical to elicit any signs or symptoms referable to cardiomyopathy or rhythm disturbance.

3. Children may be asymptomatic, despite a significant degree of cardiac dysfunction. Therefore, patients treated with anthracyclines and/or thoracic radiotherapy should be evaluated by ECG and echocardiogram every 1–5 years, with the specific interval based on age at time of exposure, cumulative dose, and use of other cardiotoxic therapies. Those younger than 5 years of age, and certainly younger than 1 year of age at time of treatment who received cumulative doses of anthracyclines of >200–300 mg/m^2 and/or thoracic radiotherapy, should receive evaluations most frequently. The Children's Oncology Group is developing a set of more specific consensus guidelines regarding risk factors and frequency of evaluations. The lifetime risk for cardiomyopathy is unknown. However, data show continued decrement in cardiac function with ongoing follow-up. Therefore, at this time, lifelong follow-up is recommended until a more defined risk period is identified.

V.   CRITERIA FOR DETERIORATING CARDIAC FUNCTION

A.   A decrease in the FS by an absolute value of 10 percentile points from the previous test (e.g., from 41–31%)
B.   An FS <29%
C.   A decrease in the RNA LVEF by an absolute value of 10 percentile points from the previous test (e.g., from 67–57%)
D.   An RNA LVEF or echocardiogram EF <55%
E.   A decrease in the RNA LVEF with stress
F.   Development of arrhythmia

VI.   MODIFICATION OF ANTHRACYCLINE THERAPY

A.   If there is a decrement of function or development of an arrhythmia during therapy, cardiac consultation should be obtained.
B.   Anthracyclines should be temporarily held pending further testing and expert opinion.
C.   Repeat testing may reveal resumption to normal and allow resumption of anthracycline.

VII. POTENTIAL CARDIOPROTECTION STRATEGIES

A. Divided dosing or continuous infusion of anthracyclines has shown to have a cardioprotective effect in some studies, but the results are not consistent across studies.

B. ICRF-187 (Dexrazoxane) is a bis-dioxopiperazine compound that readily enters cells and is subsequently hydrolyzed to form a chelating agent. It has been shown, in adults, to decrease clinical and pathologic cardiotoxicity when given immediately before the administration of doxorubicin. Smaller studies reported this for daunorubicin and epirubicin as well.
   1. ICRF-187 is currently approved for adults who have already received 300 mg/m^2 of doxorubicin; it is not yet approved for routine use in children.
   2. It is given as a rapid infusion (IV push) in a dose that is 10 times the doxorubicin dose, minutes before each dose of doxorubicin is given.

C. The level of serum cardiac troponin T (cTnT) is a sensitive marker of active myocardial injury and may be predictive of the risk for late cardiotoxicity as well.
   1. cTnT is a protein that is elevated after myocardial damage. cTnT is a thin-filament contractile protein that is released from damaged myocytes and is highly sensitive for the detection of acute myocardial infarction and unstable angina in adults.
   2. Large pediatric studies are ongoing to evaluate the role of dexrazoxane in prevention of cardiotoxicity, and of cTnT in predicting those at highest risk, but data are not currently available to support their routine use outside of research study protocols.
   3. Studies are also ongoing evaluating host-related risk factors for cardiotoxicity from either radiotherapy or anthracyclines. These include polymorphisms in enzymes involved in anthracycline metabolism or repair of radiotherapy or chemotherapy-induced DNA damage. Another area of potential investigation is that of cytokines and other biomarkers of cardiac damage seen in the general population with cardiovascular disease.

Monitoring and Management of Ototoxicity

Wendy Landier, R.N., M.S.N., CPNP, CPON
Claudine Larson-Tuttle, M.A., CCC/Audiologist

I. BACKGROUND

A. Ototoxic agents
  1. Potentially, ototoxic agents commonly used in pediatric oncology include:
     a. Platinum-based chemotherapy (e.g., cisplatin, carboplatin)
     b. Aminoglycoside antibiotics (e.g., gentamicin, tobramycin, amikacin)
     c. Loop diuretics (e.g., furosemide)
     d. Radiotherapy to ear, midline of brain, or brainstem.
  2. Mechanisms of ototoxicity
     a. Platinum-based chemotherapy and aminoglycoside antibiotics: Destruction of sensory hair cells in cochlea (usually irreversible)
     b. Loop diuretics: Possible electrolyte and/or enzymatic changes in inner ear fluids (usually transient)
     c. Radiotherapy: Serous otitis media (usually self-limiting). Fibrosis of ossicles and/or tympanic membrane; atrophy of auditory nerve and organ of Corti; cochlear sensory hair cell loss (usually irreversible)
     d. Early hearing loss, usually in high-frequency range (>2,000 Hz)
  3. Contributing factors
     a. Diminished renal function (aminoglycosides, platinum-based chemotherapy)
     b. Rapid IV administration of agent (platinum-based chemotherapy, loop diuretics)
     c. Prolonged elevated serum trough drug levels (aminoglycosides)
     d. Administration of both radiation and platinum-based chemotherapy, especially if platinum-based chemotherapy is given after radiation
     e. Presence of CNS tumor
     f. Age ≤3 years at time ototoxic agent administered

B. Incidence of ototoxicity
1. Initial hearing loss related to platinum-based therapy is usually in high-frequency ranges with stair-step progression to the speech ranges with further therapy. The extent of hearing loss is dose-related.
2. Cisplatin: 50% of patients demonstrated hearing loss in high-frequency range at 6,000 to 8,000 Hz with cumulative dose $\geq$450 mg/m^2, 25% demonstrated loss at 500 to 3,000 Hz with cumulative dose $\geq$720 mg/m^2, patients receiving cranial radiation demonstrated loss at 4,000 to 8,000 Hz average of three fewer courses than patients who did not receive radiation; 48% demonstrated significant high-frequency loss and 33% required hearing aids at median cumulative dose of 540 mg/m^2, range 400–1,860 mg/m^2.
3. Carboplatin: At cumulative dose of 1,000 mg/m^2, 57% of patients demonstrated loss at 8,000 Hz. At cumulative dose of 2,500 mg/m^2, 83% of patients demonstrated loss at 8,000 Hz, 50% demonstrated loss at 4,000 Hz, and 25% demonstrated loss at 2,000 Hz.
4. Radiotherapy-induced: Hearing loss can be sudden and involve multiple frequencies at time of onset. In one study, 11% of patients developed profound late-onset hearing loss 3–10 years after completion of therapy.

C. Symptoms
1. Tinnitus, vertigo (indicate vestibular injury and impending hearing loss)
2. Difficulty hearing in presence of background noise (indicates high-frequency hearing loss)
3. Inattentiveness, failure to turn toward sound
4. Many children have no symptoms. Audiologic testing that reveals loss in the high-frequency ranges is predictive of future loss in the speech ranges if therapy with the ototoxic agent continues, in some cases for as little as one additional course.

II. MONITORING TECHNIQUES

A. Cumulative dose calculation
1. Cisplatin
2. Carboplatin

B. History
   1. Conditions indicating child may be at increased risk of hearing loss:
      a. Prematurity (especially birth weight <1,500 grams)
      b. Low Apgar scores (≤ 4 at 1 minute; ≤ 6 at 5 minutes)
      c. Hyperbilirubinemia requiring exchange transfusion
      d. History of high-frequency ventilation
      e. History of persistent pulmonary hypertension (PPHN)
      f. Bacterial meningitis
      g. Head trauma with skull fracture or loss of consciousness
      h. Maternal use of drugs or alcohol during pregnancy
      i. Congenital infection (rubella, cytomegalovirus, herpes, toxoplasmosis, syphilis)
      j. Neurofibromatosis type II
      k. Neurodegenerative disorders
      l. Recurrent otitis media with effusion
      m. Craniofacial anomalies
      n. Prior treatment with ototoxic agents
      o. Family history of deafness
   2. Behavioral indications of possible hearing impairment (e.g., failure to attain normal speech milestones, avoidance of social interactions and/or social withdrawal, parents' suspicion that child does not hear)

C. Physical exam
   1. General indicators of increased risk of hearing impairment:
      a. Heterochromia of the iris
      b. Malformed auricles
      c. Periauricular skin tags or pits
      d. Narrow auditory canals
      e. Craniofacial abnormalities (e.g., cleft lip or palate, microcephaly)
   2. Otoscopy
      a. Auditory canal: Discharge, lesions, foreign bodies, cerumen
      b. TM: Color, landmarks, contour, perforations, mobility, fluid level
   3. CN VIII exam

    a. Rinne: AC should be $\geq 2x$ BC

    b. Weber: Sensorineural hearing loss: Lateralization to better ear if hearing loss asymmetric, to both ears if hearing loss symmetric. Conductive hearing loss: Lateralization to ear with greater conductive loss.

4. Exam may be WNL until significant hearing loss is sustained; *physical exam is not a substitute for audiologic monitoring in children at risk for hearing loss.*

D. Audiometric testing
1. Pure-tone audiometry
    a. Measures pure-tone thresholds between 250 and 8,000 Hz
    b. Behavioral modifications in administration based on developmental age:
       i.   Conventional audiometry: ≥ 5 years of age
      ii. Play audiometry: 30 months–5 years
     iii. Visual reinforcement audiometry: 9–30 months
2. Brainstem auditory evoked response (BAER, ABR):
    a. Electrophysiologic measurement of hearing recorded from responses obtained from the auditory neural pathways.
    b. Indications:
       i.   Infants <9 months of age
      ii. Older infants or children who will not cooperate with audiometric testing
    c. Child must be asleep for test; sedation is usually required for children ≥ 3 months of age.
3. Extended high-frequency audiometry
    a. Measures pure tone thresholds between 8,000 and 20,000 Hz
    b. Useful for detecting hearing loss early in course of therapy
4. Otoacoustic emissions (OAEs)
    a. Indicator of outer cochlear hair cell function
    b. Useful to validate normal hearing, but children undergoing cancer treatment require more extensive audiologic evaluation
    c. Failures with middle ear fluid, noisy environment
    d. Children with abnormal OAEs should always undergo complete audiologic evaluation

    e.   OAEs should never be used in lieu of a complete audiologic test battery except in emergent circumstances

    f.   Caution: OAEs appear normal in children with hearing loss related to carboplatin ototoxicity (carboplatin affects inner hair cells only!). OAEs should not be used to test children receiving carboplatin.

5. Word recognition testing (for children ≥5 years developmental age)

6. All audiometric testing should be performed by an experienced pediatric audiologist.

7. All testing should include the high-frequency ranges (4,000 to 8,000 Hz). Extended high-frequency audiometry (8,000 to 20,000 Hz) is advantageous for detection of changes early in the course of therapy.

III. GUIDELINES FOR MONITORING

A. Scheduling audiometric tests

1. Obtain *baseline testing* (full audiologic evaluation) for all children scheduled to receive potentially ototoxic therapy and for any child with a medical history indicative of increased risk for hearing loss.

2. Test high-risk patients *before each platinum-based chemotherapy course* (patients who meet *any* of the following criteria):

    a.   All children ≤3 years of age

    b.   All children who have received brain or ear irradiation

    c.   All children with a diagnosis of CNS neoplasm

    d.   All children concurrently receiving other ototoxic or investigational agents

    e.   All children who have received cumulative cisplatin doses above 360 mg/m^2 or cumulative carboplatin dose >1,000 mg/m^2

3. Test lower-risk patients *before every other platinum-based chemotherapy course* (patients who meet *all* of the following criteria): Children ≥4 years of age with no history of brain or ear irradiation, diagnosis other than CNS neoplasm, receiving no other ototoxic or investigational agent, and with cumulative cisplatin dose ≤360 mg/m^2 or cumulative carboplatin dose ≤1,000 mg/m^2.

4. Test *at least 3 weeks after any previously adminis-tered course* containing platinum-based chemotherapy (hearing deficits may be delayed after administration of platinum).

5. Test *6–8 weeks after final chemotherapy course.*

6. Test *if child reports* subjective decrease in hearing or increased tinnitus or dizziness.

7. Test *periodically for children treated with aminoglyco-side antibiotics and loop diuretics*–schedule to be deter-mined based on frequency and duration of treatment with these agents. Note: Amikacin requires more fre-quent monitoring, optimally 1–2 times per week during therapy.

8. Test *annually for children off-treatment* who have re-ceived platinum-based chemotherapy and/or radiation to the ear, midline of brain or brainstem. (For children >8 years of age who are able to accurately self-report symptoms, consider every-other-year monitoring.)

B. Serum trough levels

1. Determine levels 30 minutes before fourth dose of aminoglycoside antibiotic, following any change in dosage, and at least weekly during antibiotic course.

2. Avoid prolonged elevated serum trough levels of aminoglycoside antibiotics; children with renal impair-ment may require dosage and/or schedule adjustment.

IV. GRADING CRITERIA FOR OTOTOXICITY

A. Grading used as indicator for dose modification or elimina-tion of ototoxic agent from child's chemotherapy regimen. Typically, modifications are made at grades 2–3 and the ototoxic agent is eliminated at grades 3–4.

B. For disparity between ears, or in the case of a soundfield audiogram, *grading should reflect the better ear.*

C. Pediatric ototoxicity grading criteria (see Table 7.3). Au-diologic testing should include air conduction, with bone conduction added when air conduction exceeds 25dB at any frequency. In most situations, dose modification should be done for sensorineural hearing loss only. For conduc-tive hearing loss, underlying cause should be investigated and intervention provided. Dose adjustments should not be made for correctable conductive hearing loss.

Table 7.3.
Pediatric Ototoxicity Grading Criteria

Measure	0 (Normal)	1 (Mild)	2 (Moderate)	3 (Severe)	4 (Unacceptable)
			Grade		
Objective	Normal (≤25 dB, all frequencies)	≥30 dB at 8,000 Hz	≥30 dB at 4,000 Hz	30–35 dB at 2,000 Hz	≥40 dB at 2,000 Hz
Subjective	Asymptomatic	Asymptomatic	Tinnitus, vertigo, or difficulty hearing in presence of background noise	25–50% of speech signal missed. Hearing aids required	Requires services in addition to hearing aids
Dose adjustment recommendation for ototoxic agents	No change	↓dose by 25%	↓dose by 50%, consider alternative therapy	Delete if alternative therapy available, otherwise continue at 50% dose	Delete

V. PREVENTIVE MEASURES

A. Platinum-based chemotherapy and loop diuretics: Avoid rapid IV drug administration, monitor cumulative dosage, early dose modification.

B. Aminoglycoside antibiotics: Keep trough level <2.5 μg/ml for gentamicin and tobramycin and <7.5 μg/ml for amikacin.

C. Radiation: Cochlear shielding, use of high-energy linear accelerators to avoid "hot spots" in ear; 3D conformal XRT to spare cochlea; administration of platinum-based therapy before radiation and avoidance of platinum-based therapy after radiation decreases ototoxicity.

D. Chemoprotective agents: Amifostine, sodium thiosulfate

VI. MODIFICATIONS FOR TOXICITY

A. Platinum-based chemotherapy: Consider dose modification at grade 1 toxicity; consider further dose modification or alternative therapy at grade 2 toxicity.

B. Aminoglycoside antibiotics: If alternative treatment available, discontinue at grade 1 to 2 toxicity.

C. Loop diuretics: Effects are usually reversible; administer subsequent IV doses slowly (<4 mg/minute).

D. Radiation: Toxicity generally a late effect, occurring when modification of therapy is no longer possible.

VII. MANAGEMENT OF HEARING LOSS

A. Hearing aids
  1. Refer to pediatric otologist or audiologist for evaluation and fitting of appropriate hearing aids.
  2. Ensure patient returns for retesting/refitting of hearing aids every 6 months.
  3. Ensure parent learns proper cleaning and care of hearing aid and replaces battery on regular basis (most require replacement every 1–2 weeks).

B. Familiarize parents with options regarding communication methods and assistive devices
  1. Communication methods
    a. Oral/auditory-verbal

       b. Cued speech (speechreading and hand signals for clarification)

       c. Manual communication (American Sign Language)

       d. Total communication (auditory training and signed exact English)

       e. Decision regarding type of communication should be based on child's degree of hearing impairment, developmental stage, and family preference

  2. Assistive devices

       a. FM system: Allows child to receive audio output directly from another source such as a teacher's or parent's microphone and reduces interference of background noise (often available through school district for use in classrooms)

       b. Telephone amplifiers, text telephones, closed captioning, adaptive appliances

C. Familiarize parents with community and educational resources.

  1. In the United States, hearing impairment is considered a disability under PL 105-17 (Individuals with Disabilities Education Act; IDEA '97).

  2. Children from birth to age 3 eligible for family-centered or community-based services (e.g., in-home speech and occupational therapy, specialized day care placement).

       a. Parents must request services from authorized agency (e.g., developmental disabilities center; school district).

       b. Individualized Family Service Plan (IFSP) must be developed for child, outlining areas of child's deficits, or potential deficits and interventions aimed at maximizing child's abilities.

  3. Children from 3–21 years are eligible for placement in public educational system.

       a. Parents must request services from school district.

       b. Individualized Educational Plan (IEP) must be developed for child, including specific interventions (e.g., seating the child in the front of the classroom, use of FM trainer).

Hepatotoxicity and Modifications for Therapy

John Iacuone, M. D.

The liver is vital to the metabolism of many chemotherapy agents. Oncologists are concerned with liver function for a variety of reasons but two stand out: some agents can cause direct injury to the liver and some agents, by virtue of their metabolism, cause increased systemic toxicity when liver dysfunction exists during chemotherapy.

I. ASSESSMENT OF LIVER DYSFUNCTION

A. Baseline liver function can be assessed radiographically and biochemically.
1. Functional impairment is best measured by obtaining laboratory values commonly referred to as liver function tests.
    a. The most important biochemical parameters customarily monitored are alkaline phosphatase, bilirubin, gamma glutamyl transpeptidase (GGT), albumin, aspartate aminotransferase (AST), and alanine aminotransferase (ALT).
    b. Attributing causality to a chemotherapeutic agent when hepatic dysfunction is present is problematic. Antibiotics, analgesics, hepatic viruses, nutritional status, and other entities may contribute alone or cumulatively in promoting liver damage and dysfunction. Determining the appropriate modifications of chemotherapy agents in the midst of known liver abnormalities will be discussed. The National Cancer Institute has published a Common Toxicity Criteria using a 0–4 rating scale (0 = no toxicity, 4 = life threatening toxicity) (Table 7.1).
2. Ultrasound or computerized tomography can add additional information regarding structural integrity and vascular distribution.

II. HEPATOTOXICITY OF SPECIFIC CHEMOTHERAPY AGENTS

A. Alkylating agents
1. Cyclophosphamide

    a. Cyclophosphamide dosage reduction in patients with hepatic failure has not been thoroughly investigated. Because of the complexity of cyclophosphamide metabolism, toxicity, and pharmacologic effects, recommendations for dosage adjustment in the presence of hepatic failure have not been established. There are data to show that patients with hepatic failure develop more toxicity with cyclophosphamide as opposed to patients with normal hepatic function.

    b. Cyclophosphamide undergoes hepatic biotransformation in the liver to 4-hydroxycyclophosphamide, which in turn breaks down to its active form, phosphoramide mustard. Possibly due to this activation step, the overall pharmacokinetics of cyclophosphamide are not significantly altered in the presence of hepatic insufficiency.

    c. Hepatic function is rarely altered in patients receiving cyclophosphamide, Liver damage has been reported when given following azathioprine.

2. Ifosfamide

    a. Ifosfamide is enzymatically metabolized to cytotoxic compounds via hepatic microsomes; therefore, it is theoretically possible that higher doses would be necessary in patients with hepatic disease. However, since studies to establish optimal dose schedules in patients with compromised hepatic and/or renal function have not been performed, a recommended dose adjustment is not available.

    b. Elevation of hepatic enzymes has been reported during ifosfamide therapy

3. Melphalan

    a. No dose adjustment is necessary in hepatic insufficiency, melphalan is not actively metabolized but undergoes spontaneous degradation to mono- and dihydroxy products.

    b. Abnormal liver function tests, jaundice, and hepatitis have been reported following melphalan therapy.

4. Chlorambucil

    a. Chlorambucil therapy has been associated with hepatotoxicity and jaundice

B. Nitrosoureas
  1. Lomustine (CCNU)
     a. Elevations of serum transaminases, alkaline phosphatase, and/or bilirubin are usually mild and revert to normal over a brief period, although fatalities have been reported.
  2. Carmustine (BCNU)—similar issues exist.

C. Antimetabolites
  1. Cytarabine
     a. Cytarabine is reported to be partially detoxified in the liver. Therefore, it is recommended that dosage reduction be considered in patients with liver impairment.
     b. Jaundice, hyperbilirubinemia and hepatic dysfunction may occur following cytarabine therapy. Fatal veno-occlusive disease of the liver has also been reported.
  2. Fluorouracil
     a. This drug is metabolized in the liver.
     b. Given intravenously does not result in liver toxicity. However, when given intra-arterially results in hepatocellular toxicity with elevated enzymes, and bilirubin. It causes obstructive liver disease and may cause secondary sclerosing cholangitis that is irreversible. Hold dose if bilirubin >5 mg/dL.
     c. Dose may require adjustment in patients with hepatic insufficiency.

D. Mercaptopurine
  1. The dosage may need to be reduced in patients with impaired hepatic function, although no specific recommendations are provided by the manufacturer.
  2. Mercaptopurine-induced hepatotoxicity occurs most frequently with doses in excess of 2.5 milligrams/kg/day. Small cohort studies suggest an incidence ranging up to 6%. Patients presenting with drug-induced hepatic injury typically have both intrahepatic cholestasis and parenchymal cell recrosis. Jaundice generally appears within the first 1 to 2 months of therapy, although it has ranged from 1 week to 8 years after initiation of therapy. In some

cases, hepatotoxicity was associated with anorexia, diarrhea, jaundice, and ascites. Hepatic encephalopathy and deaths secondary to hepatic necrosis have occurred. Jundice has cleared upon discontinuation in some patients and reoccurred upon reintroduction. It is unknown whether the hepatic damage is the result of direct toxicity and/or a hypersensitivity reaction.

E. Thioguanine
1. Elevated liver enzymes occasionally occur with thioguanine. Reports of hepatic veno-occlusive disease (VOD) secondary to the administration of thioguanine have appeared in the literature; however, patients have also been receiving other chemotherapy agents.

F. Methotrexate
1. Dose modifications are necessary in patients with hepatic insufficiency.
2. Elevations of AST, LDH, alkaline phosphatase, and/or bilirubin may indicate drug-induced liver dysfunction. Most adverse reactions are reversible if detected early. If reactions do occur, discontinue or reduce the dosage of methotrexate and take appropriate corrective measures. These may include administration of leucovorin calcium and/or hemodialysis. Hepatic fibrosis associated with methotrexate is potentially fatal and generally occurs after prolonged use.
3. High-dose methotrexate results predicitably in elevated liver enzymes that are transient, reversible and do not result in chronic liver disease. Caution should be used in high-dose methotrexate to avoid use of other drugs which may be hepatotoxic (e.g., acetaminophen) or impair the excretion of methotrexate (e.g., salicylates or NSAID therapy).
4. In general, the drug should be held in patients with grade III-IV toxicity, to avoid greater systemic toxicity in high-dose administration.

G. Antitumor Antibiotics
1. Doxorubicin, Daunorubicin, Idarubicin
a. These agents are metabolized in the liver; thus impaired liver function results in significant systemic toxicity.

b. Doses are reduced based on abnormalities of bilirubin, AST/ALT. These modifications vary with individual protocols.
2. Dactinomycin
   a. Ascites, hepatomegaly, hepatic veno-occlusive disease (VOD), hepatitis, and liver function test abnormalities have been reported. Adverse reactions are usually reversible on discontinuance of therapy. Usual doses of dactinomycin do not produce hepatotoxicity unless other stressors are placed on the liver (i.e., concomitant irradiation).
   b. Pulsed Dactionomycin resulted in much less liver toxicity than the 5 consecutive day dosage schedule.
   c. Any increase in liver enzymes should prompt a 50% dose reduction. Gradually increase the dose as tolerated by monitoring liver function.
3. Bleomycin-metabolism is not liver dependent and no dose modifications are necessary.

H. Spindle Cell Inhibitors
   1. Paclitaxel, docetaxel—are extensively metabolized in the liver.
      a. If the bilirubin is between 1.6 and 3.0 mg/dl, give 40% of dose
      b. For bilirubin >3.0 mg/dl, hold dose.
      c. For normal bilirubin, but liver enzymes greater 2 times upper limits of normal, give 75% of dose.
   2. Vincristine
      a. Dosage modification of vincristine is recommended in patients with hepatic insufficiency.
      b. Veno-occlusive disease (VOD) of the liver and hepatotoxicity have been associated with vincristine therapy.
      c. Elevated alkaline phosphatase increases risk of systemic toxicity and dose should be reduced by 50%.
      d. Radiation and vincristine together can result in increased hepatotoxicity.
      e. In the past, modifications for elevated bilirubin levels have been commonplace. However, consideration should be given to modifying those restrictions. Currently if the bilirubin is 2–3 times upper

limits of normal, give 50% dose. Greater than 3 times normal, hold dose.

3. Etoposide
   a. Can cause severe hepatoxicity at standard doses.
   b. High-dose Etoposide can result in elevated bilirubin levels and elevated alkaline phosphatase. These abnormalities seem to occur 2–3 weeks after the administration of the chemotherapy and can take some weeks to resolve. Therefore reduce the dose by 50% for bilirubin levels 1.5–3.0 mg/dL; hold dose for bilirubin level greater than 3.0 dL.

I. Topoisomerase inhibitors
   1. Irinotecan
      a. The area under the plasma concentration-time curve is higher in patients with decreased liver function, but no formal dose adjustment recommendations have been made.
      b. Inactivated in the liver.
      c. Elevations of liver functions occur in one-fourth of patients receiving Irinotecan. Caution should be used in patients with bilirubin elevations.
   2. Topotecan
      a. Not metabolized in the liver.
      b. Topotecan can be used with bilirubin up to 10 mg/dl. About 5–8% of the patients will show mild reversible liver enzyme elevations.

J. Platinum derivatives
   1. Cisplatin
      a. Not metabolized in the liver, but can cause mild elevation of transaminase.
      b. No dose reduction is indicated based on liver disease.
   2. Carboplatin
      a. Has been implicated in VOD and liver failure when used in conjunction with Etoposide.

K. Miscellaneous agents
   1. L-asparaginase
      a. Causes disrupted protein synthesis by asparagine depletion. This results in hepatic toxicity.

b. Up to 87% of patients suffer from liver steatosis. Many liver dependent coagulation factors are depleted and can result in both bleeding and infarction with cumulative doses of aspariginase.

2. Procarbazine
    a. Is metabolized in the liver and modification of the dose is indicated in the face of liver dysfunction. Hepatic dysfunction and jaundice have rarely occurred during the administration of procarbazine. Toxicity is increased in patients with a history of hepatic dysfunction.
    b. Hold the dose if bilirubin is >5 mg/dL or ALT or AST is greater than 180 (grade III toxicity).

3. Dacarbazine (DTIC)
    a. Is associated with a hepatic vascular toxicity syndrome causing death. It is associated with eosinophilia and appears to be an allergic idiosyncratic reaction.
    b. Since the drug is metabolized in the liver, patients are more likely to experience systemic toxicity in the face of elevated liver enzymes.

4. Aldesleukin (Interleukin-2)
    a. Can cause elevated bilirubin due to intrahepatic cholestasis, coagulation disruption, and hypoalbuminemia.
    b. These changes are reversible when the drug is stopped.

Combination chemotherapy commonly used in the treatment of Acute Lymphoblastic Leukemia is hepatotoxic. Most of the liver changes are mild and do not result in serious long term sequelae. Abdominal radiation used in combination with Vincristine, or doxorubicin can result in severe toxicity and even death. Chemotherapy used simultaneously with non-chemotherapeutic agents can result in hepatotoxicity. General anesthesia, allopurinol, ketoconazole, fluconazole, ondansetron, and herbal agents may contribute to the occurrence of liver function changes.

Hepatic veno-occlusive disease is clearly associated with high-dose chemotherapy and with radiation commonly used in bone marrow transplant preparative regimes. Veno-occlusive disease results from the obliteration of small intrahepatic veins, and necrosis of centrilobular hepatocytes. The incidence is 10–20%

and mortality can be high. Treatment is generally supportive care. Wilms tumor patients have a condition unique to them that has a component of veno-occlusive disease associated with thrombocytopenia. Radiation does not seem to be a requirement for this to occur.

In summary, for many years pediatric oncologists have been very conservative in their respect for liver toxicity and subsequent dose reduction of many of the chemotherapeutic agents we use for the treatment of childhood malignancy. However as more intense regimens are developed, as metabolism of the agents we use are determined, and as we share knowledge with our adult colleagues we see that many of our drug restriction in some cases are not warranted and in other cases should be more restrictive. This is a current compendium of knowledge that will certainly be constantly changing.

Bibliography

American Academy of Pediatrics. Joint committee on infant hearing 1994 position statement. *Pediatrics* 95:152–56, 1995.

Aviles A, Herrera J, Ramo E et al. Hepatic injury during doxorubicin therapy. *Arch Pathol Lab Med* 108:912–13, 1984.

Burris HA, Fields FM. Topoisomerase inhibitors. *Hematol Oncol Clin North Am* 8:333–55, 1994.

Campbell K. *Essential Audiology for Physicians.* San Diego: Singular Publishing, 1998.

Doria MI Jr, Shepard KV, Levin B et al. Liver pathology following hepatic arterial infusion chemotherapy: Hepatic toxicity with FUDR. *Cancer* 58:855–61, 1986.

Einhorn M, Davidson I. Hepatotoxicity of mercaptopurine. *JAMA* 188:802–6, 1964.

Fanos V, Cataldi L. Amphotericin B-induced nephrotoxicity: A review. *J Chemotherapy* 12:463–70, 2000.

Giantris A, Abdurrahman L, Hinkle A, Asselin B, Lipshultz SE. Anthracycline-induced cardiotoxicity in children and young adults. *Critical Reviews in Oncology-Hematology* 27:53–68, 1998.

Gill RA, Onstad GR, Cardamone JM et al. Hepatic veno-occlusive disease caused by 6-thioguanine. *Ann Intern Med* 96:58–60, 1982.

Green DM, Hyland A, Chung CS, et al. Cancer and cardiac mortality among 15-year survivors of cancer diagnosed during childhood or adolescence. *J Clin Oncol* 17:3207–15, 1999.

Hall JW. Clinical applications of otoacoustic emissions in children. In JW Hall, *Handbook of Otoacoustic Emissions* (pp. 463–78). San Diego: Singular Publishing Group, 2000.

Hensley ML, Schuchter LM, Lindley C, et al. American Society of Clinical Oncology clinical practice guidelines for the use of chemotherapy and radiotherapy protectants. *J Clin Oncol* 17:3333–55, 1999.

Hogarty AN, Leahey A, Zhao H, et al. Longitudinal evaluation of cardiopulmonary performance during exercise after bone marrow transplantation in children. *J. Pediatr.* 136:311–7, 2000.

Huizing MT, Sewberath Misser VH, Pieters RC et al. Taxanes: A new class of antitumor agents. *Cancer Invest* 13:381–404, 1995.

Johansen HK, Gotzche PC. Amphotericin B lipid soluble formulations versus amphotericin B in cancer patients with neutropenia. Cochrane Library. (on-line) www.cochranelibrary.com.

Johnson DH, Greco FA, Wolff SN. Etoposide induced hepatic injury: A potential complication of high-dose therapy. *Cancer Treatment Reports* 67:1023–24, 1983.

Kemp G, Rose P, Lurain J, et al. Amifostine pretreatment for protection against cyclophosphamide-induced and cisplatin-induced toxicities: Results of a randomized control trial in patients with advanced ovarian cancer. *J Clin Oncol* 14:2101–12, 1996.

King PD, Perry MC. Hepatotoxicity of chemotherapy. *The Oncologist,* Vol. 6, No. 2, 162–76, April 16, 2003.

Kintzel PE. Anticancer drug-induced kidney disorders-incidence, prevention, and management. *Drug Safety* 24:19–38, 2001.

Koler RD, Forsgren AL. Hepatotoxicity due to Chlorambucil. Report of a case. *JAMA* 167:316–17, 1958.

Kortmann R-D, Kuhl J, Timmermann B, et al. Postoperative neoadjuvant chemotherapy before radiotherapy as compared to immediate radiotherapy followed by maintenance chemotherapy in the treatment of medulloblastoma in childhood: Results of the German prospective randomized trial HIT '91. *Int J Radiation Oncology Biology Physics* 46:269–79, 2000.

Landier W. Hearing loss related to ototoxicity in children with cancer. *J Pediatric Oncology Nursing* 15:195–206, 1998.

Lipshultz S, Lipsitz S, Sallan S. Chronic progressive left ventricular systolic dysfunction and afterload excess years after doxorubicin therapy for childhood acute lymphoblastic leukemia. In *Proceedings of American Society of Clinical Oncology,* 2000.

Loebstein R, Atanackovic G, Bishai R, et al. Risk factors for long-term outcome ifosfamide-induced nephrotoxicity in children. *J Clin Pharmacol* 39:454–61, 1999.

Ludwig R, Weirich A, Abel U et al. Hepatotoxicity in patients treated according to the nephroblastoma trial and study SIOP-9/GPOH. *Med Pediatric Oncology* 33:462–69, 1999.

Oettgen HF, Stephenson PA, Schwartz MK et al. Toxicity of E, coli L-aspariginase in man. *Cancer* 25:253–78, 1970.

Perry MC. Chemotherapeutic agents and hepatotoxicity. *Seminar Oncology* 19:551–65, 1992.

Puleo PR, Meyer D, Wathen C, Tawa CB, Wheeler S, Hamburg RJ, Ali N, Obermueller SD, Fernando Sorensen K, Levitt G, Bull C, et al. Anthracycline dose in childhood acute lymphoblastic leukemia: Issues of early survival versus late cardiotoxicity. *J Clin Oncol* 1591:61–68, 1997.

Rollins BJ. Hepatic veno-occlusive disease. *Am J Med* 81:297–306, 1986.

Shaunak S, Munro JM, Weinbren K et al. Cyclophosphamide induced liver necrosis: A possible interaction with azathioprine. *A J Med,* New Series 252:309–17, 1988.

Skinner R, Pearson ADJ, English MW, Price L, Wyllie RA, Coulthard MG, Craft AW. Cisplatin dose rate as a risk factor for nephrotoxicity in children. *Brit J Cancer* 77:1677–82, 1998.

Steinherz LJ, Steinherz PG, and Tan C. Cardiac failure and dysrhythmias 6–19 years after anthracycline therapy: A series of 15 patients. *Med Pediatric Oncology* 24:352–61, 1995.

Stewart DJ, Dulberg CS, Mikhael NZ, et al. Association of cisplatin nephrotoxicity with patient characteristics and cisplatin administration methods. *Cancer Chemother Pharmacol* 40:293–308, 1997.

Sutherland CM, Krementz ET. Hepatic toxicity of DTIC. *Cancer Treat Rep* 65:321–322, 1981.

vanWarmerdam LJ, Rodenhuis S, ten Bokkel Huinink WW, Maes RA, Beijnen JH. Evaluation of formulas using the serum creatinine level to calculate the optimal dosage of carboplatin. *Can Chem Pharm* 37:266–70, 1996.

Weber BL, Tanyer G, Poplack DG et al. Transient acute hepatotoxicity of high-dose methotrexate therapy during childhood. *NCI Monograph* 5:207–12, 1987.

8

The Management of Drug Extravasation

John S. Murphy, B. Pharm., and
Claudia Deffenbaugh, Pharm.D.

I. DEFINITIONS

A. Extravasation
Extravasation is the unintentional instillation or leakage of a vesicant or irritant agent into the perivascular and subcutaneous spaces during parenteral administration (see Table 8.1). It may result when an intravenous (IV) cannula slips from a vein into adjacent tissue or when fluid leaks from a vein via a puncture or around a cannula site.

B. Vesicant
An agent that, when extravasated, can produce ulceration and local necrosis (often severe).

C. Irritant
An agent that, when extravasated, produces burning or inconsequential inflammation without necrosis.

II. PREVENTION

Appropriate administration techniques designed to prevent drug extravasation from occurring in the first place are the most important factors in the prevention of extravasation injury. These procedures should be available at each location where chemotherapy is administered. Procedures to minimize the likelihood of extravasation include:

A. The employment of knowledgeable and highly skilled personnel.

B. The use of centrally placed venous access devices. (If peripheral lines are used, the time of venipuncture, the flow

Table 8.1.
Vesicant and Irritant Chemotherapy Agents

Vesicant
  Amsacrine*
  Cisplatin (>20ml, ≥0.5 mg/ml)
  Dactinomycin
  Daunorubicin
  Doxorubicin
  Idarubicin
  Mechlorethamine HCl
  Mitomycin C*
  Paclitaxel
  Plicamycin*
  Vinblastine
  Vincristine
  Vindesine*
  Vinorelbine
Irritant
  Carboplatin
  Carmustine
  Cisplatin (<0.5 mg/ml)
  Dacarbazine*
  Doxil
  Etoposide
  5-Fluorouracil*
  Ifosfamide
  Irinotecan
  Melphalan
  Mitoxantrone*
  Pentostatin*
  Streptozocin*
  Teniposide
  Topotecan

Note: All investigational chemotherapy agents should be considered vesicants unless known to be otherwise.
* Agents rarely used in pediatrics.

characteristics, condition and location of the IV site, blood return, and patient comfort must be assessed.)

C. The avoidance of "risky" cannulation sites. These include the lower extremities, veins over joints, wrists, any area of flexion, the antecubital area, superficial tendons, and ligaments. Candidate veins should be prominent, easily accessible, and visible at all times without any evidence of compromised circulation.

D. Routine use of vasodilatory procedures (e.g., hot packs).

E. Checks of IV line patency before, during, and after the administration of a vesicant drug. The IV line should be flushed with enough saline (5–10 mL), before and after the infusion of the vesicant drug, to test line patency. During the infusion, the line should be tested periodically for blood return. The frequency of testing will depend on the concentration of the vesicant and the duration of the procedure. Infusions running into a side arm of a fast-running drip, over an hour, will need less frequent testing than an IV push, which might require a blood return test after each 1–2 mL.

F. Secure taping of cannulas to prevent excessive "in and out" motion, which can enlarge the vein entry site, increasing the likelihood of extravasation.

G. Minimization of venous exposure to "high-risk" drugs by adequate dilution or injection into the side arm of a fast-running, additive-free, IV solution.

H. Avoidance of the use of "pump-controlled" or "continuous" infusions of vesicant drugs into peripheral lines.

I. Maximization of patient cooperation by:
    1. Encouraging a confident, yet relaxed, approach to the patient by highly competent personnel.
    2. Performing cannulation procedures in a well-lit environment with all the appropriate equipment readily at hand.
    3. Displaying an awareness of high levels of patient anxiety and having in place appropriate measures to deal with it.
    4. Instructing patients of the need to report, immediately, any untoward sensations associated with the injection/ infusion.

III. RECOGNITION AND MANAGEMENT OF EXTRAVASATION (Table 8.2)

A. Rationale
    Should an extravasation occur, the aim of all management plans is to minimize long-term damage. All efforts, therefore, are directed toward minimizing tissue contact time. A

Table 8.2.
Signs and Symptoms of Extravasation

- Change in quality or rate of infusion.
- Signs of swelling, erythema, or any change at the injection site.
- Symptoms of pain, burning, stinging, or other discomfort at IV site.
- No blood return.

Table 8.3.
Vesicant Chemotherapeutic Agents for which Specific Antidotes Have Been Recommended

Fluid/Medication Extravasated	Warm/Cold Compress	Antidote/ Recommendation
DNA intercalaters Amsacrine (M-AMSA) Daunorubicin (Cerubidin)[†] Doxorubicin (Adriamycin)[†] Idarubicin (Idamycin)[†]	Cold; apply immediately for 30–60 minutes, then alternate on/off every 15 minutes for 24 hours.	Dimethyl Sulfoxide (DMSO) 50–99% 1. Topical application of 1.5 mL to area of extravasation every 6 hours for 14 days. 2. Allow to air dry after application; do not cover.
Alkylating agent Mitomycin		
Vinca alkaloids and epipodopyllotoxins Etoposide (VP-16, Vepesid)* Teniposide (VM-26, Vumon)* Vinblastine (Velban) Vincristine (Oncovin) Vindesine (Eldisine) Vinorelbine (Navelbine)	Warm; apply immediately for 30–60 minutes, then alternate on/off every 15 minutes for 24 hours.	Hyaluronidase (Wydase)** 1. Add 1 mL NS to 150-unit vial to make 150-units/mL concentration. 2. Inject 5 subcutaneous injections of 0.2 mL each, in and around the edge of extravasation.
Alkylating agents and others Mechlorethamine (Mustine HCl nitrogen mustard) Cisplatin (Platinol) (>20 mL, ≥0.5mg/mL)	None	Sodium Thiosulfate 1. Mix 1.6 mL of a 25% sodium thiosulfate with 8.4 mL sterile water to make 1/6 molar solution. 2. Inject 5 subcutaneous injections of 0.2 mL each, in and around the edge of extravasation.

*For most epipodopyllotoxin extravasations, hyaluronidase is not necessary, as these drugs are irritants rather than vesicants.

**If hyaluronidase is not available, use warm compresses only. Formula for extemporaneous compounding may be found in IJPC:5(4) July/Aug 2001.

†Recent studies investigating the systemic use of dexrazoxane as an antidote to anthracycline extravasation have shown it to be effective for up to 6 hours after subcutaneous anthracycline injections in mice. Two patients with large subcutaneous infiltrations of doxorubicin or epirubicin received intravenous dexrazoxane 1000 mg/m2 within 5 hours of the extravasation, 1000 mg/m2 on day 2 and 500 mg/m2 on day 3. All resolved without sequelae (*J Clin Oncol* 18 (16):3064, 2000; *Clin Cancer Res* 6(9):3680–86, 2000; *Ann Oncol* 12(3):405–10, 201).

truly standardized and universally accepted management plan does not exist; however, with disagreement as to the most appropriate course of action continuing, management is usually based on a limited number of animal experiments and anecdotal reports appearing in the literature, as well as personal experience.

Only those steps that appear to have attained near "universal" acceptance are listed below.

B. Procedure for suspected extravasation:
1. Stop the administration of the agent immediately, *but do not remove the needle/cannula.*
2. If possible, attempt to draw back 3–5 mL of blood/drug solution into the tubing/needle with the aim of removing as much as possible of the infiltrated drug.
3. Using a 25–27g needle attached to a 1mL TB syringe, aspirate (from several sites) any subcutaneous "bleb" of drug solution remaining after the completion of step 2.
4. With the needle/cannula still in place, instill the specific antidote using a 25–27g needle attached to a 1mL TB syringe. At least 5 separate volumes of 0.2 mL of the appropriate antidote should be injected subcutaneously around the edge of the extravasation site. (See Tables 8.3 and 8.4.)
5. Remove the needle/cannula.
6. Cleanse the site with antiseptic and allow to dry.
7. Apply cold packs or hot packs, for periods of 15 minutes, every 6 hours for 24 hours as appropriate. (See Tables 8.3 and 8.4.)
8. Apply a designated "topical" agent if appropriate. (See Tables 8.3 and 8.4.)
9. Elevate the extremity above the level of the heart using pillows, a sling, or stockinette dressings. Elevation should be maintained, ideally, for up to 48 hours.
10. Document the incident. This may include marking and/or photographing the site as well as completing an incident report. The ongoing resolution of the extravasation should be documented in the progress notes.
11. Order medication for symptomatic relief. Oral medications including analgesics, sedatives or anxiolytics, and antihistamines may be of value in individual cases.

Table 8.4.
Noncytotoxic Infusions/Agents That May Cause Problems If
Extravasated

Fluid/Medication Extravasated	Warm/Cold Compress	Antidote/Recommendation
Calcium Dextrose Parenteral nutrition Potassium	Cold; apply immediately for 30–60 minutes, then alternate on/off every 15 minutes for 24 hours.	Hyaluronidase (Wydase)* 1. Add 1 mL NS to 150-unit vial to make 150 units/mL concentration. 2. Inject 5 SC injections of 0.2 mL each, in and around the edge of extravasation

Note: Concentrated solutions of electrolytes (e.g., potassium or calcium salts) can cause serious problems if extravasated.

* If hyaluronidase is not available, use warm compresses only. The formula for extemporaneous compounding may be found in "Hyaluronidase Injection." Formulations Section. *Intl J Pharmaceutical Compounding* 5(4): 303, July/August 2001.

12. Apply an appropriate dressing to protect the area from infection. Dress the site with a light dressing to avoid undue pressure or rubbing, which might irritate the wound. Where dimethylsulfoxide (DMSO) is used topically, the area should be allowed to air dry. If appropriate, a light, dry sterile and totally nonocclusive covering dressing may be used to protect the site.

13. Re-evaluate the site no later than 24 hours after the extravasation. If the signs and symptoms are progressing despite conservative treatment, initiate a surgical referral as soon as possible. (The role of "early" surgery to remove the drug-laden tissue may reduce later necrosis. Solid consensus on the importance of traditional debridement and plastic surgery in the management of serious extravasation does exist.)

14. Ensure adequate follow-up observation of the extravasation site.

Bibliography

Beckwith C, Tyler L. *Cancer Chemotherapy Manual, March 2001.* Facts and Comparisons, University of Utah; 25–34, 2001.
Bertelli G, Gozza A, Forno GB, Vidili MG, Silvestro S, Venturini M, Del Mastro L, Garrone O, Rosso R, Dini D. Topical dimethylsulfoxide for

the prevention of soft tissue injury after extravasation of vesicant cyto-toxic drugs: a prospective clinical study. *J Clin Oncol* 13(11): 2851–55, 1995.

Clark BS, Gallegos E, Bleyer WA. Accidental intramuscular vincristine: lack of untoward effects and recommendations for management. *Med Pediat Oncol* 28:314–15,1997.

"Hyaluronidase Injection." Formulations Section. *Intl J Pharmaceutical Compounding* 5(4): 303, July/August 2001.

Langer SW, Sehested M, Jensen PB. Dexrazoxane is a potent and specific inhibitor of anthracycline induced subcutaneous lesions in mice. *Ann Oncol* 12(3):405–10, 2001.

9

Side Effects of Radiation Therapy

Richard S. Pieters, M.D., Karen Marcus, M.D., and Robert B. Marcus, Jr., M.D.

Radiation therapy has inherent side effects, early (during or immediately after treatment, termed *acute*), intermediate (weeks to months after treatment, termed *subacute*), and late. Early and intermediate effects are temporary, while late effects tend to be permanent. In general, tissues are most vulnerable to late effects during periods of rapid proliferation. Severity of late effects is not related to severity of acute effects, but both can be minimized by careful fractionation and definition of treatment volume. Medical measures can also be taken to minimize or prevent the occurrence of either early or late effects and to manage those that do occur.

General Principles: Management of Side Effects of Radiation Therapy

I. EARLY EFFECTS

    A. Nutritional support
        1. Nutritional support during radiation therapy is vital for prevention of cachexia, immune compromise, and inability to repair normal tissue damage.
            (See Chapter 13 on nutritional support.)
        2. Initial assessment of nutritional status
            a. Weight loss probably indicates negative nitrogen balance, which must be corrected.
            b. Counsel the patient and family regarding unusual or idiosyncratic dietary habits to ensure a nutritionally complete diet.

3. Caloric need during radiation therapy is approximately 110% of baseline.
4. An enteral diet is preferable to a parenteral one.
   a. Oral diet modifications
      i. Taste may change secondary to the tumor or to treatment, which may alter diet.
      ii. If mucosa of upper GI tract is being irradiated, a soft, bland diet may be required (no spices or acidic, hot, or cold food or drink).
      iii. Standard oral supplements must be used if caloric requirements cannot be met otherwise (Sustacal, Ensure, Carnation Instant Breakfast).
   b. Nasogastric tube feeding is probably required if 10% weight loss occurs during treatment.
5. Intravenous hyperalimentation is indicated if the patient is unable to tolerate oral or nasogastric feeding.

B. Management of hematologic and immunologic toxicity
   Radiation therapy of any part of the body can suppress blood counts, particularly white cells and platelets. Patients who have received chemotherapy, previously or concurrently, or whose treatment volume encompasses a significant percentage of marrow, are at particular risk.
   1. See Chapter 1 on the prevention of infection.
   2. Follow protocol guidelines for interruption of therapy due to hematologic toxicity.
   3. In the absence of protocol guidelines, consider rate of decrease in counts and clinical situation; consider holding treatment for ANC $<1000/mm^3$, or platelets $<75,000/mm^3$.
   4. The role of hematopoietic stimulating factors during radiation therapy is not established.

C. Management of radiation-induced nausea and vomiting
   Radiation-induced nausea and vomiting can be difficult to prevent. Nausea can be seen with radiation of the head or the stomach; occasionally it is seen when other parts of the body are irradiated. The mechanisms are different, requiring different interventional approaches.
   1. Management of nausea and vomiting due to cranial radiation
      (See section on Cranial Radiation.)

2. Management of nausea and vomiting due to direct effect on the stomach
   a. Etiology is not well understood.
   b. Treatment
      i. Sipping decarbonated cola drinks may relieve symptoms.
      ii. Antiemetic medications:
   Promethazine
      (1) Dose: Children (>10 kg, or >2yr) 0.5 mg/kg, PO or PR, t.i.d.-q.i.d., maximum 25 mg per dose
      (2) Available: Tablets: 12.5, 25 mg
          Syrup: 6.25 mg/5 ml or 25 mg/5 ml
          Suppository: 12.5, 25 mg
   Metoclopramide
      (1) Dose: 1–2 mg/kg PO q.i.d. (Premedicate with diphenhydramine to reduce extra pyramidal syndrome)
      (2) Available: Tablets: 5 mg, 10 mg
          Syrup: 5 mg/5 ml
   Cisapride
      (1) Dose: Children: 0.2–0.3 mg/kg/dose PO t.i.d.-q.i.d.
      (2) Available: Tablets:10, 20 mg
          Suspension: 1 mg/ml
   Ondansetron
      (1) Dose: <4yr: 2 mg/dose
          4–11 years: 4 mg/dose
          Teenagers: 8 mg/dose
          Usually administered PO, Q4-6h, starting 1 hour before radiation daily.
      (2) Available: Tablets: 4, 8 mg
   Prochlorperazine, the most common antiemetic used in adults, should be avoided in children because of a reported increased incidence of extrapyramidal side effects.
3. Management of nausea and vomiting due to radiation of other parts of body
   a. Etiology: This is believed to be due to delayed gastric emptying.
   b. Treatment: Cisapride and Metoclopramide may facilitate gastric emptying.

II. LATE EFFECTS

A. Growth problems
  1. Neuroendocrine effect of irradiation of hypothalamic pituitary axis. See section of this chapter on neuroendocrine effect of cranial radiation.
  2. Direct effect on irradiated bone and soft tissue
     a. Effect is age and dose dependent
        i. Irradiated bones may be smaller or shorter than nonirradiated bones.
        ii. Spinal irradiation may affect height, and may exacerbate kyphosis/scoliosis.
     b. Irradiated muscle may atrophy.
  3. Management of growth problems
     a. Consider growth hormone replacement.
     b. Monitor for scoliosis and kyphosis.
     c. Consider early plastic surgical intervention for correction of facial deformities sufficient to cause psychosocial distress.
     d. Psychosocial support

B. Soft tissue fibrosis over a joint
  1. Etiology
     Scarring after high-dose radiotherapy; the risk is increased if the field also includes a radical surgical site.
  2. Prevention
     If possible, plan surgical incisions to allow the radiation oncologist to avoid treatment of a full joint.
  3. Treatment
     Daily range-of-motion exercises for the rest of the patient's life.

C. Peripheral edema
  1. Etiology
     a. Lymphatic obstruction
     b. Venous insufficiency.
  2. Prevention
     Place incisions vertically, not transversely in extremities, to allow radiation oncologist to treat entire scar without treating entire circumference of extremity.

D. Carcinogenesis
  1. Risk factors for second malignant neoplasm (SMN) due to radiation therapy

Table 9.1.
Tissues at Risk for Secondary Neoplasm

Tissue Radiated	Second (Malignant) Neoplasm	Signs and Symptoms	Usual Time Interval to Occurrence (years)
Bone marrow	leukemia (acute myelogenous)	fatigue, petechiae	7–10; rare past 15
Bone and soft tissues	sarcoma	pain, mass	≥ 8
Neck, mediastinum	thyroid adenoma	nodule	<10
	thyroid carcinoma	nodule, mass	≥ 10
Chest	breast carcinoma	mass, characteristic mammographic lesions	≥ 8
	lung cancer	cough, mass on chest X-ray	≥ 8
Skin	melanoma	characteristic lesion	≥ 8
	atypical basal cell carcinoma	characteristic lesion	3–20
Brain	brain tumor	headache, vomiting, ataxia	≥ 8
Upper airways	atypical squamous cell carcinoma	pain, bleeding, mass, ulceration	≥ 8

a. Relative risk of SMN due to radiation therapy is not yet well defined, as it varies from report to report, and by original disease, age at treatment, and site treated.

b. Children treated for one malignancy have increased risk of developing SMN, even in absence of radiation therapy.

c. Genetics (heredity) plays a role.
   i. Patients with basal cell nevus syndrome often develop basal cell cancers in irradiated field 6 months–3 years after treatment.
   ii. Patients with familial retinoblastoma are at increased risk of SMN, even after surgery alone.

d. About two-thirds of SMNs are found in field of radiation therapy.

   Bone and soft tissue sarcoma are considered radiation induced only if they occur in the radiated treatment volume.

    e. Tissue sensitivity to carcinogenesis from radiation varies:

       i.   Thyroid and breast are at risk after low doses.

      ii.   Lung, liver, and lymphoid tissue are at risk after moderate dose.

     iii.   Bone and muscle are at risk after higher dose.

    f. Tissue stage of development alters risk; proliferating cells are most at risk. Girls whose breast tissue is irradiated between ages 10–16 years (during pubertal development) have greatest increase in risk of developing breast cancer; risk declines as age at treatment increases thereafter.

    g. Sex

        Risk of SMN is higher for females than males, even excluding breast cancer.

  2. Management

    a. Discourage smoking in survivors, especially if respiratory tract has been irradiated.

    b. Examination of at-risk tissues: those in radiation treatment volume. (See Table 9.1.)

    c. Scrupulous breast follow-up for women whose breasts received radiation during adolescence

       i.   Monthly breast self-examination

      ii.   Regular clinical breast examinations

     iii.   Early annual mammography (exact age to start is controversial)

Side Effects of Skin Radiation

I. MANAGEMENT OF EARLY SKIN TOXICITY

All radiation treatments treat skin. Severe skin reactions, sufficient to interrupt treatment, may occur at any site; intertriginous areas are most at risk.

  A. Prevention

    1. Avoid heat or cold, sun exposure, sun blocks, and perfumes or perfumed ointments during treatment.

    2. At most, use gentle soap on radiated surface. Preferably, rinse with lukewarm water and gently pat dry with soft towel avoiding soap altogether.

3. Do not place adhesive or medical tape on irradiated fields.
   a. If tape is absolutely required, use paper tape.
   b. If tape is present on irradiated skin, soak it off.
4. Avoid scratching.
   a. Corn starch applied generously, as desired, will provide some relief; wash it off frequently with luke-warm water.
   b. Diphenhydramine (1 mg/kg per dose PO; maximum 5 doses per day) may decrease itching.
   c. Close observation by care provider.
   d. Keep fingernails clipped short.
   e. The patient may need to sleep with stockings over hands to prevent scratching while asleep.
   f. Do not scrub off radiation field marks; when treatment is complete, allow them to wear off.
B. Treatment
   1. For dry desquamation:
      a. Use Sween Cream, Aquaphor, or aloe vera lotion 4–6 times per day to affected area.
      b. Rub in gently until gone. It is acceptable to use cream or lotion before radiation treatments as long as it is rubbed into the skin so that minimal residual medication is present to provide bolus.
      c. Can be started as early as start of radiation.
   2. For moist desquamation:
      a. Clean gently; air dry then apply either gentian violet, Biolex, or silver sulfadiazine
      b. Gentian violet solution USP; apply sparingly 2–3 times per day.
         or
      c. Biolex Spray and Gel to affected area 4 times per day.
      d. For large areas or failure to respond to above, use silver sulfadiazine topical antibiotic cream, 1% 2 times per day

II. MANAGEMENT OF LATE SKIN REACTION
A. Permanent increased sensitivity to sun
   1. Dose dependent
   2. Sensitivity is greatest in first year after radiation.

B. Treatment
   1. Avoid prolonged sun exposure.
   2. Use sun block scrupulously.
   3. Remind patient and family that a layer of cloth provides an SPF of only about 7.

Side Effects of Cranial Radiation

I. EARLY EFFECTS

A. Nausea
   1. Etiology
      Nausea secondary to brain irradiation is due to brain edema with increased intracranial pressure.
   2. Prevention
      If peritumoral edema is present, start steroid treatment at least 4 hours before starting radiation; otherwise, just before radiation is acceptable. If only a small amount of tumor remains (either after surgery or chemotherapy) and minimal edema is present, no steroids are usually needed.
   3. Treatment
      Dexamethasone
      a. For adults and teenagers, loading dose of 1 mg/kg IV, then 4–6 mg IV or PO q.i.d., and then taper after completion of radiation. For younger children, dose can be individualized; 0.1 mg/kg/dose q6h (maximum 48 hours) is a reasonable initial dose, and then taper can be started.
      b. Available: Tablets: 0.25, 0.5, 1, 1.5, 2, 4, 6 mg
         Injection: 4, 10, 20, 24 mg/ml
         Elixir: 0.5 mg/ 5ml
         Oral solution: 0.1, 1 mg/ml

II. INTERMEDIATE EFFECTS

A. Delayed somnolence syndrome
   1. Presentation
      Extreme sleepiness occurring several weeks to approximately 6 months after cranial radiation.
   2. Etiology
      Believed to be due to transient demyelinization.

3. Treatment
   a. Self-limiting; very gradually improves over several weeks to months.
   b. Wake patient to eat, to maintain adequate nutrition.
   c. Corticosteroids may shorten duration.
      Dexamethasone, dose as above, taper gradually.

B. Headache/nausea
   1. Presentation
      a. Rare, occurring several weeks to approximately 6 months after cranial radiation.
      b. Severe headache with associated nausea
   2. Etiology
      Unknown
   3. Treatment
      a. Also self-limiting with gradual improvement
      b. Corticosteroids diminish severity of symptoms and may shorten duration
         Dexamethasone, as above.

III. LATE EFFECTS

A. Cognitive impairment
   1. Age at treatment, dose, and volume dependent.
   2. Variability between individual patients is great.
   3. Mathematical skills more often affected than verbal abilities.
   4. Management
      a. Early and regular neuropsychological testing.
      b. Parents need to be informed of their child's legal rights to special educational help when indicated.

B. Neuroendocrine
   1. Etiology
      a. Damage is dependent on dose to pituitary and hypothalamus.
      b. Etiology is unknown; may be vascular insufficiency or late mitotic death.
      c. Hormones vary in sensitivity to radiation.
         i. Growth hormone is most sensitive; first to be affected.
         ii. Gonadotrophins and ACTH are intermediate.
         iii. TSH is least sensitive, last to be affected.
         iv. Transient hyperprolactinemia is seen

    d. Anterior pituitary hormones are at risk; no posterior pituitary damage has been observed.

    e. Hypothalamus appears to be the site of damage.

    f. Premature onset of puberty
Effect is age and sex dependent.

       i. Females: Youngest girls at age of irradiation have earliest onset of puberty.

      ii. Males: Pubertal onset earliest in those irradiated between 3–6 years of age.

2. Management

    a. Early referral and annual endocrine evaluation in follow-up are indicated to minimize effect on eventual height.

    b. Consider growth hormone replacement for those who have received >2700 cGy to pituitary hypothalamic axis.

    c. For brain tumor patients, wait 2 years after therapy.

    d. Early puberty shortens time available for growth hormone treatment, and the early pubertal growth spurt may mask fact of ultimate short stature.

Side Effects of Head and Neck Radiation

I. **ACUTE EFFECTS**

  A. Radiation mucositis

    1. Prevention

       a. Orthodontic braces should be removed before treatment.

       b. If a metal dental prosthesis or filling is in place, cover it with substance such as chewing gum, dental rolls, dental wax, or fluoride carriers to avoid local scatter of electrons.

       c. Observe scrupulous oral hygiene; brush after each meal; rinse frequently as below.

    2. Treatment

       a. Rinse mouth with a lukewarm solution of 1 tablespoon of salt and 1 tablespoon of baking soda in a quart of water *and/or* diluted hydrogen peroxide solution for several minutes, 5 or 6 times a day.

       b. Consider UlcerEase

          i. Use 5–10 cc, swish, or gargle 15 seconds, then spit out.

      ii. May be used q2 hours while awake.

      iii. Use with caution in child under 6, or one who is unable to avoid swallowing medication.

c. The patient should avoid spicy foods, very warm, very cold, or acidic food or drink, and exposure to tobacco smoke.

d. On mouth care, see Chapter 14.

e. Vigorously address patient's nutritional status.

      i. Mucositis will discourage adequate nutrition.

      ii. Mucositis will resolve only when patient is in positive nitrogen balance.

      iii. See section above and Chapter 13 on nutritional support.

f. Recipes vary for a prophylactic anti-inflammatory/antibiotic solution; here is a representative one:

      Tetracycline syrup, 2 g. OR Erythromycin syrup 2 g

      Nystatin oral suspension, 2 million U

      Hydrocortisone 50 mg

      Mix in distilled water with flavoring to make 120 cc

      Take 5 cc, swish and swallow q.i.d.

g. Take a 3–4 or day weekend off treatment. If mucositis is severe, a longer break until healing is well under way, may be necessary. However, long breaks (more than a week) may compromise tumor control and are not recommended. Once healing has started, it will usually continue despite resumption of radiation therapy.

h. Pain management

      i. Acetaminophen 10 mg/kg (max. 650 mg) and/or codeine 0.5–1 mg/kg (max. 10–20 mg) PO q4h.

      ii. A solution of diphenhydramine and Maalox in equal parts has been effective as a soothing mouthwash; small amounts can be swallowed without ill effect. Do not exceed maximum Benadryl dose of 5 mg/kg/day.

      iii. Use 2% viscous xylocaine in an older child who can expel the material as a swish and gargle before and during meals as needed. Be aware of the increased risk of cardiac arrhythmia from xylocaine in the pediatric patient; adding 2% xylocaine to above diphenhydramine/Maalox solution (1:1:1) is also useful.

    iv. Severe mucositis may require systemic opiates. (See Chapter 11 on Pain Management, section III, B, 3.)

B. Radiation candidiasis
1. Prevention
Scrupulous oral hygiene; unfortunately, this is of limited efficacy.
2. Diagnosis
Clinical evidence of candidal infection is sufficient to start treatment.
3. Treatment
  a. Candidal infection must be managed immediately and vigorously.
  b. Each of the following has been used with success:
    i. Fluconazole
Dose: Children: Loading: 10 mg/kg PO or IV, then 3–6 mg/kg PO QD
Teenagers: Loading: 200 mg PO or IV, then 100 mg PO QD Available: Tablets: 50,100, and 200 mg
Injection: 2 mg/ml
Suspension: 10 mg/ml; 40 mg/ml
OR
    ii. Nystatin oral suspension
Dose: Infants and young children: swab and swallow
Older children: 1–2 ml q.i.d., swish and swallow
Teenagers: 5 ml swish and swallow q.i.d.
Available: Suspension: 100,000 U/ml
OR
    iii. Clotrimazole troche
Dose: 10 mg (1 troche) sublingually, 5 times daily.
OR
    iv. For refractory cases: Ketoconazole
Dose: Children: 5 mg/kg PO per day, rounded up to the nearest 50 mg (maximum 10 m/kg per day, divided b.i.d.).

Teenagers: 200–400 mg PO QD or divided b.i.d.
Available: Tablets: 200 mg
Suspension: 100 mg/ml

   c.   Once a candidal infection has occurred during radiation therapy, it is important to continue oral candidal treatment as prophylactics against recurrence until the end of radiation therapy.

C. Sialadenitis
1. Painful inflammation of salivary glands in direct radiation beam occurs occasionally, at variable intervals, after the start of radiation.
2. This condition is usually self-limiting, as it disappears when the affected glands cease to function.
3. Treat symptomatically with anti-inflammatory agents.

D. Loss of taste
1. Most noticeable in patients with tongue in treatment field, but may occur during treatment of nasal cavity and nasopharynx and in patients receiving mantle field irradiation.
2. Some patients complain of metallic taste, others of cardboard taste of all food.
3. Eventually, sense of taste disappears.
4. Reassure patient/parents that this is usually temporary; taste returns at least partially to normal, but may take months after treatment.

E. Ear
1. Otitis Externa
   a. Etiology
      i. Skin reaction
      ii. Superimposed infection
   b. Management
      i. See skin care section of this chapter.
      ii. Wicks
      iii. Otic antibiotics
      iv. Steroid creams.
2. Decreased hearing/sensation of water in ear
   a. Etiology
      Eustachian tube swelling, obstruction.
   b. Treatment

    i. Diphenhydramine
Dose: Children: (1 mg/kg per dose PO; maximum 5 doses per day)
Teenagers: 10–50 mg/dose PO q6-8h
Available: Tablets: 25, 50 mg
Syrup: 12.5 mg/5ml

    ii. Consider inserting tympanic tubes.

II. LATE EFFECTS

A. Dry mouth
1. Etiology
   a. Doses > approximately 3,000 cGy in conventional fractionation obliterate salivary function in treated glands.
   b. Severity of dry mouth depends on volume of salivary glands irradiated.
2. Prevention
   Two radioprotective agents have been approved for use in adults, amofostine and pilocarpine hydrochloride to decrease severity of dry mouth in adults; this use in pediatrics has not been established and should be used in children only when specified by the individual protocol.
3. Treatment, since prevention is not often possible:
   a. Life-long scrupulous oral hygiene.
   b. Carry water at all times for sipping.
   c. Consider Pilocarpine Hydrochloride, as above
      i. Available: 5 mg tablets
      ii. Use consistently t.i.d. for at least a month before assessing response.
      iii. Safety and efficacy of this drug in children has not been established; off protocol, this should only be used in older adolescents.
   d. Sugarless chewing gum helps many patients.
   e. Fat: a teaspoon of corn oil or olive oil PRN, especially at bedtime, has been reported to help.
   f. Room humidifier should be used at night in winter.

B. Radiation caries
1. Etiology
   Dry mouth leading to altered oral flora; this is not a direct effect of radiation on the teeth.

    2.   Prevention
       Life-long scrupulous oral hygiene. (See Chapter 14 on mouth care.)

C. Osteoradionecrosis
This complication is seen less commonly in pediatric patients than would be expected from experience in adults, but it is so devastating when it occurs, that prevention is vital.

    1.   All patients requiring radiation to the mouth or parotid glands should be seen by a dentist as soon after diagnosis as possible to start a rigorous program of dental prophylaxis.
    2.   Healthy teeth should not be removed.
    3.   Permanent teeth in poor condition requiring removal in the foreseeable future, should be removed before treatment.
    4.   After dental extractions, radiotherapy must be delayed approximately 2 weeks for healing.
    5.   Dental prophylaxis. (See Chapter 14 on mouth care.)
    6.   Prophylactic antibiotics should be administered for all dental work performed after head and neck radiation therapy.

D. Ocular
    1.   Cataracts
       a.   Etiology
          i.   Direct effect of radiation to the lens
          ii.   Dose dependent; greater than 200 cGy in single fraction or 500 cGy fractionated to the lens virtually assures cataract development.
          iii.   Busulfan and steroids can exacerbate cataractogenesis.
       b.   Treatment
          Surgical removal of lens.
    2.   Dry eye
       a.   Etiology
          i.   Loss of lacrimal gland function
          ii.   Dose dependent; > approximately 3,000 cGy in conventional fractionation may lead to permanent loss of lacrimal gland function.
          iii.   Severity of dry eye depends on volume of gland treated; sparing minor glands can diminish problem.

          iv. Dry eye can cause corneal ulceration and severe pain.
- b. Treatment
  - i. Over-the-counter eyedrops during the day, preservative-free are preferred, such as Carboxymethylcellulose 1.0% ophthalmic solution.
  - ii. Over-the-counter viscous lubricant or white petrolatum/mineral oil lubricant ophthalmic ointment at bedtime.
  - iii. Early ophthalmologic evaluation is vital to prevent complications of dry eye.
  - iv. Painful, sightless dry eye can lead to enucleation as last resort.
- 3. Retinitis
  - a. Etiology
    - i. Apparently vasculitis: microangiopathy
    - ii. Dose and fraction size dependent
    - iii. Latency 6 months–3 years
    - iv. Can lead to neovascular glaucoma.
  - b. Treatment
    - i. Not well understood
    - ii. Appears similar to diabetic retinopathy, so similar management seems reasonable.
    - iii. Therefore, laser treatment has been used.
    - iv. Early referral to retinal ophthalmologist is indicated if retina receives >5,000 cGy in conventional fractionation. Patients should be referred during treatment and reevaluated by the ophthalmologist routinely at 6-month intervals after treatment.

E. Auditory
- 1. Etiology
  - a. Radiation alone rarely damages hearing.
  - b. Cisplatin concomitantly or after radiation to middle ear can increase hearing loss.
  - c. Cisplatin before radiation is not as ototoxic.
  - d. Hearing loss progresses gradually up to 6 years after radiation.

F. Neuroendocrine
See section on neuroendocrine effect of cranial radiation.

Management of Late Effects of Thyroid Irradiation

I. HYPERTHYROIDISM

    A. Not dose-related.

    B. Occurs up to 18 years after irradiation.

    C. Can occur in patients on thyroid hormone replacement.

II. GRAVES OPHTHALMOPATHY

    A. Etiology is not known.

    B. Does not require patient to be biochemically hyperthyroid.

III. THYROTOXICOSIS

    A. Etiology is not known.

    B. Condition is transient; progresses rapidly to overt hypothyroidism.

IV. HYPOTHYROIDISM

    A. About 50% of patients treated with mantle radiation for Hodgkin disease become subclinically hypothyroid; therefore, thyroid function studies should be obtained at least annually if the lower neck has been irradiated.

    B. Elevated TSH levels are occasionally transient.

    C. Consider treatment for subclinical hypothyroidism.

    D. Incidence of progression from subclinical to overt hypothyroidism is unknown.

    E. Thyroid hormone replacement therapy.

    F. Hypothyroidism may increase risk of accelerated atherosclerosis.

V. THYROID NODULAR DISEASE

    A. Detection
        1. Careful palpation of thyroid at all follow-up examinations.
        2. Thyroid scans, biopsy of suspicious nodules.

    B. 10–20% of nodules are malignant.

Side Effects of Thoracic Irradiation

I. EARLY EFFECTS

A. Esophagitis
1. Prevention
   a. Sucralfate slurry, starting on the first day of irradiation has been suggested to decrease incidence and severity.
      i.   Dose: 10–20 mg/kg/dose PO q.i.d.
      ii. Available: Suspension: 100 mg/ml.
   b. Ranitidine HCl has also been suggested to decrease severity.
      i.   Dose: Infants and children: 4–5 mg/kg/24h, divided, b.i.d. or t.i.d.
           Teenagers: 150 mg b.i.d. or 300 mg QHS
      ii. Available: Tablets: 75 mg (over the counter), 150 mg, 300 mg.
           Syrup: 15 mg/ml.
2. Presentation
   a. Substernal pain on swallowing, sensation of lump in throat, sore throat
   b. Symptoms begin about 2 weeks into course of thoracic radiation therapy.
   c. Symptoms usually ease after radiation to esophagus stops, or even decrease when oblique fields start.
3. Treatment
   a. Treat identically to oral mucositis.
   b. If dysphagia persists or there is evidence of oral candidiasis, start candidal treatment (see above).
   c. If the dysphagia is severe, a break from radiation treatment may be necessary.

II. INTERMEDIATE EFFECTS

A. Radiation pneumonitis
1. Presentation
   a. Presents either during radiation therapy or up to about 6 months after treatment is completed.
   b. Shortness of breath, dyspnea on exertion, cough.
   c. Fever is rare.

      d. Radiographic changes in most patients:
          Infiltrates within irradiated volume of lung.
      e. Decreased vital capacity and diffusing capacity.
      f. Actinomycin D and Adriamycin may reactivate.
      g. Abrupt steroid withdrawal may reactivate.
2. Treatment
      a. Bed rest
      b. Prednisone
          i. Dose: 0.5–2 mg/kg/day, max. 80 mg/24h, divided t.i.d.-q.i.d.
          ii. Available: Tablets:1, 2.5, 5, 10, 20, 50 mg
          Syrup: 1 mg/ml (5% alcohol)

III. LATE EFFECTS

A. Cardiac
1. Late cardiac complications
      a. Acute myocardial infarction
      b. Acute pericarditis
      c. Constrictive pericarditis
2. Risk factors
      a. Dose, volume, and exact target dependent.
          i. Proximal coronary arteries tend to be in high-dose mediastinal fields.
          ii. Pericardial problems require that most of the heart be in treatment volume; rare today.
      b. Age dependent: risk decreases as child's age at treatment increases.
      c. Acute pericarditis may be precipitated by abrupt steroid withdrawal.
      d. Malignant hypertension can exacerbate arteriosclerosis in irradiated vessels precipitating myocardial infarction in patients at risk.
3. Presentation
      a. Acute myocardial infarction
          Remember this risk in patients after chest irradiation who present with chest pain or congestive failure.
      b. Acute pericarditis
          Pain
      c. Constrictive pericarditis
          Chest pain, poor exercise tolerance, normal heart size

B. Pulmonary fibrosis
1. Presentation
a. Radiographs: scarring in field of radiation, sometimes with retraction.
b. Rarely symptomatic
c. Reduced diffusing capacity.

Side Effects of Abdominal Irradiation

I. **EARLY EFFECTS**
Nausea
(See Chapter 9, General Principles: Management of Side Effects
of Radiation Therapy, section IC2.)

II. **LATE EFFECTS**

A. Renal toxicity
1. Hypertension
a. Etiology
i.   Parenchymal damage
ii. Extrarenal vascular damage
b. Treatment
i.   Partial or total nephrectomy.

B. Bowel toxicity
(See the following section on late effects of pelvic radiation.)

Management of Acute and Late Effects of Pelvic Irradiation

I. **EARLY EFFECTS**

A. Radiation enteritis
Radiation enteritis is seen as a result of radiation to the
pelvis or lower abdomen.
1. Diagnosis
Radiation enteritis usually presents as diarrhea with
frequent watery, soft stools and sometimes with cramping pain.
2. Prevention
If the patient has a full bladder for as many radiation
treatments as possible, incidence and severity of radiation enteritis will decrease.

3. Treatment
   a. Diet
      i. Restrict the roughage, or residue, in the diet.
      ii. If this is not successful, restrict fat.
      iii. If this is still not successful, restrict lactose; milk products can still be used if lactase-treated milk is provided (Lactaid, sweet acidophilus milk).
      iv. An elemental diet, which is absorbed in the upper small bowel to put the bowel at rest, may help.
      v. The patient's weight must be maintained as adequate nutrition is required to recover from radiation enteritis.
   b. Drug: Loperamide
      i. Avoid in the presence of significant abdominal distention.
      ii. Dose: 2–6 yr (13–20 kg): 1 mg PO t.i.d.
          6–8 yr (20–30 kg): 2 mg PO b.i.d.
          8–12 yr (>30 kg): 2 mg PO t.i.d.
          Teenagers: 2 mg after each loose stool to max of 16 mg/24h
      iii. Available: Caps: 2 mg
           Tablets: 2 mg
           Syrup: 1 mg/5 ml
   c. Radiotherapy may have to be interrupted for severe enteritis.
   d. If the above measures fail, admit the patient to the hospital for appropriate diagnostic evaluation, parenteral fluids, and other indicated therapies.

B. Proctitis
   1. Presentation
      a. Perianal inflammation.
      b. Exacerbated by diarrhea or constipation.
   2. Treatment
      a. Treat diarrhea/constipation.
      b. Sitz baths after each bowel movement.
      c. Lukewarm water sprayed into anus may help.
      d. Consider cortisone enemas.
      e. Pain management.

C. Acute radiation cystitis
Acute radiation cystitis manifests as urinary frequency and dysuria. Anthracyclines or actinomycin-D given with bladder radiation increases the risk of hemorrhagic cystitis.
1. Diagnosis
   a. Symptoms are identical to those of urinary tract infection.
   b. Urinalysis with clean-catch urine culture and sensitivity are mandatory to rule out infection.
2. Prevention
If patient has a full bladder for as many radiation treatments as possible, incidence and severity of radiation cystitis will decrease.
3. Treatment
   a. If urinalysis and culture are negative:
      i. Phenazopyridine HCl for topical analgesic effect
Dose: 6–12 yr: 12 mg/kg per day PO divided, t.i.d.
Teenagers: 100–200 mg PO t.i.d.
Available: Tablets: 95, 100, 200 mg
OR
      ii. Urispas (100–200 mg PO t.i.d. or q.i.d. if the child is >12 years old) to relieve urinary spasm. If obstruction of the bladder outlet is a risk, avoid Urispas because of its anticholinergic effect.
      iii. Oxybutynin chloride
Dose: <5 years old, 0.28 mg/kgh PO b.i.d.-q.i.d.
>5 years old, 5 mg PO b.i.d. or t.i.d
Available: Tablets: 5 mg
Syrup: 5 mg/5 ml
      iv. Interrupt radiation therapy only for gross hematuria.

II. LATE EFFECTS

A. Fertility
1. Female
   a. Preservation of ovarian function is dose dependent: about 500 cGy seems to be enough to sterilize adult women.

    b. Age dependent: younger girls have better chance of preservation of function at a given dose.

    c. Prevention: Ovarian transposition and marking with metallic clips to place ovaries outside of radiation field and allow radiation oncologist to verify their location.

    d. Treatment: Cryopreservation of oocytes is under investigation.

2. Male

    a. Preservation of testicular function is dose dependent

    b. Hormone function less sensitive than fertility.

    c. Oligospermia or azospermia may recover after 18–24 months.

    d. Treatment: Consider sperm banking when radiation therapy is planned to or near testes.

3. Treatment for endocrine dysfunction from gonadal radiation

    a. If gonadal damage is expected, screen gonadotropins and sex hormones regularly after age of expected puberty is reached.

    b. Monitor growth velocity and total growth closely.

    c. Early endocrine consultation

    d. Hormonal replacement as indicated

B. Radiation enteritis

1. Etiology

    a. Dose, volume dependent

    b. Vascular damage

    c. Risk increased by diabetes underlying bowel disease

    d. Risk increased by prior abdominal surgery

2. Presentation

    a. Diarrhea, bloody stool

    b. Small bowel obstruction

    c. Fistulization

3. Treatment

    a. For diarrhea:
Low-fat, low-residue, gluten, cow's milk protein, and lactose-free diet

    b. For bleeding:

      i. Rest bowel

      ii. Consider photo or laser coagulation of telang-
iectatic, bleeding vessels.

      iii. Consider temporary colostomy.

      iv. Removal of bleeding segment of bowel is last resort.

    c. For small bowel obstruction:

      i. Complete bowel rest

      ii. Surgical bypass

    d. For fistulization:

      i. Rule out tumor recurrence

      ii. Surgical repair

C. Chronic radiation cystitis

  1. Prevention

    Treat with full bladder, if possible, to minimize volume of bladder wall treated.

  2. Presentation

    Chronic radiation cystitis is an infrequent late complication secondary to telangiectasia of blood vessels and can cause hemorrhagic cystitis with dysuria and frequency; at cystoscopy, telangiectatic mucosa is found.

  3. Treatment

    a. Hydrate to ensure good urine flow and observe, to be certain, the outlet is not obstructed.

    b. Conservative management: acidify the urine with cranberry juice or vitamin C until the pH is <6.

    c. Hyperbaric oxygen therapy may be considered.

    d. Installation of formalin or acetylcysteine solutions.

    e. Cystectomy is the last resort.

Bibliography

Bhatia S, Robison LL, Oberlin O, et al. Breast cancer and other second neoplasms after childhood Hodgkin's disease. *N Engl J Med* 334:745–94, 1996.

Budtz-Jorgensen E. Etiology, pathogenesis, therapy and prophylaxis of oral yeast infections. *Acta Odontol Scand* 48:61–69, 1990.

Green DM. *Long-Term Complications of Therapy for Cancer in Childhood and Adolescence.* Baltimore: Johns Hopkins University Press, 1989.

Haie-Meder C, Mlike-Cabanne N, Michel G, Briot E, et al. Radiotherapy after ovarian transposition: ovarian function and fertility preservation. *Int J Radiation Oncology Biol Phys* 25:419–24, 1993.

Horning SJ, Adhikari A, Rizk N, et al. Effect of treatment for Hodgkin's disease on pulmonary function: results of a prospective study. *J Clin Oncology* 12:297–305, 1994.

Late effects of cancer treatment. In Halperin EC, Constine LS, Tarbell NJ, Kun LE, eds., *Pediatric Radiation Oncology*, 2nd ed. New York: Raven Press, 1994.

Littley MD, Shalet SM, Beardwell CG. Radiation and the hypothalamic pituitary axis. In Gutin PH, Leibel SA, Sheline GE, eds., *Radiation Injury to the Nervous System*. New York: Raven Press, 1991.

Mulhern RK, Ochs J, Jun LE. Changes in intellect associated with cranial radiation therapy. In Gutin PH, Leibel SA, Sheline GE, eds., *Radiation Injury to the Nervous System*. New York: Raven Press, 1991.

Parson JT, Bova FJ, Fitzgerald CR, et al. Tolerance of the visual apparatus to conventional therapeutic irradiation. In Gutin PH, Leibel SA, Sheline GE, eds., *Radiation Injury to the Nervous System*. New York: Raven Press, 1991.

Sher ME, Bauer J. Radiation induced enteropathy. *Am J Gastroenterol* 85:121–28, 1990.

Simon AR, Roberts MW. Management of oral complications associated with cancer therapy in pediatric patients. *ASDC J Dent Child* 58:384–89, 1991.

10

Chemotherapy-induced Nausea and Vomiting

Donna L. Betcher, R.N., M.S.N., CPNP, Dana Bond, R.N., M.N., CPNP, Kevin Graner, R.Ph., and Alan Lorenzen, Pharm.D., BCOP

Nausea and vomiting associated with cancer treatment remain important concerns for patients and medical personnel. Although new drugs have been developed which have improved the quality of life for many patients, nausea and vomiting remain a major problem for some patients.

The management of nausea and vomiting is complicated by the complex sequence of visceral and somatic events coordinated by a vomiting center in the medulla. The vomiting center may be stimulated through drugs, pathologic conditions, or radiation. Cortical stimulation can be affected by psychic factors such as unpleasant scenes or odors. Motion, nausea, and gastrointestinal irritation can also contribute to this complex problem.

Poor control of nausea and vomiting can lead to dehydration, electrolyte abnormalities, and the need for hospital admission to correct these problems.

I. TYPES OF NAUSEA AND VOMITING ASSOCIATED WITH CHEMOTHERAPY

A. Anticipatory nausea and vomiting
   1. Usually defined as nausea and vomiting occurring prior to the administration of chemotherapy agents. It may occur during or after the administration of the chemotherapy as well but usually before the average onset of emesis. May occur in patients who experienced poor control of acute or delayed nausea and vomiting in initial or prior chemotherapy cycles.

2. Nausea and vomiting is a conditioned response where the hospital or clinic environment, medical personnel, or other treatment related visual, auditory, or olfactory cues trigger the onset of emesis.
3. Anticipatory nausea and vomiting is usually unresponsive to antiemetic agents for the treatment of acute or delayed nausea. Behavior modification may be useful in preventing anticipatory nausea and vomiting.
4. Some factors may predispose the patient to anticipatory nausea and vomiting, including a history of motion sickness. Efforts should be directed at preventing nausea and vomiting by administering the most effective antiemetics with the initial course of emesis-producing chemotherapy.

B. Acute nausea and vomiting.
1. Nausea and vomiting that occurs within the first 24 hours after administration of chemotherapy; combination chemotherapy usually causes an increase in acute nausea and vomiting.
2. The pathophysiology appears different from that which causes delayed nausea and vomiting.

C. Delayed nausea and vomiting.
1. Begins at least 24 hours after administration of cancer chemotherapy; the timing is arbitrary and may occur earlier in some patients.
2. It is more likely to occur when the stimulus for emesis is strong and/or acute vomiting is poorly controlled.

D. Breakthrough nausea and vomiting.
1. Occurs despite preventive therapy.
2. Requires the use of rescue therapy.

E. Radiation therapy induced nausea and vomiting.
1. Nausea and vomiting caused by radiation therapy varies with the treatment administered.
2. The primary factors to consider include the site of radiation, the dose, the dose rate and field size.
3. Patients more commonly experience nausea and vomiting when the gastrointestinal (GI) tract is target of radiation therapy or when patients receive total body irradiation.

4. The risk of nausea and vomiting can be reduced by not scheduling chemotherapy concurrently with radiation therapy or by utilizing a fractionated radiation schedule.

5. The onset, peak and duration of nausea and vomiting will vary for patients undergoing radiation therapy and the antiemetic regimens need to be individualized for optimal control.

II. CONSIDERATIONS WHEN PRESCRIBING ANTIEMETICS

A. Emetogenic potential of the chemotherapy agent

1. The extent of nausea and vomiting caused by the chemotherapeutic agent depends on the drug's inherent emetogenic properties as well as the dose and schedule of administration.

2. The emetogenic potential of chemotherapy drugs can be rated as very high, high, moderate, mild, or very mild. These are listed in Table 10.1.

3. Emetogenicity rating is based on the percentage of patients who will vomit if not premedicated.

4. Combination chemotherapy is usually more emetogenic than single agents.

5. Emetogenicity is dose related (e.g., stem cell transplant conditioning regimens are more emetogenic than standard doses).

6. IV boluses and short infusions are more emetogenic than continuous infusions (peak effect).

B. Emetogenic agent and dose schedule selection.

1. The severity and frequency of nausea and vomiting varies with the agent administered. By understanding the onset and duration of nausea and vomiting from single agent or combination chemotherapy an effective antiemetic regimen can be developed.

2. Table 10.2 lists the onset of emesis and the duration of emesis for some commonly used chemotherapeutic agents, adapted from American Society of Health-System Pharmacists (ASHP) guidelines.

3. The selection and dose schedule of antiemetic agents that prevent acute and delayed nausea and vomiting is essential in limiting the potential adverse effects of chemotherapy administration.

Table 10.1.

Emetogenicity of Chemotherapeutic Agents

Level 1: Very Mild (less than a 10% frequency)
  Bleomycin
  Busulfan (oral, <4 mg/kg/day)
  Chlorambucil (oral)
  Corticosteroids
  Fludarabine
  Hydroxyurea
  Interferon
  Melphalan (oral)
  Mercaptopurine
  Methotrexate ($\leq$50 mg/m^2)
  Thioguanine (oral)
  Vinblastine
  Vincristine
Level 2: Mild (10–30% frequency)
  Asparaginase
  Cytarabine (<1 g/m^2)
  Docetaxel
  Doxorubicin hydrochloride (<20 mg/m^2)
  Etoposide
  Gemcitabine
  Methotrexate (>50 mg/m^2; <250 mg/m^2)
  Mitomycin
  Thiotepa
  Topotecan
Level 3: Moderate (30–60% frequency)
  Cyclophosphamide (IV, $\leq$750 mg/m^2)
  Dactinomycin ($\leq$1.5 mg/m^2)
  Doxorubicin hydrochloride (20–60 mg/m^2)
  Idarubicin
  Ifosfamide
  Methotrexate (250–1,000 mg/m^2)
  Mitoxantrone ($\leq$15 mg/m^2)
Level 4: High (60–90% frequency)
  Carboplatin
  Carmustine (<250 mg/m^2)
  Cisplatin (<50 mg/m^2)
  Cyclophosphamide (>750 mg/m^2 to $\leq$1,500 mg/m^2)
  Cytarabine ($\geq$1 g/m^2)
  Dactinomycin (>1.5 mg/m^2)
  Doxorubicin hydrochloride (>60 mg/m^2)
  Irinotecan
  Melphalan (IV)
  Methotrexate ($\geq$1,000 mg/m^2)
  Procarbazine (oral)
Level 5: Very High (more than a 90% frequency)
  Carmustine (>250 mg/m^2)
  Cisplatin ($\geq$50 mg/m^2)
  Cyclophosphamide (>1,500 mg/m^2)
  Dacarbazine ($\geq$500 mg/m^2)
  Lomustine (>60 mg/m^2)
  Mechlorethamine

Source: Adapted from American Society of Health-System Pharmacists, 1999.

Table 10.2.
Onset and Duration of Emesis

Agent	Onset of Emesis (hr)	Duration of Emesis (hr)
Asparaginase or Pegasparagase	1–3	N.A.
Bleomycin	3–6	N.A.
Busulfan	N.A.	N.A.
Carboplatin (200–400 mg/m^2)	2–6	1–48
Carmustine	2–6	4–24
Chlorambucil (oral)	48–72	N.A.
Cisplatin	1–6	>24
Corticosteroids	N.A.	N.A.
Cyclophosphamide	6–12	6–36
Cytarabine (>1000 mg/m^2)	6–12	3–5
Dacarbazine	2–6	6–24
Dactinomycin	2–6	12–24
Daunorubicin	2–6	<24
Docetaxel	N.A.	N.A.
Doxorubicin	2–6	6–24
Etoposide	3–6	6–12
Fludarabine	N.A.	N.A.
Fluorouracil	3–6	3–6
Gemcitabine	N.A.	N.A.
Hydroxyurea	6–12	N.A.
Idarubicin	N.A.	N.A.
Ifosfamide	3–6	6–12
Interferon-beta	N.A.	N.A.
Irinotecan	2–6	6–12
Lomustine	3–6	6–12
Mechlorethamine	0.5–2	6–24
Melphalan (oral)	6–12	N.A.
Mercaptopurine	4–8	N.A.
Methotrexate	4–12	3–12
Mitomycin	2–6	18–24
Mitoxantrone (<15 mg/m^2)	N.A.	N.A.
Paclitaxel	N.A.	N.A.
Procarbazine (oral)	24–27	Variable
Semustine	3–6	6–12
Teniposide	3–6	6–12
Thioguanine	4–8	N.A.
Thiotepa	6–12	Variable
Vinblastine	4–8	N.A.
Vincristine	4–8	N.A.

N.A. = not available.

C. Patient-related factors
    1. Prior chemotherapy and the degree of previous antiemetic control have an effect on the incidence and severity of nausea/vomiting.
    2. Psychosocial factors such as history of depression predispose to nausea and vomiting.
    3. Susceptibility to motion sickness or morning sickness predisposes to more nausea and vomiting.
    4. Children and adolescents have more nausea and vomiting from chemotherapy than adults do. Children often receive very aggressive chemotherapy and radiation allowing for the high cure rate for many pediatric tumors.

D. Rate and route of administration.
    1. The onset, amount, and interval of chemotherapy induced nausea and vomiting can be affected by the rate of administration of the chemotherapy agent.
    2. The incidence of nausea and vomiting for regimens with continuous infusion administration of the chemotherapy agents usually the greatest in the first 24 hours of treatment and decreases steadily with each subsequent day. Many patients experience little or no nausea and vomiting by the end of multiple day continuous infusion regimen therapy.
    3. Nausea and vomiting occurs more frequently when chemotherapy is administered rapidly than when it is administered slowly.

E. Administration of drugs and the circadian or biological clock.
    1. The administration of some chemotherapeutic agents in accordance with the circadian or biological cycle may affect the severity and incidence of chemotherapy-induced nausea and vomiting.
    2. It has been documented that cisplatin chemotherapy initiated during the early morning causes patients to experience more nausea and vomiting than those who receive the same dose during the evening (after 6 pm).

F. Delayed and anticipatory nausea and vomiting
    1. Behavioral techniques may assist in the prevention and treatment of anticipatory or delayed nausea and vomiting.

2. Some effective interventions that have been used include behavioral modifications, guided imagery, hypnosis, and distraction.

III. PHARMACOLOGIC THERAPY FOR NAUSEA AND VOMITING

Agents used in the prevention of nausea and vomiting include both true antiemetics and ancillary agents. The antiemetics can be classified on the basis of the site of action or pharmacologic class. Antiemetic agents fall into several drug classes. These classes include antihistamines, anticholinergics, benzodiazepines, butyrophenones, cannabinoids, corticosteroids, phenothiazines, 5-HT_3 (serotonin) antagonists, and miscellaneous gastrointestinal drugs. Ancillary agents are used to potentiate the effects of true antiemetics, to treat anxiety, or to induce sleep. The 5-HT_3 antagonists, developed in the 1980s, are the most effective and widely used agents in the prevention of nausea and vomiting in cancer patients. Selection of an appropriate antiemetic regimen should be based on the emetogenic potential of the chemotherapeutic agents used and then modified based on the patient's response. Table 10.3 summarizes some commonly used antiemetics.

A. 5-HT_3 (serotonin) antagonists
   1. The 5-HT_3 antagonists have become the standard antiemetics used for chemotherapy-induced nausea and vomiting. Three agents in this drug class are currently available in the United States: ondansetron (Zofran, GlaxoSmithKline), granisetron (Kytril, Roche), and dolasetron (Anzemet, Aventis). All agents selectively block the serotonin receptors. Concomitant administration with corticosteroids is considered first-line therapy for treatment of acute nausea and vomiting from moderate to very high-risk emetogenic chemotherapy.
   2. 5-HT_3 receptors are found centrally in the chemoreceptor trigger zone and peripherally at vagal nerve terminals in the intestines. It is not known whether the action is mediated centrally, peripherally, or a combination of both actions. Emesis caused by chemotherapy and radiation appears to be associated with the release of serotonin from enterochromaffin cells in the small intestine. Blocking these nerve endings in the intestinal

Table 10.3.

Overview of Antiemetic Agents

Medication	Dosage	Side Effects	Comments
5-HT$_3$ (Serotonin) antagonist			
Ondansetron (Zofran)	Oral	Headache, asthenia, lightheadedness, dizziness, asymptomatic prolongation of electrocardiographic interval, constipation, diarrhea, abdominal pain, ataxia, fever, tremor, transient serum transaminase elevations, sedation, fatigue, warm sensation on IV administration	Oral therapy is considered as efficacious as IV therapy and less costly.
	Child 4–11 years: 4 mg before chemotherapy and every 4 hours for 2 doses		Single-dose regimens preferred over multiple-dose regimens in adult patients.
	Alternative therapy: single 12 mg dose before chemotherapy		Antiemetic of choice for prophylactic therapy in pediatric and adult patients receiving chemotherapy with emetic potential of levels 3 through 5 (in combination with a corticosteroid).
	Child >11 years and adults: 8 mg before chemotherapy and every 4 hours for 2 doses.		
	Alternative therapy: single 24 mg dose before chemotherapy.		
	Intravenous		At equipotent doses, ondansetron, dolasetron, and granisetron are equally efficacious.
	Child >3 years: 0.15 mg/kg/dose before chemotherapy and every 4 hours for 2 doses		Use in combination with corticosteroids for delayed emesis in adult and pediatric patients.
	Adult: 8–12 mg before chemotherapy and every 4 hours for 2 doses		
	Alternative therapy: single 24–32 mg dose before chemotherapy		

Granisetron (Kytril)	Oral *Adult*: 2 mg before chemotherapy and every day or 1 mg twice daily Intravenous *Child >2 years*: 20–40 mcg/kg before chemotherapy *Adult*: 10 mcg/kg before chemotherapy		
Dolasetron (Anzemet)	Oral *Child >2 years*: 1.8 mg/kg before chemotherapy *Adult*: 100–200 mg before chemotherapy Intravenous *Child >2 years*: 1.8 mg/kg before chemotherapy *Adult*: 100 mg or 1.8 mg/kg before chemotherapy		
Corticosteroid Dexamethasone	Oral/Intravenous *Child*: 10 mg/m^2/dose (maximum 20 mg) before chemotherapy and 5 mg/m^2/dose (maximum 10 mg) every 6–12 hours as needed *Adult*: 20 mg before chemotherapy and 10–20 mg every 4–6 hours as needed	Anxiety, insomnia, dyspepsia, hyperglycemia, euphoria, behavioral changes, agitation, perineal burning after rapid IV infusion	Can be used as a single agent in prophylactic therapy for adult and pediatric patients receiving chemotherapy regimens with level 2 emetic potential. Should be added to 5-HT$_3$ receptor antagonist for adults and pediatric patients receiving chemotherapy with emetic potential of levels 3 through 5. Oral therapy as safe and effective as IV therapy.

cont.

Table 10.3.
continued

Medication	Dosage	Side Effects	Comments
Methylprednisolone	Oral/Intravenous *Child*: 0.5–1 mg/kg/dose before chemotherapy and every 4 hours for 2 doses		Use for breakthrough nausea and vomiting in adult and pediatric patients. Use with metoclopramide or 5-HT$_3$ receptor antagonist for delayed emesis in adult patients. Use with lorazepam, 5-HT$_3$ receptor antagonist or chlorpromazine for delayed emesis in pediatric patients.
Benzodiazepine Lorazepam	Oral/Intravenous *Child*: 0.03 mg/kg/dose every 6–8 hours as needed. Maximum 2 mg/dose. *Adult*: 1–2 mg/dose every 6 hours as needed	Sedation, amnesia, behavior changes	May be effective to reduce anticipatory vomiting. Use for breakthrough nausea and vomiting in adult and pediatric patients Use in combination with dexamethasone for delayed emesis in pediatric patients

Class / Drug	Dose	Side effects	Use
Phenothiazine Chlorpromazine	Oral *Child >6 months*: 0.5 mg/kg/dose every 4–6 hours as needed. Maximum dose 40 mg/day if <5 years; 75 mg/day if 5–12 years. Intravenous *Child >6 months*: 0.5 mg/kg/dose every 6–8 hours as needed. Maximum dose 40 mg/day if <5 years; 75 mg/day if 5–12 years.	Sedation, extrapyramidal effects	Use for breakthrough nausea and vomiting in adult and pediatric patients Use in combination with dexamethasone for delayed emesis in pediatric patients
Promethazine Phenergan	Oral/Intravenous *Child*: 0.25 mg–1 mg/kg/dose every 4–6 hours as needed. Maximum 25 mg/dose. *Adult*: 12.5–25 mg/dose every 4 hours as needed	Sedation, extrapyramidal effects	Use for breakthrough nausea and vomiting in adult and pediatric patients Use in combination with dexamethasone for delayed emesis in pediatric patients
Benzamide Metoclopramide	Oral/Intravenous *Adult*: 2 mg/kg/dose IV every 2–4 hours for 2–5 doses. Delayed emesis: 0.5 mg/kg/dose or 30 mg IV every 4–6 hours for 3–5 days.	Sedation, diarrhea, extrapyramidal effects	Use for breakthrough nausea and vomiting in adult patients. Use in combination with dexamethasone in delayed emesis in adult patients.
Butyrophenone Haloperidol	Oral/Intravenous *Adult*: 1–4 mg every 6 hours	Sedation, hypotension, tachycardia, extrapyramidal effects	Use for breakthrough nausea and vomiting in adult patients.
Cannabinoid Dronabinol	Oral *Adult*: 2.5–10 mg every 6 hours	Euphoria, dysphoria, drowsiness, dry mouth, anxiety, irritability, confusion	Use for breakthrough nausea and vomiting in adult patients.

mucosa prevents signals to the chemoreceptor trigger zone in the central nervous system.

3. Each of the 5-HT$_3$ receptor antagonists can be administered parenterally or orally 30 minutes before initiation of emetogenic chemotherapy. The oral dosage forms have been shown to be equivalent to the IV forms. They are generally well tolerated in both adults and children with minimal side effects. They usually do not cause sedation and only rarely cause an extrapyramidal reaction due to lack of interaction with dopamine receptors. Headache and diarrhea are listed as the most common adverse effects. All share a number of characteristics including a wide therapeutic margin, minimal toxicity, a threshold response with little or no dose response, and high cost.

B. Corticosteroids
1. The use of corticosteroids is considered first-line therapy in combination with 5HT$_3$ receptor antagonists for the treatment of acute nausea and vomiting caused by moderate to very high-risk emetogenic chemotherapy.
2. Corticosteroids are also recommended for the treatment of delayed nausea and vomiting. The most commonly used corticosteroid agents for the treatment of nausea and vomiting are dexamethasone and methylprednisolone.
3. The mechanism of antiemetic action is not well known. One theory suggests corticosteroids act as antiemetics by inhibition of cortical input into the vomiting center; others focus on inhibition of prostaglandin synthesis or interference with cellular permeability.
4. The agents can be administered parenterally and orally.
5. The side effects of chronic corticosteroid administration are numerous and preclude the long-term use of these drugs in the management of chronic nausea and vomiting. The most common side effects with short-term administration include central nervous system stimulation (agitation, euphoria, mood changes, and insomnia), transient hyperglycemia, dyspepsia, and perineal burning after rapid IV administration. The agents are well tolerated in the short term.

C. Phenothiazines
1. The phenothiazines were the first agents to be routinely used as antiemetics in oncology. The piperazine phenothiazine derivatives such as thiethylperazine (Torecan) and prochlorperazine (Compazine) are considered more potent antiemetics than aliphatic derivatives such as chlorpromazine (Thorazine) and promethazine (Phenergan). Phenothiazines are used for the prevention and control of severe nausea and vomiting caused by toxins, radiation, cytotoxic agents, and pre- and postoperative nausea and vomiting. These agents have been replaced as first-line therapy by the 5-HT$_3$ receptor antagonists, but serve as useful alternatives and rescue therapy when first-line regimens fail.
2. The mechanism of action for phenothiazines is thought to be mediated by blocking postsynaptic dopamine receptors in the mesolimbic system and increasing dopamine turnover by blockade of the D$_2$ somatodendritic autoreceptor. Dopamine blockade in the medullary chemoreceptor trigger zone accounts for the antiemetic activity. These agents also possess moderate anticholinergic activity that may add to their effectiveness as antiemetics. Blockade of alpha-adrenergic receptors produces sedation, muscle relaxation, and cardiovascular effects such as hypotension, reflex tachycardia, and minor changes in ECG patterns. Phenothiazines usually do not inhibit emesis caused by the action of drugs at the nodose ganglion or by the local actions on the GI tract.
3. Antagonism of dopamine receptors in the chemoreceptor trigger zone also leads to the extrapyramidal side effects such as dystonic reactions, pseudo-Parkinsonism, and akathisia (restlessness). Hypotension is most common with parenteral therapy and is usually short-lived when therapy is discontinued. Phenothiazines can lower the seizure threshold and should be used with caution in patients with seizure disorders. Dystonic reactions may be effectively treated or prevented with antihistamines such as diphenhydramine or with anticholinergics agents such as benztropine. Lorazepam may be a more effective treatment for patients experiencing akathisia.

D. Substituted benzamide
   1. Metoclopramide was the first agent specifically approved for the treatment of chemotherapy-induced vomiting. High IV doses (1–3 mg/kg/dose) are required to prevent nausea and vomiting caused by chemotherapy drug administration. Use of high-dose metoclopramide for moderate to highly emetogenic chemotherapy has essentially been replaced by the 5-HT$_3$ receptor antagonists.
   2. The principal mechanism of action for metoclopramide is complex. It blocks dopamine receptors, specifically, the D$_2$ subtype, in the chemoreceptor trigger zone as do other antiemetics such as the phenothiazines. Antiemetic effects of metoclopramide are the result of central dopamine antagonism and weak 5-HT$_3$ receptor antagonism. High doses are required to produce the inhibition of the 5-HT$_3$ receptors in the GI tract and chemoreceptor trigger zone, especially for highly emetogenic chemotherapy. Metoclopramide is administered orally and parenterally; the high-dose therapy is usually given intravenously.
   3. The adverse effects caused by metoclopramide generally involve the CNS and GI tract and are usually mild, transient, and reversible after discontinuance of the drug. Extrapyramidal reactions may occur and are mediated via blockade of central dopaminergic receptors involved in motor function. Extrapyramidal reactions occur most frequently in children and young adults and after IV administration of high doses required with highly emetogenic chemotherapy. The risk of extrapyramidal side effects is much higher than with the phenothiazines and butyrophenones; diphenhydramine is routinely administered with high-dose metoclopramide to prevent extrapyramidal side effects and continued for 24 hours after the drug is stopped. Parkinsonian symptoms, including tremor, rigidity, and akinesia, can occur and may be associated with usual or excessive doses or with decreased renal function. The incidence of drowsiness, fatigue, and lassitude rises to 70% with dosages of 1–2 mg/kg/dose.

E. Butyrophenones
   1. The butyrophenones have been used as alternative agents for the treatment of nausea and vomiting when

other first-line agents have failed. The two agents most often used are haloperidol (Haldol) and droperidol (Inapsine). These agents have antiemetic activity that is generally less efficacious than the serotonin receptor antagonists and corticosteroids. These agents have more side effects because they are less selective than the $5\text{-}HT_3$ receptor antagonists and should be reserved for patients intolerant of, or refractory to, serotonin receptor antagonists and corticosteroids.

2. The antiemetic activity of the butyrophenones results from blockade of postsynaptic dopamine type 2 receptors (D_2) in the mesolimbic system and increasing dopamine turnover by blockade of the D_2 somatodendritic autoreceptor similar to the phenothiazines. This dopamine blockade occurs in the chemoreceptor trigger zone. These agents also possess weak anticholinergic and alpha-adrenergic receptor blocking effects.

3. The most common adverse effects of butyrophenones include sedation, mild to moderate hypotension, and sinus tachycardia. Droperidol may produce Q-T interval prolongation. Extrapyramidal symptoms can be observed and consist of a dystonic reactions, akathisia, or oculogyric crisis. Extrapyramidal symptoms occur more frequently with haloperidol and appear to result from the blockade of the D_2-receptor. Extrapyramidal symptoms are less common with IV administration than with oral or IM administration. Risk factors include younger age and the use of large dosages. Akathisia may respond to dose reduction or concomitant administration of a benzodiazepine (usually lorazepam). Dystonic reactions may be effectively treated or prevented with antihistamines such as diphenhydramine or with anticholinergics agents such as benztropine.

F. Cannabinoids
1. Dronabinol (Marinol) is indicated for the relief of nausea and vomiting secondary to cancer chemotherapy in patients who have failed to respond to first-line antiemetics. It is also used as an appetite stimulant in cancer and AIDS patients. In acute chemotherapy-induced emesis, there is no group of patients for whom agents of lower therapeutic index are appropriate as first-line antiemetic drugs. Dronabinol is effective

against very mild to moderate chemotherapy and is comparable to the efficacy of the phenothiazines. Dronabinol should be reserved for patients intolerant of or refractory to 5-HT$_3$ receptor antagonists and corticosteroids.

2. Dronabinol, a synthetic form of tetrahydrocannabinol (THC), has a complex mechanism of action that is not well defined. THC has a high affinity to binding sites in the brain and liver, and is believed to inhibit prostaglandin synthesis or cortical input to the vomiting center and interaction with endogenous opiate receptors in the vomiting center. Dronabinol is also an adrenergic blocker; the relationship between prostaglandins or the adrenergic system and control of emesis remains unclear. Peak concentrations of Dronabinol and the main active metabolite occur about 2–3 hours after oral administration. Excretion is mainly fecal via the bile with a half-life of approximately 30 hours.

3. The most common adverse effects of dronabinol include sedation, euphoria or dysphoria, increased appetite, and anticholinergic effects, especially dry mouth. Other possible CNS effects include anxiety, irritability, and confusion. THC increases the heart rate and should be used with caution in patients with cardiac dysfunction. There is a marked reddening of the conjunctivae. THC also produces change in REM sleep patterns; nightmares are rare, but can be observed. Euphoria is not required for successful antiemetic activity. Increased appetite is often a desirable side effect in cancer patients.

G. Benzodiazepines
1. Benzodiazepines, most commonly lorazepam (Ativan), have been widely given for the control of chemotherapy-induced nausea and vomiting, both in combination and as single agents. Benzodiazepines have limited antiemetic activity. Benzodiazepines possess potent anxiolytic, sedative, and amnestic actions making them useful in the prevention and treatment of anticipatory nausea and vomiting. An effective combination includes a 5-HT$_3$ receptor antagonist, a

corticosteroid, and/or a benzodiazepine. Lorazepam should be viewed as an adjunctive agent and is not recommended as a single antiemetic regimen.

2. The mechanism of action of the benzodiazepines is not fully understood. It is believed to inhibit limbic and cortical input into the vomiting center. Anxiolytic and paradoxical CNS stimulatory effects of benzodiazepines may result from release of previously suppressed responses (inhibition). These agents are capable of producing all levels of CNS depression—from mild sedation to hypnosis to coma.

3. The most common adverse effects of benzodiazepines are dose-dependent sedation and amnesia. These agents rarely produce respiratory depression. Most adverse CNS effects are a direct extension of the pharmacologic activity and include drowsiness, ataxia, fatigue, confusion, weakness, dizziness, vertigo, and syncope. Some patients experience behavioral changes, which may include bizarre or abnormal behavior, agitation, panic, hyperexcitability, auditory and visual hallucinations, paranoid ideation, panic, delirium depersonalization, agitation, sleepwalking, and disinhibition manifested as aggression, excessive extroversion, and/or antisocial acts. Decreased inhibition may be similar to that observed with alcohol or other CNS depressants. Physical and psychological dependence is rare with short-term use of benzodiazepines.

H. Antihistamines
1. Antihistamines have been given both as antiemetics and as adjunctive agents to prevent dystonic reactions caused by dopamine antagonists (phenothiazines, metoclopramide, and butyrophenones). Drugs such as diphenhydramine or hydroxyzine are the most commonly used agents. Diphenhydramine can prevent extrapyramidal reactions caused by the dopamine antagonists; the development of 5-HT$_3$ serotonin receptor antagonists as the standard of care has replaced the need for antihistamine therapy. Antihistamines should be viewed as adjunctive agents when dopamine antagonists are used. They are not recommended as single agents emesis control.

2. The mechanism of action of antihistamines is by blocking H_1-receptor sites, preventing the action of histamine on the cell. They do not chemically inactivate or physiologically antagonize histamine; they do not prevent the release of histamine. They do not block the stimulating effect of histamine on gastric acid secretion, which is mediated by H_2-receptors on the parietal cells. The antiemetic and anti-motion sickness actions appear to result from their central anticholinergic and CNS depressant properties in the chemoreceptor trigger zone.

3. The most common adverse effects of antihistamines vary in incidence and severity. CNS effects include sedation (ranging from mild drowsiness to deep sleep), dizziness, and lassitude. Children may experience paradoxical excitement characterized by restlessness, insomnia, tremors, euphoria, delirium, and even seizures. Adverse GI effects include epigastric distress, anorexia, nausea, vomiting, diarrhea, or constipation. Anticholinergic effects include dryness of mouth, nose, and throat; dysuria; urinary retention; visual disturbances; insomnia; tremors; nervousness; irritability; and facial dyskinesia.

IV. NUTRITIONAL SUGGESTIONS TO MINIMIZE NAUSEA AND VOMITING

Regardless of what pharmacologic intervention has been undertaken to prevent nausea and vomiting, reinforce common sense with caregivers regarding food intake.

A. Try foods such as:
   1. Clear liquids, ice chips
   2. Toast, crackers, and pretzels
   3. Sherbet, yogurt
   4. Fruits and vegetables that are soft or bland
   5. Baked/broiled skinless chicken
   6. Angel food cake

B. Avoid foods that are:
   1. Fatty, greasy, or fried
   2. Spicy, hot
   3. Characterized by strong odor

C. Try the following ideas:
   1. Eat small amounts frequently and avoid overeating.
   2. Offer liquids throughout the day except at mealtime.
   3. Serve beverages chilled.
   4. Serve foods at room temperature or cooler; hot foods may add to nausea.
   5. Avoid serving food one to two hours before chemotherapy or radiation treatments.

Bibliography

American Society of Health-System Pharmacists. ASHP Therapeutic Guidelines on the Pharmacologic Management of Nausea and Vomiting in Adult and Pediatric Patients Receiving Chemotherapy or Radiation Therapy or Undergoing Surgery. *Am J Health-Syst Pharm* 56:729–64, 1999.

Hebel S, ed. *Drug Facts and Comparisons*. St. Louis: Facts and Comparisons, 2002.

Hesketh PJ, Kris MG, Grunberg SM, et al. Proposal for classifying acute emetogenicity of cancer, chemotherapy. *J Clin Oncology* 15:103–9, 1997.

Lacy C, ed. *Drug Information Handbook, 2002–2003*. Hudson: Lexicomp, Inc., 2002.

McEvoy G, ed. *American Hospital Formulary Service Drug Information, 2002*. Bethesda: American Society of Health-System Pharmacists, 2002.

Taketomo CK, Hodding JH, Kraus DM. *Pediatric Dosage Handbook*. Ninth Ed. Lexicomp; 2002–2003.

U.S. Department of Health and Human Services, Public Health Service, National Institutes of Health. *Eating hints, recipes, and tips for better nutrition during cancer treatment*. Publication 92-2079, July 1992.

U.S. Department of Health and Human Services, Public Health Service, National Institutes of Health. *Managing your child's eating problems during cancer treatment*. Publication 92-2038, December 1991.

11

The Management
of Pain

William T. Zempsky, M.D., Neil L. Schechter, M.D.,
Arnold J. Altman, M.D., and Steven J. Weisman, M.D.

Most children with cancer will be at risk for significant pain at some time during the course of their illness. Pain may be a product of the disease itself or the result of medical intervention in the form of diagnostic procedures, surgery, chemotherapy, or radiation therapy. An adequate standard of care requires that the clinician systematically assess and effectively manage pain on a routine basis for all children with cancer.

I. THE ETIOLOGY OF PAIN IN CHILDHOOD CANCER

Pain in childhood cancer has a number of possible etiologies. Because the epidemiology of childhood cancer is different from that of adult cancer, the pain experiences of children are different from those of adults. Pain in children with cancer can be from one or more of the following categories: (1) cancer-related, (2) procedure-related, (3) treatment-related, (4) another etiology unrelated to the cancer or its treatment. In children, unlike adults, the majority of cancer pain is caused by procedures and treatments with far less stemming from the disease itself. Many pediatric malignancies are both rapidly progressing and rapidly responding diseases. Thus, the patterns of pain seen in children are very different from those seen in adults in whom chronic pain related to metastasis or neural plexus inflammation predominate. Because most children have more than one type of pain, a pain problem list is often helpful.

    A. Cancer-related pain
        1. Bone pain is most common. It may be generalized as in leukemia or localized to specific sites as in bony metastases.

2. Compression of central or peripheral nervous system structures is also relatively common (i.e., headache from increased intracranial pressure or back pain associated with spinal cord compression).
3. Also, organ invasion or viscus obstruction causes disease-related pain.

B. Procedure-related pain
   1. For many children, this is the most feared aspect of the disease.
   2. Pain ranges in severity from the significant pain associated with bone marrow aspirations and lumbar punctures to the milder pain associated with venipuncture, venous cannulation, and reservoir access.
   3. Anxiety associated with the procedure is sometimes worse than the pain.

C. Treatment-related pain
   1. Chemotherapy-related pain
      a. Mucositis
      b. Peripheral neuropathy
      c. Aseptic necrosis of bone
      d. Steroid-induced myopathy
   2. Radiation therapy-related pain
      a. Mucositis
      b. Radionecrosis
      c. Myelopathy
      d. Brachial/lumbar plexopathies
      e. Peripheral nerve tumors
   3. Postsurgical pain
      a. Acute postoperative pain
      b. Post-thoracotomy pain
      c. Postamputation pain

D. Pain unrelated to cancer
   1. The diagnosis of cancer does not make a child immune to the other pain problems that children experience.
   2. Pain associated with trauma, with traditional childhood illnesses such as otitis and pharyngitis, and common recurrent pain syndromes such as migraine and recurrent abdominal pain syndrome are as likely to occur in children with cancer as in the general population.

II. THE MANAGEMENT OF PAIN ASSOCIATED WITH DIAGNOSTIC PROCEDURES

One of the goals of pain management during pediatric procedures is to make the child comfortable so that the child (and parents) will not dread the subsequent procedures. Thus, success is not a matter of merely restraining the child sufficiently to allow the procedure to be performed. Measures to control pain and anxiety should be considered an integral part of patient management. It is imperative that aggressive pain management be part of the initial diagnostic evaluation since this may help prevent future difficulties with these and other procedures.

A. General principles
 1. In general, avoid unnecessary tests.
 2. Consolidate blood work so that all necessary studies are obtained at the same time; use central lines when possible.

B. Environment and behavioral management
 1. Procedures (e.g., bone marrow aspiration, lumbar puncture) should never be performed in the patient's bed but in an appropriately outfitted treatment room. For less-invasive procedures (port access, venipuncture, IV access), consider the patient's preference.
 2. The environment of the treatment room should be relatively calm, quiet, and child friendly.
 3. The treatment room should have distraction equipment (bubble columns, light wands, etc.), as well as video, and stereo availability.
 4. Child Life personnel should be available to assist with comforting and distracting the child. The Child Life personnel can also assist in training the parents and staff in these techniques.
 5. A parent (or parent substitute) should be encouraged to attend the procedure and to actively participate in assisting the child. This should not demand that the parent restrain the child in any way. Instead, the parent should provide comfort or lead the child in any of a variety of distracting behavioral interventions.
 6. Techniques for behavioral management should be age specific and include stroking, swaddling, or pacifier use

for infants. Older change can be managed using distraction measures, imagery, and hypnosis. (Please see references for a full review of these techniques.)

C. Sedation
1. Standards for administration, monitoring, and documenting sedation as developed by the American Academy of Pediatrics or the American Society of Anesthesiology should be followed (see references).
2. One practitioner with advanced pediatric airway management skills should be entirely devoted to the evaluation and monitoring of the patient undergoing sedation.
3. Patients should be NPO for clear liquids at least 2 hours before the procedure and NPO for solid foods at least 6 hours before the procedure. There must be a time-based record that documents vital signs and levels of sedation at appropriate intervals. All patients should be monitored for pulse oximetry, blood pressure, heart rate, response to verbal command, and adequacy of pulmonary ventilation. ECG monitoring may be indicated for patients undergoing moderate or deep sedation.
4. *Warning:* Before administering a sedative or opioid agent, ensure the immediate availability of oxygen, naloxone, flumazenil, and resuscitative equipment for the maintenance of a patent airway and support of ventilation. Pulse, respiration, blood pressure, and pulse oximeter measurements should be monitored by a person specifically assigned to this task.

D. Pharmacologic intervention
1. Topical anesthetics
   a. Consider topical anesthetics before all invasive procedures. Available topical anesthetics include:
      i. EMLA Cream: combination of lidocaine and prilocaine. Requires 1 hour application time (2 hours even better). Safety has been documented in neonates (reduce amount applied to 1 gm).
      ii. ELAmax Cream: Liposomal lidocaine. 30-minute application time. No neonatal studies currently.

      iii. Numby Stuff: Lidocaine iontophoresis. 10-minute application time. Active drug transport using low-level electric current. Iontophoretic delivery system required.

      iv. Vapocoolant sprays: Effective on contact. Useful for IM injections. Efficacy not proven for intravenous access.

   b. Supplementation of topical anesthesia with infiltration of the deeper tissues with 1% lidocaine is helpful. Buffering of lidocaine with $NaHCO_3$ (9 parts lidocaine: 1 part $NaHCO_3$ USP) may alleviate some of the burning discomfort associated with the lidocaine injection. For procedures performed without EMLA cream, buffered 1% lidocaine should be used for the skin as well as deeper structures. The dose of lidocaine should not exceed 5 mg/kg (0.5 ml/kg).

2. Sedation and analgesia
   a. Age 0–6 months
      i. Consider using a 22g lumbar-puncture needle for both bone marrow aspiration and lumbar puncture.
      ii. All neonates should receive topical and/or local anesthesia before lumbar puncture and bone marrow aspiration.
      iii. The use of opioids and sedatives for sedation in this age group may be difficult. If analgesia is deemed necessary, consider small doses of a single medication. Completion of the procedure under general anesthesia or deep sedation by an anesthesiologist should be considered.
      iv. Sucrose analgesia
         (1) 12–25% sucrose intraorally 1–2 minutes before procedure has been shown to provide analgesia.
         (2) Dose is 1–2 cc of sucrose either instilled with a syringe or applied to a pacifier.
         (3) Use of sucrose does not obviate the need for other methods of sedation and analgesia.

b. Age >6 months
  i. In patients who do not have an established IV route and in whom an IV line would not otherwise be indicated, try the oral route first. In patients who already have an IV in place, use IV sedation.
  ii. Use a combination of a sedative (for anxiety) and an opioid (for analgesia). Sedatives alone are inadequate.
  (1) Sedatives
      Midazolam (Versed) IV solution: 0.5–1.0 mg/kg, orally 20–30 minutes before the procedure or 0.05–0.1 mg/kg, IV, 3–4 minutes before the procedure. When deemed appropriate, midazolam can also be administered rectally at a dose of 0.5 mg/kg 5–10 minutes before the procedure. If IV access is available, half the original dose may be repeated if the child is not adequately sedated when the procedure begins. When using midazolam (or other benzodiazepines), flumazenil (Romazicon), a benzodiazepine reversing agent should be available–the dose of flumazenil is 0.01 mg/kg (max. dose 0.2 mg) by slow IV push.

      AND

  (2) Opioid
      Fentanyl 0.001 mg/kg (1 µg/kg) IV over 1–2 minutes, 3–5 minutes before the procedure. Half the original dose can be repeated if the child is not adequately sedated when the procedure begins.
      OR
      Morphine sulfate 0.15–0.2 mg/kg orally 20–30 minutes before the procedure or 0.05 mg/kg IV over 1–2 minutes, 10 minutes before the procedure.
3. Agents such as ketamine, propofol, and nitrous oxide are used in some institutions for sedation in children undergoing painful procedures. All of these agents may

best be employed by clinicians with advanced pediatric airway skills.

   a.   Ketamine is a dissociative anesthetic agent. Dose of ketamine is 1–1.5 mg/kg IV. Additional doses of ketamine should be titrated in 0.5 mg/kg increments. Side effects include hypersalivation, increased cerebral blood flow, and hallucinations. Recent literature has documented the safety of ketamine for use during procedural sedation. Ketamine may be given with atropine (0.01 mg/kg) to decrease secretions. Use of ketamine with versed has not been shown to decrease the incidence of hallucinations or emergence phenomena.

   b.   Propofol is an IV diisopropylphenol general anesthetic agent, which can easily result in loss of all protective reflexes, markedly decreases systemic vascular resistance, and can cause severe myocardial depression. Propofol is given as a bolus dose 0.5–1.0 mg/kg and then as a continuous infusion of 50–200 mcg/kg/min. Advantages of propofol include rapid onset of action and rapid recovery. Propofol should be used in conjunction with opiates for painful procedures.

   c.   Nitrous oxide is a clear, odorless inhaled anesthetic agent that is analgesic as well as amnestic. It can be administered in oxygen and has been employed for painful procedures. It can induce general anesthesia with loss of protective reflexes. In addition, it must be used with a dedicated scavenging system to prevent environmental contamination. Advantages of nitrous oxide include ease of administration, no need for IV access, rapid onset of action, and rapid recovery.

4.   Consider general anesthesia if efforts at sedation are inadequate or if multiple painful procedures (e.g., bilateral bone marrow aspirations and biopsies) are to be performed.

III. THE MANAGEMENT OF PAIN ASSOCIATED WITH DISEASE

As with all forms of pain, the management of pain in the child with cancer requires a thorough investigation to establish a specific etiology. In the pediatric oncology setting, pain may be due to tumor infiltration or invasion of a number of structures including bone, soft tissues, viscera, and nerves. Pain may also reflect treatment-related toxicity (e.g., vincristine neuropathy) or complications (e.g., infection). Once the mechanism for the pain is identified, more effective specific (e.g., local radiation therapy) and systemic therapy may be offered. The mainstay of the treatment of pain due to refractory tumor is administering analgesic medications. Behavioral interventions should be incorporated into the pain treatment plan of disease-related cancer pain.

A. General principles for the use of analgesics
  1. When feasible, try the oral route first.
  2. The goal should be to provide a level of comfort that the patient finds satisfactory; the patient should be the judge of adequate analgesia.
  3. Tailor the dosages of opioid analgesics to the clinical effect rather than excessively adhering to "standard doses." The "right" dose is that sufficient to achieve relief of pain without undue toxicity.
  4. Effective use of opioids requires careful attention to, and management of, side effects (e.g., pruritus, constipation, dysphoria).
  5. Disease-associated pain may be acute or chronic. For acute pain, rapid dose escalation and weaning is indicated. For chronic pain, long-acting opiates with the availability of breakthrough medications are appropriate.

B. Pharmacologic management
  1. Mild pain
    a. Initial management involves the use of nonopioids
      i. Acetaminophen (Tylenol). Suggested dosage: 10–20 mg/kg PO q4h. Maximum single dose: 1000 mg. Maximum 24 hr cumulative dose 4000 mg.
      ii. Nonsteroidal anti-inflammatory drugs (NSAIDs) (see Table 11.1) The Cox-2 inhibitors cause significantly less gastritis and antiplatelet activity than traditional NSAIDS, which make them the preferred mode of therapy for many oncologic conditions.
    b. If pain is not relieved by the higher range of recommended doses, consider adding opioids or other modalities.

Table 11.1.

Recommended Starting Doses for Analgesic Medications

Medication	Dose (mg/kg)	Route	Schedule
Nonsteroidal anti-inflammatory drugs			
Acetaminophen	10–15	PO	q4h
	15–20	PR	q4h
Choline-magnesium salicylate	10–15	PO	q6–8h
Ibuprofen	5–10	PO	q6h
Rofecoxib	0.6 mg/kg (adult dose 25 mg)	PO	qd
Ketorolac	0.5	IV	q6h
Opioids			
Codeine	0.5–1	PO	q4h
Fentanyl	0.001–0.002 (1–2 μg/kg)	IV	q1–2h
	0.002–0.004 (2–4 μg/kg)	IV	qh continuous infusion
Hydromorphone	0.02	IV	q3–4h
	0.1	PO	q4h
Methadone	0.1	IV	q4h × 2–3 doses; then q8–12h
	0.3–0.7/day	PO	Divide into 3 equal doses
Morphine	0.08–0.1	IV	q2–3h
	0.03–0.05	IV	qh continuous infusion
	0.2–0.3	PO	q4h
Morphine (MS Contin)	0.3–0.6	PO	q12h long acting
Oxycodone	0.15	PO	q4h
Oxycodone (Oxycontin)	0.15	PO	q12h long acting
Adjuvants			
Amitriptyline	0.1–0.2	PO	qday at bedtime; advance to 0.5–2.0 mg/kg/day
Gabapentin	Initial 5 mg/kg or 300 mg	PO	qday at bedtime; advance dose to t.i.d.
Methylphenidate	0.1–0.2	PO	qdose; slowly advance dose as tolerated
Dextroamphetamine	0.1–0.2	PO	qdose; slowly advance dose as tolerated

Note: For all medications, dosages should be modified based on individual circumstances. Many of these agents have not yet received specific approval for infants and younger children. Certain doses are based on extrapolation from adult doses or from unpublished experience. For nonintubated infants aged 4 months or less, reduce initial opioid doses to 1/3–1/4 of the recommended doses. Administer opioids with the patient in a location that permits close observation and immediate intervention. For the management of severe ongoing acute or chronic pain, increase opioid doses until comfort is achieved or until side effects prohibit further dose escalation.

2. Moderate pain
   a. Continue acetaminophen or NSAID, ketorolac may be given for those patients who cannot tolerate oral medication.
   b. If pain is not controlled with the above, add a weak opioid (e.g., codeine). A standard starting dose of codeine is 0.5–1.0 mg/kg PO q4h; this may be increased to 1–2 mg/kg q4h.
   c. If pain is not ameliorated, codeine may be replaced by a stronger agent such as oxycodone (Roxicodone)—0.1–0.15 mg/kg q3-4h, oxycodone/acctaminophen (Percocet), or morphine (see III.B.3.B). A controlled release preparation of oxycodone (OxyContin) or morphine (MSContin) is also available, although the use of these medications in children is limited by their weight and ability to swallow pills. A short-acting opiate should be prescribed in conjunction with long-acting opiate to treat breakthrough pain.
   d. Tylenol with codeine and hydrocodone (Lortab) are both available in liquid form.
3. Severe pain
   a. Continue acetaminophen or NSAID in conjunction with a strong opioid.
   b. Morphine is the first-line opioid in most settings.
      i. The oral dose of 0.3 mg/kg q4h can be started.
      ii. After an appropriate dose of short-acting morphine is determined, timed-release tablets (MSContin) are convenient for patients who can swallow them. The recommended starting dose is 0.3–0.6 mg/kg PO q12h, but should be determined by the total amount of short-acting morphine required to achieve comfort. Methadone is also an effective long-acting agent that has the advantage of being prepared in liquid and tablet forms. A short-acting opiate should be prescribed in conjunction with long-acting opiate to treat breakthrough pain.
      iii. If the oral route is not feasible, continuous IV or SC infusions are effective.
      iv. Continuous morphine infusion (see Table 11.2) is the preferred means of providing analgesia.

Table 11.2.
Pediatric Pain Management with Morphine

	Initial Bolus	Continuous Infusion	Repeat Bolus	How to Increase Patient Comfort		Other Issues
				Increase Continuous Infusion	Discontinue MS Infusion*	
Infants <6 months old (corrected)	0.03 mg/kg over 30 min	0.01–0.02 mg/kg/h	0.02 mg/kg/h over 30 min	Increase rate by 10–15%.	Decrease IV by 50%, add acetaminophen with codeine 0.2–0.4 mg/kg.	1. Naloxone at bedside with syringe and needle. Respiratory depression/arrest dose 0.1 mg/kg. 2. Vital signs (HR, RR, BP) q30 min for first 2 hours, then respiratory rate and sedation scale q2h.
All children >6 months old (corrected age)	0.08–0.1 mg/kg over 30 min	0.04–0.05 mg/kg/h	0.05 mg/kg over 30 min	Increase rate by 10–15%.	Decrease IV by 50%, add acetaminophen with codeine 0.5–1.0 mg/kg PO q4h or morphine 0.2 mg/kg PO q4h.	3. If bolus given or rate increased, vital signs q30 min × 4. 4. IV access at all times. 5. Pulse oximeter is recommended, especially in children under 6 months (corrected age). 6. Bag, mask 0₂ set-up, and tubing should be readily available on the floor.

*Usually 24 to 72 hours postop, begin weaning IV medications and begin PO medications.

Note that Table 11.2 describes a "bolus/ raised rate" method for infants younger than 6 months (corrected age) and for all children over 6 months. This "bolus/raised rate," increasing the rate by 10–15%, can be repeated every 1–2 hours until the pain is relieved. Each time the dose is increased, pain assessments and vital signs should be done every 30 minutes for 2 hours, followed by a return to assessments every 2 hours.

v. Patient-controlled analgesia (PCA) is available for age-appropriate children. Although its use has been described in children as young as 5 years of age, most children should be 7–8 years of age to be able to cognitively understand the mechanism of action of PCA.

It can be used with a background continuous infusion. PCA is often started at a dose of 0.01–0.02 mg/kg q6-10 minutes with or without a basal infusion at 0.01–0.02 mg/kg/h. Consultation with anesthesiology or a pain service may be required.

vi. To change opioids: If changing between short half-life opioids (i.e., morphine to hydromorphone), start new opioid at 50% of equianalgesic dose. Titrate to desired effect. If changing from short to long half-life opioid (i.e., morphine to methadone), start at 25% of equianalgesic dose and titrate to desired effect.

vii. It is necessary to taper opioids for any patient taking them for over 1 week. Decrease dose by 50% × 2 days; then taper by 25% q2 days. Opioid may be stopped when dose is equianalgesic to an oral morphine dose of 0.3 mg/kg/day (for patient <50 kg) or 15 mg/day (for patient >50 kg). Methadone is useful to wean patients on high-dose opioids.

c. Transdermal fentanyl

i. This route allows for the continuous administration of fentanyl at one of four different dosing strengths (25–50–75–100 mcg/h). Steady state is reached 8–12 hours after the patch is applied.

   ii. Because this patch comes in only four sizes, it has limited applicability to children who are opiate naivé, as they would receive excessive opiate, even with the smallest patch. Its use is not recommended for children under 12 years of age.

   iii. The transdermal patch may be considered for patients with relatively stable pain who are unable to take medications by the oral route and in whom IV access is limited.

  d. Transmucosal fentanyl (Actiq)

   i. Transmucosal fentanyl is effective for breakthrough pain in adult subjects.

   ii. Starting dose is 200 mcg, dose can be titrated upward depending on effect.

   iii. There are limited data on the use of transmucosal fentanyl for this purpose in children.

4. Neuropathic pain (e.g., "phantom limb," vincristine neuropathy, herpes zoster, burning sensation)

  a. Tricyclic antidepressants

   i. Tricyclics have several uses in the management of children's cancer pain. Although classically regarded as best for pain of a burning character, tricyclics are regarded by many as the agent of first choice for most forms of persistent or neuropathic pain.

   ii. Tricyclics are typically begun with a very small single daily dose an hour before bedtime with Amitriptyline (Elavil) being the most commonly used. Starting dosages for amitriptyline and imipramine are 0.1–0.2 mg/kg at bedtime. The dose may be increased by 50% every 2–3 days up to 0.5–2.5 mg/kg at bedtime, although many patients will not tolerate the larger doses. Common side effects include dry mouth and somnolence; less common side effects, seen mostly with larger doses, are disorientation, urinary retention, constipation, and tachyarrhythmia. Hypertension may develop in patients with neuroblastoma. These side effects can frequently be managed by a temporary reduction and then a gradual increase in the dosage.

   iii. Use great caution in prescribing tricyclics to patients who have a history of palpitations or tachyarrhythmia or who have an increased risk for cardiac dysfunction (e.g., after the administration of anthracyclines). ECGs should be obtained at baseline and during ongoing therapy to assess the effects of the medication.

  b. Anticonvulsants

Anticonvulsants are used for neuropathic pain, especially when it is of a shooting or stabbing character. Gabapentin (Neurontin) has become the predominant anticonvulsant used for neuropathic pain (see Table 11.1). Predominant side effects with gabapentin include somnolence (especially at initiation of therapy) and increased appetite. Other new anticonvulsants used in neuropathic pain include topiramate (Topomax), oxcarbazepine (Trileptal), and levetiracetam (Keppra).

5. Specific pain problems
  a. Mucositis
    i. Mucositis can often cause severe pain; therapy should include both local and systemic measures.
    ii. Local measures
      (1) MagicMouthwash (Benadryl/Maalox ± Lidocaine)
      (2) Sulcrafate
      (3) Capsaicin: active ingredient in chili peppers
Burning sensation results in desensitization
Available as a gum
      (4) Gelclair
  b. Phantom limb pain
    i. Symptoms can last for months after amputation.
    ii. Use of regional anesthesia yields mixed results.
    iii. Use epidural acutely.
    iv. Opiates plus anticonvulsants chronically.

IV. THE MANAGEMENT OF POSTOPERATIVE PAIN

The goal of postoperative pain management is to keep the patient as comfortable as possible without compromising his or her safety. In addition to being more humane, adequate pain management will decrease hypoventilation and atelectasis secondary to splinting, allow increased patient mobility in the early postoperative period, and improve the patient's general state of well being, which may have important immunologic and healing consequences.

A.   General principles
  1.   The responsibility for patient comfort should be shared by the medical, surgical, and nursing services.
  2.   Pain assessment is critical for good pain management; scheduled assessments including bedside charting should be incorporated into the pain plan.
  3.   Pharmacologic management should use PO or IV routes; avoid IM injections. Analgesic administration should be done on a fixed, not PRN, schedule.
  4.   Behavioral approaches (distraction, hypnosis, self-control techniques) have demonstrated efficacy and should be incorporated into the care plan in conjunction with the Child Life therapist and/or psychological providers.

B.   Pharmacologic management
  Use of wound infiltration with local anesthetics by the surgeon, regional nerve blocks, or use of indwelling catheters for postoperative pain management are highly recommended. Epidural and regional plexus catheters can provide extremely effective and safe postoperative analgesia.
  1.   Mild pain: Examples might include the discomfort seen after placement of a central line or a simple biopsy of a superficial structure (lymph node).
    a.   Oral: Acetaminophen with codeine (1 mg/kg codeine) or nonsteroidal anti-inflammatory drug (see Table 11.1).
    b.   Parenteral: Morphine sulfate (0.08–0.1 mg/kg IV) every 2–3 hours ± ketorolac (0.5 mg/kg) every 6 hours.
  2.   Moderate and/or severe pain: Examples might include appendectomy, incision and drainage of a deep

abscess, complex orthopedic procedure, exploratory laparotomy, or thoracotomy.

a. Regional analgesia: Epidural or plexus catheters can be used to infuse local anesthetics with or without opioids. In some circumstances, the anesthesiologist may use a single-shot technique such as a single-shot caudal injection of bupivacaine and morphine. Alternatively, a single-shot axillary block may be placed. More commonly, an epidural catheter can be placed to permit bolus and continuous infusion delivery of low-dose solutions of opioids with or without local anesthetics.

b. Parenteral analgesia
   i.   Morphine infusions: (See Table 11.2).
   ii. Patient-controlled analgesia: (See section III.B.3.c.IV).
   iii. All patients should be carefully reassessed for pain on a regular basis to determine the need for continued infusion or PCA therapy. In general, with major surgical procedures, children will benefit from analgesia for at least 48–72 hours.
   iv. Discontinuing continuous morphine:
        (1) Timing: Usually 48–72 hours after surgery, if the patient is comfortable.
        (2) Transition to oral medications: Discontinue the infusion 30–60 minutes after an oral dose of acetaminophen with codeine or oral morphine.
        (3) If pain relief is inadequate on oral analgesics, resume IV therapy at previous doses.
        (4) Oral analgesics should be scheduled around the clock or in a "reverse PRN" fashion (the nurse checks and offers the analgesic for pain every 3–4 hours).
   v.   Monitoring: Bedside charting of pain assessments should be recorded along with respiratory rate and an assessment of the level of sedation every 2 hours. Many clinicians will employ continuous pulse oximetry for monitoring during continuous opioid therapy.

3. Safety guidelines for postoperative pain management:
   a. Naloxone (Narcan) should be readily available.
   b. Oxygen should be available at the bedside.
   c. Respiratory depression: (See sections V.B and C).
   d. All continuous infusions should be delivered by infusion pump. Specific, easy-to-program pain management pumps are available from several manufacturers.
   e. Infants less than 6 months old (corrected postgestational age) should be in a location that permits close observation and monitoring.
   f. For infants less than 4 months old, reduce opioid doses to 1/3 to 1/4 of the usual childhood doses.

V. THE MANAGEMENT OF OPIOID SIDE EFFECTS

A. Somnolence
   1. Reduce opioid doses to the minimum required to produce adequate analgesia.
   2. Stimulants are useful in situations in which opioid administration is limited by somnolence.
      a. Both dextroamphetamine and methylphenidate have been shown to provide additive analgesia with a reduction in somnolence in patients with cancer. They are generally prescribed b.i.d., at morning and noon, in starting doses of 0.1–0.2 mg/kg. Evening dosing should be avoided because it may lead to sleep disturbances. After prolonged dosing, these medications should be tapered gradually to avoid withdrawal reactions.
      b. Caffeine has been advocated for use for analgesia in a similar fashion and is a component of many proprietary headache remedies.
   3. If somnolence persists and is not desired by the patient, consider the use of regional analgesic techniques.

B. Respiratory depression
   Depression of respiration usually correlates reliably with the level of sedation, except in the very young infant.
   1. Constant monitoring of the patient is essential. When the patient is sleeping or left unattended, pulse oximetry can be used.

2. For respiratory depression, full pharmacologic reversal is often not necessary. Administration of oxygen and reduction of the next dose of opioid may be all that is necessary. If the respiratory depression is more severe, support the airway, provide supplemental oxygen, and administer naloxone to the point of reversal of respiratory slowing without compromising pain relief. It is important to recognize that rapid infusion of a large dose of naloxone can precipitate withdrawal with the dramatic onset of severe pain and sympathetic instability in the child. Therefore, the naloxone dose should be 0.5–1 mcg/kg every 2 minutes titrated to effect, provided that the patient is maintaining adequate oxygenation and ventilation.

C. Respiratory arrest
   1. Begin ventilatory assistance and call for help (Code).
   2. Administer naloxone, 0.1 mg/kg IV, IM, or SC for infants and children <5 yr (or <20 kg). Older children (or those >20 kg) may be given 2 mg. Repeat in 1–5 minutes for 2 or 3 doses until effective. This can be repeated every hour as needed.
   3. Deliver 100% oxygen, support the airway, and closely monitor the patient. The effect of naloxone may not outlast the effect of the opioid and the patient may again become somnolent or apneic.

D. Nausea and vomiting
   Exclude primary conditions (e.g., bowel obstruction).
   1. Antiemetics currently used for opioid-induced nausea and vomiting are: Metaclopramide (Reglan), 0.2 mg/kg orally or 0.1 mg/kg IV q6h and ondansetron (Zofran), 0.1 mg/kg up to 4 mg q6h, naloxone, 0.001 mg/kg; if effective, can be administered by continuous infusion [see section IVE]).
   2. Phenothiazines and butyrophenones are indicated in the treatment of nausea and vomiting. With the exception of methotrimeprazine (Levoprome), the neuroleptics provide little or no analgesia. They sedate and may mask the outward expression of pain more than they diminish the intensity of pain experienced. Commonly used agents include: chlorpromazine (Thorazine), 0.15–0.5 mg/kg IV or PO q6h, perphenazine (Trilafon),

0.05–0.1 mg/kg IV or 0.1 mg/kg PO q6h, promethazine (Phenergan), 0.25 mg/kg q6h, droperidol, 0.01 mg/kg up to 0.625 mg q4-6h.

3. The doses of these agents for the treatment of opioid-induced nausea appear to be much smaller ($^1/_5$-$^1/_2$×) than those required to treat chemotherapy-induced nausea.

E. Pruritus
Administer diphenhydramine (Benadryl) 0.5–1.0 mg/kg IV or PO q4-6h or naloxone 0.001 mg/kg q1-2 min for 2 or 3 doses until the effect is obtained. Naloxone can be successfully administered by continuous infusion after these doses. Infusions at 0.0005–0.001 mg/kg/h can successfully reverse the peripheral annoying side effects of the opioids without causing reversal of the analgesic effects. In addition, trying other opioids such as dilaudid or fentanyl, which does not release histamine, can be helpful with itching.

F. Urinary retention
Apply warm compresses over the bladder. The patient should ambulate, if possible. Patients who are adequately hydrated and have not voided in 8 hours and/or who begin to experience discomfort must be straight catheterized. Some of these patients will require the placement of a urinary drainage catheter. A continuous infusion of naloxone, or the use of an agonist-antagonist nalbuphine (0.1 mg/kg), can be tried in this situation.

G. Constipation
Patients who receive opioids for more than 24 hours should be started on a stool softener such as Kondremul (1–2 teaspoons at night or b.i.d.), Senekot (1 pill or 1 teaspoon of granules) at bedtime, or Peri-Colace Syrup (1–3 teaspoons) at bedtime.

VI. NURSING RESPONSIBILITIES

A. General postoperative care
1. During the first 24–48 hours after surgery, it is very important to maintain a constant level of analgesia to provide pain relief for the patient. If a continuous infusion is not ordered, the nurse must make a special effort to offer and provide PRN pain medications.

Assessments of the pain level should be done at least every 4 hours and medications administered accordingly. Offering pain medications "around the clock" is often the best way to provide adequate pain relief.

2. Use nonpharmacologic interventions as appropriate. (If there is a concern whether an intervention is safe for a specific patient, check the patient's orders and, if there is still doubt, check with the physician.)

   a. Reposition the patient
   b. Use basic comfort measures (e.g., blankets, closed curtains).
   c. Relieve thirst from dry mouth.
   d. Use distraction (e.g., television, movies, music).
   e. Use parents, Child Life, and volunteers to comfort the patient.

3. If all of the above have been used and the patient is still in pain, then notify the appropriate physician.

B. Continuous infusion of opioids

   1. The respiratory rate and level of sedation will be assessed and documented every half hour when the infusion begins. If the assessments are stable after the 2 hours, then the respiratory rate and the level of sedation will be assessed every 2 hours. The acceptable respiratory rate for a given patient must be determined on an individual basis reflecting the patient's age and clinical status.

   2. If the rate of opioid is increased or a bolus is given, the respiratory rate and level of sedation (see below) will be assessed and documented every half hour for 2 hours. If the assessments are stable after that time, the respiratory rate and level of sedation will be assessed every 2 hours.

   3. Sedation scale
   0 = none; the patient is alert.
   1 = mild; the patient is occasionally drowsy but easy to arouse.
   2 = moderate the patient is frequently drowsy and sleeping but still easy to arouse.
   3 = severe; the patient is somnolent and difficult to arouse.

   4. If the patient's sedation level is 3, turn off morphine drip (maintain IV access); stimulate and encourage the

patient to breathe deeply; stay with the patient and have another nurse call the physician.

5. If the rate of opioid is decreased, the respiratory rate and level of sedation will continue to be assessed and documented every 2 hours, but pain assessment should be increased to ensure that the patient is still receiving enough analgesic.

6. If all of the above have been used and the patient is still in pain, notify the appropriate physician.

Bibliography

American Academy of Pediatrics, Committee on Drugs. Emergency drug doses for doses for infants and children and naloxone use in newborns; clarification. *Pediatrics* 83:803, 1989.

American Academy of Pediatrics, Committee on Drugs. Guidelines for monitoring and management of pediatric patients during and after sedation for diagnostic and therapeutic procedures. *Pediatrics* 89:1110–15, 1992.

American Academy of Pediatrics, Committee on Drugs. Guidelines for monitoring and management of pediatric patients during and after sedation for diagnostic and therapeutic procedures: Addendum. *Pediatrics* 110:836–38, 2002.

American Society of Anesthesiology, Task Force on Sedation and Analgesia by Non-Anesthesiologists. Practice guidelines for sedation and analgesia by non-anesthesiologists. *Anesthesiology* 96:1004–17, 2002.

Berde C, et al. Report of the Subcommittee on Disease-Related Pain in Childhood Cancer. *Pediatrics* 86:1990 (suppl).

Collins JJ, Weisman SJ. Management of pain in childhood cancer. In Schechter NL, Berde CB, Yaster M, eds., *Pain in Infants, Children, and Adolescents*, 2nd ed. Philadelphia: Lippincott Williams & Wilkins, 2003, pp. 517–38.

Committee on Palliative and End of Life Care for Children and their Families, Institute of Medicine. *When Children Die: Improving Palliative and End of Life Care for Children and Their Families*. Washington, D.C.: National Academies Press, 2003.

Goldman A, Frager G, Pomietto M. Pain and palliative care. In Schechter NL, Berde CB, Yaster M, eds., *Pain in Infants, Children, and Adolescents*, 2nd ed. Philadelphia: Lippincott Williams & Wilkins, 2003, pp. 539–62.

World Health Organization. *Cancer Pain Relief: With a Guide to Opioid Availability*, 2nd ed. Geneva: WHO, 1996.

World Health Organization. *Cancer Pain Relief and Palliative Care in Children*. Geneva: WHO, 1998.

12

Oncologic Emergencies

Edythe A. Albano, M.D., and Eric Sandler, M.D.

Pediatric oncologic emergencies arise as a result of space-occupying lesions, metabolic or hormonal derangements, and cytopenias. They can be the presenting feature of a new malignancy or can arise during treatment or recurrence. All of these conditions are reversible if recognized and treated appropriately in a timely manner.

I. METABOLIC COMPLICATIONS

A. Tumor lysis syndrome
   1. Overview
      a. Acute tumor lysis syndrome is a consequence of the rapid release of intracellular metabolites (uric acid, potassium, and phosphorus) in quantities that exceed the excretory capacity of the kidneys.
      b. Renal failure, hyperkalemia, and hypocalcemia (secondary to hyperphosphatemia) are common complications.
   2. Etiology
      a. Tumor lysis syndrome is seen in tumors with a high growth fraction and that are exquisitely sensitive to chemotherapy.
      b. Burkitt's lymphoma and T cell leukemia-lymphoma syndrome and/or hyperleukocytosis are the most common causes. Evidence for tumor lysis can be found before beginning therapy (because of spontaneous tumor degradation) and from 1–5 days after the initiation of treatment.
   3. Evaluation
      a. Perform repeated physical examinations.

221

b. Measure urine output, blood pressure, and weight 1–3 times daily.
c. Monitor serum creatinine, uric acid, calcium, phosphate, sodium, and potassium every 4–8 hours until the risk is over.
d. If patient remains oliguric, ultrasound study of the kidney may be useful to rule out tumor infiltration or obstructive uropathy.

4. Prevention
a. Urine output should be maintained at 5 ml/kg/h before initiating chemotherapy and at 3 ml/kg/h after chemotherapy is begun, and verified every 2–4 hours; if urine output falls, institute corrective measures promptly (more fluids and/or diuretics).
b. Assure adequate hydration by replacing calculated deficits; intravenous (IV) fluid (e.g., D5 ¼ NS) at *3000 ml/m²/day (125 ml/m²/h); may need to increase fluids further to maintain urine output. Do not administer IV potassium until the tumor lysis is controlled.*
c. Diuresis with lasix (0.5 to 1 mg/kg/dose IV) or mannitol as 25% solution (provided circulating fluid volume and renal function are adequate); 1 gm/kg IV initially over 5–10 minutes followed by 0.5 gm/kg q4-6h as necessary to achieve desired urine volume.
d. Allopurinol 300 mg/m²/day PO divided t.i.d. May be given intravenously (200 mg/m²/day) if necessary.
e. Alkalinization of urine pH between 6.5 and 7.5 with $NaHCO_3$ (120 meq/m²/day) IV will increase the solubility of urates; pH >7.5 should be avoided as it is associated with precipitation of hypoxanthine as well as calcium phosphate crystals.

5. Management
a. Hyperuricemia (>8 mg/dl): An elevated uric acid results from nucleic acid breakdown. Urates can precipitate in the acid environment of the kidney causing renal failure.
    i.   Allopurinol 300 mg/m²/day divided t.i.d. PO.
    ii. IV allopurinol (200 mg/m²/day as a single dose or divided b.i.d., t.i.d., or q.i.d.) is available if patients are unable to take oral medications.

    iii. Recombinant urate oxidase (Rasburicase) (0.15–0.2 mg/kg/day) catalyzes the oxidation of uric acid to allantoin, a highly water-soluble metabolite readily excreted by the kidneys. It can achieve rapid reduction of uric acid level. Rasburicase should be avoided in patients with glucose-6-phosphate dehydrogenase deficiency.

b. Hyperphosphatemia (≥ 6.5 mg/dl): Lymphoblasts have four times the phosphate content of normal lymphocytes. When the calcium-phosphate product exceeds 60, calcium phosphate precipitates in microvasculature and renal tubules. This can lead to renal failure.

    i.   Low-phosphate diet

    ii. Aluminum hydroxide 150 mg/kg/day. Use should be limited to 1–2 days to avoid cumulative aluminum toxicity.

    iii. Urine output maintained at ≥ 3ml/kg/h.

c. Hyperkalemia (>6.0 meq/L): Potassium can be elevated because of tumor lysis or secondary to renal failure. Hyperkalemia leads to ventricular arrhythmias and death.

    i.   No IV potassium until tumor lysis is controlled.

    ii. Calcium administration is the fastest means of reversing the cardiac effects of hyperkalemia. Onset of action is within minutes, but the duration of action is only about a half hour. Administer in life-threatening arrhythmias as calcium chloride 10–30 mg/kg by *slow* IV infusion. (Do not administer in the same line as sodium bicarbonate.)

    iii. Sodium bicarbonate at 1–2 meq/kg IV will drive potassium into the cell. For every increase in 0.1 pH units, potassium decreases about 1 meq/L. Onset of action is within half an hour and duration of activity is for several hours.

    iv. Insulin and glucose administration will also move excess potassium into the cell. Glucose is administered continuously at 0.5 gm/kg/h with insulin 0.1 unit/kg/h. Serum glucose should be monitored closely and infusion rates adjusted appropriately. In an emergency, glucose alone can facilitate potassium entry into the cell (1 ml/kg of D50 in a central line). Onset is within 20–30 minutes and duration of activity lasts several hours.

    v. Kayexalate removes 1 meq potassium/L per gm resin over 24 hours; given as 1 gm/kg/dose orally every 6 hours with sorbitol 50–150cc. This is *not* an emergency intervention. The duration of action depends on the rate of endogenous potassium release.

  d. Hypocalcemia (ionized calcium <1.5 meq/L): This occurs secondary to hyperphosphatemia as a compensatory mechanism to maintain the calcium phosphate product at 60.

    i. For *symptomatic* hypocalcemia, administer 10 mg/kg of calcium chloride in a drip over 1 hour with EKG monitoring.

    ii. Discontinue administration when symptoms resolve.

  e. Dialysis: Indications include fluid overload with congestive heart failure, symptomatic hypocalcemia or hyperphosphatemia, hyperkalemia with QRS interval widening (generally occurs with potassium >6 meq/L), and elevated creatinine with poor urine output.

  f. Institute hyperleukocytosis interventions if appropriate (see section II).

B. Hypercalcemia
  1. Overview
    a. Hypercalcemia, a paraneoplastic syndrome, has been reported in patients with leukemias, lymphomas, rhabdomyosarcoma, neuroblastoma, Ewing sarcoma, Wilms tumor, and rhabdoid tumors of the kidney.
    b. Mechanisms postulated to be the cause for the hypercalcemia are the following.
      i. Production by the tumor of a parathyroid hormone-related protein

Table 12.1.
Signs and Symptoms of Hypercalcemia

Neurologic	Gastrointestinal	Cardiovascular	Genitourinary
Headache	Nausea	Hypertension	Polyuria
Irritability	Vomiting	Bradycardia	Polydipsia
Seizures	Anorexia	Arrhythmia	Nocturia
Lethargy	Constipation		
Hypotonia	Ileus		
Coma	Abdominal pain		

       ii. Production by the tumor of bone-resorbing substances (lymphotoxin and tumor necrosis factor)

      iii. Elevation of 1,25 dihydroxyvitamin D

      iv. Production of parathyroid hormone

  c. All the above cause excess release of calcium from bone into the blood. This results in polyuria and dehydration leading to diminished glomerular filtration with increased renal absorption of calcium, worsening the hypercalcemia.

2. Evaluation

  a. The normal value of calcium corrected for albumin is 9–11 mg/dl (4.5–5.5 mEq/L). Mild hypercalcemia can be defined as 12–14 mg/dl (6–7 mEq/L) and severe hypercalcemia is >15 mg/dl (7.5 mEq/L). Add 0.8 mg/dl to total calcium for every gram per liter reduction of serum albumin.

  b. Non-protein bound ionized calcium is of greater physiologic importance and does not need correction for serum protein.

  c. Signs and symptoms of hypercalcemia are shown in Table 12.1.

3. Management

  a. Mild hypercalcemia

      i. Administer IV hydration with normal saline (3,000 ml/m^2/day) and encourage oral intake. High fluid volume promotes the excretion of calcium, and saline interferes with the reabsorption of calcium in the proximal tubule of the kidney.

          ii. Furosemide 1–2 mg/kg IV t.i.d. or q.i.d. blocks the reabsorption of calcium in the ascending loop of Henle.

          iii. Monitor electrolytes frequently.

          iv. Maintain exercise and movement.

    b. Severe hypercalcemia

          i. Increase IV hydration in gradual stages to 6,000 mL/m^2/d and continue furosemide as above. Patients should be monitored carefully for volume overload and for precipitous falls in serum potassium.

          ii. Administer bisphosphonates such as pamidronate 60 mg IV over 4 hours once for children over 50 kg (dose should not exceed 30 mg if there is renal failure). May repeat in 7 days as necessary. The dosage for smaller children has not been established. Action results in an inhibition of bone resorption.

          iii. For lymphoproliferative disorders, steroids (prednisone 2 mg/kg/day PO), or its equivalent, may decrease serum calcium over several days of use.

          iv. Calcitonin, gallium nitrate, indomethacin, and mithramycin have all been used with some success but should be tried only if the above fails.

          v. Oral or IV phosphates seem to have more toxicity than benefit. They decrease bone resorption and can increase extraosseous bone formation, possibly leading to increased renal toxicity. If they are used, monitor carefully.

          vi. For patients refractory or resistant to other methods of treatment, dialysis, either peritoneal or hemodialysis, can be used.

C. Syndrome of inappropriate antidiuretic hormone (SIADH)

    1. Overview

        Antidiuretic hormone (ADH or arginine vasopressin) causes the resorption of free water at the renal collecting duct; thus, it is an important mechanism in regulating the volume and osmolality of extracellular fluid.

        a. ADH is released from the pituitary gland when osmoreceptors in the hypothalamus detect increased osmolality of the serum.

b. Secretion of ADH also occurs when volume receptors in the left atrium, carotid sinus, and aortic arch detect decreased effective circulating volume.

c. Volume depletion stimulates the secretion of ADH regardless of serum osmolality.

2. Etiology

SIADH results from the release of ADH in the absence of increased serum osmolality or volume depletion. It may occur with the following:

a. Malignancies (e.g., leukemia, lymphoma, Ewing sarcoma, and brain tumor)

b. Drugs (e.g., vIncristine, vinblastine, barbiturates, and opiates). Cyclophosphamide produces an SIADH-like syndrome by acting directly at the kidney tubule to enhance the absorption of free water.

c. Head trauma

d. Infection of the central nervous system (CNS) or lungs

e. Pain and/or stress

f. Surgery

3. Evaluation

The urine is not maximally diluted and has a paradoxically high urinary sodium concentration (>20 mEq/L) despite hyponatremia and low serum osmolality. Volume depletion, nephrotic syndrome, adrenal insufficiency, hypothyroidism, and congestive heart failure are absent.

4. Management

a. Treatment of the underlying disorder

b. Mild disease

   i. Fluid restriction, equaling urine output

   ii. Normal maintenance of Na+ intake

c. Severe hyponatremia (120–125 mEq/L) without life-threatening symptoms

   i. Furosemide 1 mg/kg promotes a free water diuresis.

   ii. Replace urine loss milliliter for milliliter with normal saline.

   iii. Demeclocycline 6.6–13.2 mg/kg divided into 2 doses (maximum 600–1,200/day) inhibits the action of ADH on renal tubules by interfering with the formation and action of cyclic adenosine monophosphate.

    d. Life-threatening neurologic symptoms (convulsion and stupor)
       i. Furosemide 1 mg/kg promotes a free water diuresis.
      ii. To correct sodium to 120 mEq/L, give 200 mL/m^2 of 1.5% NaCl in 6–8 hours, and then more slowly to normal over 24–72 hours.
     iii. It is important to avoid a rapid correction of serum sodium. Hypertonic sodium causes a sodium diuresis and may exacerbate the loss of sodium. Neurologic deterioration and death have occurred with too rapid correction of serum Na+.

D. Hypokalemia
  1. Overview
    a. Normal serum potassium is 3.5 to 5.5 meq/L; EKG changes are seen at <2.5 meq/1.
    b. The principle effects are on cardiac rhythm with symptoms occurring most commonly when the cause is acute.
    c. Patients may develop ileus or muscle weakness.
  2. Etiology
    a. Renal wasting secondary to drugs is the usual etiology in pediatric cancer patients.
    b. Commonly administered agents associated with tubular potassium loss include amphotencin B, antipseudomonal penicillins, aminoglycosides, ifosphamide, cisplatin, loop diuretics, and glucocorticoids.
  3. Evaluation
    a. A semiquantitative assessment of potassium needs per day can be determined by the potassium content of the patient's spot urine and the 24-hour urine output.
    b. Serum magnesium must be assessed as potassium cannot be conserved without adequate magnesium.
  4. Management
    a. Oral therapy is indicated for chronic hypokalemia
      i. Normal potassium requirements:
         Newborn: 2–6 meq/kg/day

Child: 2–3 meq/kg/day
Adult: 40–80 meq/day
ii. Oral supplementation for prevention of hypokalemia during diuretic therapy:
Child: 1–2 meq/kg/day (divided in 2 doses)
Adult: 20–40 meq/day (divided in 2 doses)
iii. Oral replacement therapy of hypokalemia:
Child: 2–5 meq/kg/day (divided into 2–4 doses)
Adult: 40–100 meq/day (divided into 2–4 doses)
b. IV replacement is indicated for an acute fall, particularly below 2.5 meq/L, or if the patient cannot take an oral supplement.
   i. Potassium infusion (for rapid correction)
      (1) May be given over 1–2 hours in concentration of 1 meq KCl/5 ml NS.
      (2) Infusion rate should not exceed 0.5 meq/kg/h (maximum dose 10–15 meq/h).
      (3) EKG monitoring throughout IV potassium replacement is essential.
      (4) Avoid (or minimize) dextrose in infusions as it tends to drive K+ into cells.
   ii. Potassium infusion (for chronic correction)
      (1) Concentrations >40 meq/L administered via peripheral vein are irritating, painful, and can cause phlebitis.
      (2) Concentrations as high as 80–100 meq/L are acceptable in a central line, but must be monitored carefully.
      (3) Avoid (or minimize) dextrose in infusions, as it tends to drive K+ into cells.
c. Potassium-sparing diuretics such as amiloride or aldactone may help conserve potassium.

II. HYPERLEUKOCYTOSIS

A. Overview
Hyperleukocytosis is defined as a total peripheral white blood cell count >100,000/mm^3.
B. Etiology
Hyperleukocytosis occurs in 9–13% of children with acute lymphoblastic leukemia, 5–20% of children with acute

nonlymphoblastic leukemia, and in virtually all children with chronic myelogenous leukemia.

C. Pathogenesis
1. Blood viscosity
   Hyperleukocytosis increases blood viscosity and is associated with aggregation of leukemic cells in the microcirculation.
2. Respiratory failure
   a. Stasis of leukemic blasts in the pulmonary vasculature can cause an oxygen diffusion block.
   b. Release of intracellular contents of leukemic cells in the pulmonary vessels and interstitium can cause diffuse alveolar damage.
   c. This is seen almost exclusively in AML patients.
3. Hemorrhage
   a. Central nervous system, gastrointestinal, pulmonary, and pericardial hemorrhages can occur with devastating results.
   b. Hemorrhage is significantly more common in AML than ALL. The mortality from CNS hemorrhage in AML patients with WBC counts >300,000/mm^3 approaches 60%.
   c. Complicating coagulation defects are particularly common with M3 (acute promyelocytic leukemia) M4 and M5 AML.
   d. Metabolic complications also occur, primarily related to tumor lysis, and are more common with ALL.
4. Evaluation
   a. Signs and symptoms of hypoxia and acidosis should be elicited such as dyspnea, blurred vision, headache, somnolence, and confusion.
   b. Physical examination may show papilledema.
5. Management
   a. Avoid nonessential transfusions. Do not raise the hemoglobin >8–10 g/dl.
   b. Leukapheresis or exchange transfusion has been proposed for rapidly lowering WBC counts, particularly when WBC counts are >300,000/mm^3.
   c. Keep platelets >20,000/mm^3; transfusing platelets does not add appreciably to blood viscosity.

   d. Specific antileukemic therapy should be instituted as soon as life-threatening complications have been corrected.

   e. Consider whole-brain irradiation at 400cGy in an attempt to prevent intracranial hemorrhage in patients with AML. This is a controversial therapy whose value has not been proven.

   f. Aggressive management of metabolic abnormalities and any underlying coagulopathy associated with the leukemia.

   g. Institute precautionary measures for tumor lysis syndrome: hydration, alkalinization, and allopurinol.

III. SUPERIOR MEDIASTINAL SYNDROME / SUPERIOR VENA CAVA SYNDROME

A. Overview
1. Superior vena cava syndrome (SVCS) refers to the signs and symptoms resulting from compression of the superior vena cava.
2. Superior mediastinal syndrome (SMS) occurs when tracheal compression also occurs.

B. Etiology
1. Malignant tumors are the most common primary cause of SMS in children.
2. Tumors arising from the anterior mediastinum and/or involving middle mediastinal lymph nodes such as non-Hodgkin lymphoma, Hodgkin's disease, leukemia, and germ cell tumors compress the thin walled, low pressure vena cava and its tributaries impairing venous return to the heart and increasing venous pressure distal to the obstruction, specifically in the head, neck, and upper thorax.
3. Intravascular thrombosis occurs in 50% of cases.
4. Obstruction of small and large airways occurs and edema further compromises air flow.

C. Evaluation
1. Common symptoms include cough, dyspnea, chest pain, and orthopnea. Anxiety, confusion, somnolence,

headache, visual disturbances, and syncope are less common but reflect a more profound impairment in physiology.

2. A supine position often worsens symptoms. Symptoms often progress rapidly over a few days.

3. On physical examination, facial edema and possibly conjunctival edema are noted. Plethora or cyanosis of the face, neck, and upper extremities; distention of chest wall and other collateral veins, diaphoresis, wheezing, and stridor are all signs of SMS.

4. A chest radiograph confirms the clinical picture. More detailed evaluation with computed tomography (CT), echocardiography, and pulmonary function studies may be needed to accurately define the degree of impairment and the anesthetic risk.

5. Carefully consider and evaluate before administering sedation or anesthesia since severe morbidity and even mortality can be the end result.

   a. Establishing a tissue diagnosis is essential for planning definitive therapy; however, children with SMS often tolerate sedation/anesthesia poorly.

      i. With anesthesia, abdominal muscle tone increases, respiratory muscle tone decreases, bronchial smooth muscle relaxes, and lung volumes are greatly reduced. Even with intubation these patients sometimes cannot be ventilated.

      ii. Venous return is further reduced by the peripheral vasodilitation caused by sedation and sometimes cannot be restored.

   b. Attempt to make the diagnosis by the least invasive methods. A complete blood count (CBC) or bone marrow aspirate may yield the diagnosis of lymphoma or leukemia. A pleurocentesis or pericardiocentesis, if an effusion is present, may yield diagnostic material. Serum alpha-fetoprotein or beta-human chorionic gonadotropin hormone can identify some germ cell malignancies. In a cooperative older child, a peripheral lymph node biopsy under local anesthesia can be performed without sedation.

D. Management
When symptoms are life-threatening, prebiopsy empiric therapy may be necessary.
1. Radiation is the most common emergency therapy using daily dosages of 200–400cGy. A small radiation field concentrating on the trachea and superior vena cava is sufficient. Improvement can be seen within 12 hours. Histologic distortion and an inability to make a correct diagnosis is a potential complication. Anticipate radiation-induced edema. Both these problems can be minimized with small fields.
2. IV steroids (methylprednisolone 50 mg/m^2/day divided 4 times daily) can reduce a lymphoid mass. Empiric chemotherapy may be necessary. Anticipate histologic distortion and tumor lysis.
3. Observe in an intensive care unit.
4. Elevate the patient's head and give supplemental oxygen.
5. Avoid overhydration, but maintain adequate circulating blood volume.
6. Avoid upper extremity venipunctures (which can bleed excessively due to high intravascular pressure).
7. Institute tumor lysis syndrome precautions (see section IA).

IV. PERICARDIAL TAMPONADE

A. Overview
Pericardial tamponade is a rare complication usually associated with mediastinal tumors, congestive heart failure, or infection. It occurs when extrinsic pressure prevents normal left ventricular output.

B. Symptoms
1. Precordial pain
2. Hypotension
3. Diminished heart sounds
4. Dyspnea
5. Pulses paradoxus
X-ray may reveal an enlarged heart and echocardiogram will reveal pericardial fluid collections.

C. Management
Immediate aspiration of fluid from pericardial sac. If recurrent, patient may need surgical treatment.

V. PLEURAL EFFUSION

A. Overview
   1. Pleural effusion is usually due to tumor involvement of the pleural surface.
   2. It may also occur with infection or with obstruction of venous or lymphatic drainage, sympathetic response to tumor in chest or abdomen, heart failure, or fluid overload. Hemothorax may occur as a complication of central venous line placement.
   3. The most common associated tumors include lymphomas, osteogenic sarcoma, soft tissue sarcoma, and neuroblastoma.

B. Signs and symptoms
   1. Respiratory symptoms (dyspnea)
      a. Pleuritic chest pain
      b. Decreased breath sounds on auscultation

C. Management
Diagnostic and therapeutic thoracentesis for symptomatic effusions. If recur, place chest tube. Analyze fluid for cytology, cultures, protein, and LDH.

VI. NEUROLOGIC EMERGENCIES

A variety of neurologic emergencies can arise in children with cancer. They can be seen at the time of presentation during therapy or at relapse. The etiologies are numerous and include a direct effect of tumor or treatment sequelae. A detailed history with attention to the natural course of the malignancy and knowledge of the treatment is critical, as is a thorough neurologic examination.

A. Compression of the spinal cord
   1. Overview
      a. Spinal cord compression causes severe neurologic morbidity. Prompt recognition of this process

with appropriate intervention may prevent these complications.

b. Back pain occurs in 80% of children with spinal cord compression. Any child with cancer plus back pain should be considered to have spinal cord compression until proven otherwise.

2. Etiology

a. Sarcomas, lymphomas, neuroblastoma, and leukemia at diagnosis or with relapse.

b. Although a tumor may involve the vertebral body and secondarily compress the cord, it is more likely to cause spinal cord compression by infiltrating through intervertebral foramina from a paraspinous location.

3. Evaluation

a. A detailed neurologic examination with particular attention to extremity strength, reflexes, and tone. Percussion of the spine may elicit localized tenderness. Determination of a sensory level should be attempted.

b. Close observation may be appropriate for the child with localized back pain and a normal neurologic exam. Evaluate persistent pain with a magnetic resonance imaging (MRI) scan.

c. For the child with an abnormal neurologic finding, an MRI of the entire spine is essential. There is probably no role for plain films, as fewer than half of children have abnormalities on this study.

4. Management

a. Administer dexamethasone 1–2 mg/kg IV as a single loading dose (10 mg maximum dose) followed by 1.5 mg/kg/day divided every 6 hours (maximum dose 4 mg) to reduce edema. Neurologic function may improve with steroids but spinal cord decompression still needs to be carried out.

b. For chemosensitive tumors such as lymphoma, leukemia, and neuroblastoma, administer appropriate chemotherapy in addition to steroids.

c. For spinal cord compression secondary to nonchemosensitive tumors that are radioresponsive, administer radiation therapy in addition to steroids.

    i. The entire tumor volume should be included in the radiation field plus one vertebral body above and below the lesion.

    ii. Even in patients with a short life expectancy, radiation should be initiated, as loss of function is devastating to quality of life.

    d. Decompressive laminectomy is indicated only to establish a histologic diagnosis, for radioresistant and chemoresistant tumors, and for rapid neurologic deterioration.

    e. For spinal cord compression secondary to osteoporosis and vertebral collapse, laminectomy and fixation may be necessary.

B. Acute change in mental status

  1. Etiology

    a. Metastatic disease, primary CNS infection (bacterial, fungal, viral), sepsis/disseminated intravascular coagulation (DIC), and metabolic abnormalities are the most common causes of acute alterations in consciousness.

    b. Although uncommon, acute changes in mental status can occur with chemotherapy drugs such as Ifosfamide, methotrexate, and high-dose cytarabine.

  2. Evaluation

    a. In an emergency, evaluate vital signs, breathing pattern, pupil size with responsiveness to light, extraocular movements, spontaneous movements, and response to stimuli for evidence of herniation.

    b. Monitor for signs of increased intracranial pressure such as papilledema and focal neurologic deficits.

    c. Obtain glucose, electrolytes, renal and hepatic function, and a DIC screen to rule out metabolic or hemorrhagic causes. Transfuse platelets if count $<20,000/mm^3$, or $<50,000/mm^3$ in a recently postoperative brain tumor patient or brain tumor patient with significant residual disease.

    d. After the patient is stabilized, obtain an emergency CT scan if a mass lesion is suspected or the initial evaluation fails to identify the cause for the acute change in mental status.

e. Once a mass lesion has been ruled out and coagulopathy corrected, perform a lumbar puncture and order cerebrospinal fluid protein, glucose, cytology, and appropriate cultures.
3. Management
    a. Correct life-threatening cardiorespiratory abnormalities.
    b. Manage increased intracranial pressure with hyperventilation to pCO_2 of 20–25 mm Hg, IV dexamethasone (1–2 mg/kg) IV as a loading dose followed by 1.5 mg/kg/day divided every 6 hours (maximum dose 4 mg) and mannitol 20% at 0.5–1 gm/kg by slow IV infusion.
    c. Correct metabolic abnormalities and coagulation defects.
    d. Treat potential infectious etiologies appropriately. If bacterial meningitis is a possibility, administer emergency antibiotic therapy at presentation.

C. Seizure
1. Etiology
    a. Etiology is similar to that of acute change in mental status. (See section VI.B.1.)
    b. Metastatic disease late in the course of illness and therapy complications are most common.
    c. Antineoplastic drugs such as vincristine, intrathecal methotrexate, cisplatin, and L-asparaginase or the antibiotic Imipenem can cause seizures.
    d. Cranial radiation may increase seizure potential.
2. Evaluation
    a. Evaluation is similar to that for acute change in mental status.
    b. MRI may show abnormalities not seen on CT, particularly ones related to CNS damage from therapy.
    c. An electroencephalogram (EEG) may localize the focus of seizure origin or show activity not suspected clinically.
3. Management
    a. Prolonged seizure requires emergency management with cardiopulmonary support and anticonvulsant administration intravenously.

        i. Administer lorazepam (Ativan), which has a longer duration of activity than diazepam, at 0.05 mg/kg (max. 4–6 mg) IV over 2 minutes.

       ii. Administer phenytoin 10 mg/kg IV at 1 mg/kg/ min.

  b. Antiepileptic medications are often not required after a seizure. With correction of the underlying abnormality, they can be discontinued quickly, particularly if the follow-up EEG is normal and there is no focal neurologic abnormality on imaging studies or persistent deficit on examination.

     Consider the consequences of continuing anticonvulsant agents that interfere with the metabolism of chemotherapeutic agents.

D. Cerebrovascular accident

  1. Overview

    A cerebrovascular accident (CVA) usually presents as acute impairment in motor function, speech, and/or impaired mental status. Seizures are a common accompaniment.

  2. Etiology

    a. CVAs may be due to direct or metastatic spread of tumor, chemotherapeutic agents, CNS infection, hemorrhage, or thrombosis. Embolic causes are rare.

    b. At initial diagnosis, CVAs are most commonly associated with disease-related coagulation abnormalities, while on-therapy CVAs are usually drug related.

    c. At the end stages of disease, DIC, tumor or infection can be associated with stroke.

    d. Radiation-induced vascular damage is associated with strokes months to years after treatment.

  3. Evaluation

    a. After the child has been stabilized, perform CT or MR imaging with and without contrast.

    b. If the initial scan is normal, a repeat study in 7–10 days may be needed.

    c. Evaluate coagulation status with CBC, DIC screen, including d-dimer, antithrombin III, protein C, and protein S.

    d. Once a mass lesion has been ruled out and coagulation abnormalities corrected, proceed with lumbar puncture.

    e. MR angiography or arteriography can help diagnose partial sagital sinus thrombosis or radiation vasculopathy.

  4. Management

    a. Supportive care is the mainstay of therapy; corticosteroids (dexamethasone) to reduce edema and mannitol to decrease intracranial pressure are warranted. (See section VIB.)

    b. Treatment of DIC includes platelet and FFP infusions and possibly low-dose heparin; however, the use of anticoagulation for venous thrombosis is controversial. (See Chapter 5 on Hemorrhagic and Thrombotic Complications in Children with Cancer.)

    c. Some investigators recommend the twice daily infusion of FFP or antithrombin III concentrate for L-asparaginase-associated CVAs.

VII. THE ACUTE ABDOMEN

The classic physical examination findings of an acute abdomen in a neutropenic patient are muted; however, pain is virtually always present. Steroids also mask the signs and symptoms of an acute abdomen. Physical examination at frequent intervals is essential for detecting subtle changes.

  A. Appendicitis

Although rare, appendicitis is often associated with a delayed diagnosis and poor outcome including death. It should always be considered in the differential diagnosis of typhlitis unresponsive to medical management and vincristine toxicity.

  B. Typhlitis

    1. Overview

Typhlitis is a necrotizing colitis of the cecum with inflammation, often involving surrounding tissue, and seen in neutropenic cancer patients, particularly those with leukemia.

2. Etiology

The pathophysiology is related to the disruption of intestinal mucosa from chemotherapy and bacterial invasion of bowel wall in the setting of neutropenia.

3. Evaluation

a. Perform a careful and thorough physical examination.

b. Blood cultures are positive occasionally and are usually gram-negative enteric organisms.

c. Obtain radiographic studies such as plain radiograph (three views of the abdomen), abdominal ultrasound, and/or CT scanning. Air in bowel wall, generally cecum, thickened bowel wall, and soft tissue mass are findings of typhlitis.

4. Management

a. Medical management is generally the mainstay of therapy and includes bowel rest, broad-spectrum antimicrobial coverage (consider double gram-negative coverage as well as anaerobic coverage), and supportive care.

b. Vasopressors are occasionally needed and hypotension at presentation is associated with a poor outcome.

c. Indications for surgery include free air, hemorrhage, and persistent hypotension.

C. Hemorrhagic pancreatitis

1. Overview

In the setting of abdominal pain, vomiting, and preceding treatment with L-asparaginase, pancreatitis should be considered.

2. Evaluation

a. An elevated serum amylase, lipase, and/or urinary amylase/creatinine ratio 1.5–2.0 times normal may be considered to be consistent with pancreatitis.

b. Ultrasound and/or CT scanning of the abdomen should be obtained.

c. Serial studies may be necessary, particularly to monitor for abscess development pancreatic dissolution or pseudocyst formation.

3. Management
   a. Bowel rest, nasogastric drainage, antibiotic coverage of bowel flora, fluid replacement, and hyperalimentation are necessary.
   b. Surgical drainage may be required if an abscess develops, pancreatic dissolution occurs, or a pseudocyst persists.
   c. Further administration of asparaginase is contraindicated.

Bibliography

Antunes NJ, DeAngelis LM. Neurologic consultation in children with systemic cancer. *Pediatr Neurol* 20:121, 1990.

Basade M, Dhar AK, Kulkarni SS, et al. Rapid cytoreduction in childhood leukemic hyperleukocytosis by conservative therapy. *Medic Pediatr Oncol* 25:204–7, 1995.

Bertsch H, Rudoler S, Needle MN, et al. Emergent/urgent therapeutic irradiation in pediatric oncology: patterns of presentation, treatment and outcome. *Med Pediatr Oncol* 30:101, 1998.

Bilsky MH, Lis E, Raizer J, et al. The diagnosis and treatment of metastatic spinal tumor. *Oncologist* 4:459, 1999.

Byrne TN. Spinal cord compression from epidural metastases. *N Engl J Med* 327:614–19, 1992.

Escalante CP. Causes and management of superior vena cava syndrome. *Oncol* 7:61–68, 1993.

Jones DP, Mahmoud H, Chesney RW. Tumor lysis syndrome: pathogenesis and management. *Pediatr Nephrol* 9:206–12, 1995.

Kelly RE Jr, Isaacman DJ. Thoracic emergencies. In: Fleisher GR, Ludwig S eds. *Textbook of Pediatric Emergency Medicine,* 4th ed. Philadelphia: Lippincott Williams & Wilkins, 1999; p. 1539.

Levi M, Cate HT. Disseminated intravascular coagulation. *N Engl J Med* 341:586, 1999.

Loblaw DA, Laperriere NJ. Emergency treatment of malignant extradural spinal cord compression: an evidence-based guideline. *J Clin Oncol* 16:1613, 1998.

Pui C-H, Mahmoud HH, Wiley JM, Woods GM, et al. Recombinant urate oxidase for the prophylaxis or treatment of hyperuricemia in patients with leukemia or lymphoma. *J Clin Oncol* 19:697–704, 2001.

Sahu S, Saika S, Pai SK, et al. L-asparaginase (Leunase) induced pancreatitis in childhood acute lymphoblastic leukemia. *Pediatr Hematol Oncol* 17:433, 1998.

Smalley RY, Guaspari A, Haase-Shatz S, Anderson SA, et al. Allopurinol: Intravenous use for prevention and treatment of hyperuricemia. *J Clin Oncol* 18:1758–63, 2000.

Wetzstein, GA. Tunor lysis syndrome: A treatment guide. *Oncol Special Ed* 5:31–34,2002.

Young G, Shende A. Use of pamidronate in the management of acute cancer-related hypercalcemia in children. *Med Pediatr Oncol* 30:117, 1998.

13

Nutritional Support

Nancy Sacks, M.S., R.D., CNSD, Karen Ringwald-Smith, M.S., R.D., LDN, and Gregory Hale, M.D.

The goals for nutrition intervention in the pediatric oncology patient are to prevent or reverse nutritional deficits, promote normal growth and development, minimize morbidity, and maximize the quality of life. Factors contributing to the origin and progression of cachexia in a young patient with cancer are shown in Figure 13.1.

I. CALORIE AND PROTEIN REQUIREMENTS

A. Recommended Dietary Allowances (RDAs) (see Table 13.1) can be used to determine estimated calorie and protein needs. Since the RDAs were developed as recommendations for healthy populations rather than sick individual patients, adjustments are usually necessary to maintain appropriate growth in sick patients. The allowances may need to be increased 15–50% to compensate for previous weight loss, malnutrition, or increased needs due to metabolic demands.

B. The estimation of basal metabolic rate (BMR) developed by the World Health Organization (see Table 13.2) may be more appropriate in acutely ill patients for determining energy requirements.

C. Premature infants may require 120 kcal/kg or more due to increased needs for growth.

II. INDICATIONS FOR SUPPLEMENTAL NUTRITION

A. To prevent malnutrition

B. Specific childhood cancers associated with the poorest prognoses tend to have the most intense cancer treatment regimens and; therefore, are most likely to be associated with the development of protein energy malnutrition.

Fig. 13.1.
Factors Contributing to the Origin and Progression of Cachexia in a Child with Cancer

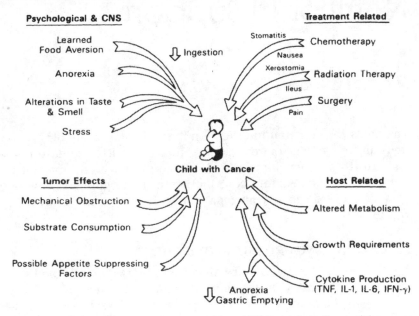

Source: Alexander, Rickard, and Godshall, 1997, p. 1170. Reprinted with permission.

Table 13.1.
Recommended Daily Allowances for Calories and Protein

Category	Age (years)	Protein (g/kg/day)	Calories (kcal/kg/day)
Infant	0.0–0.5	2.2	108
	0.5–1.0	1.6	98
Child	1–3	1.2	102
	4–6	1.1	90
	7–10	1.0	70
Male	11–14	1.0	55
	15–18	0.9	45
Female	11–14	1.0	47
	15–18	0.8	40

Table 13.2.
Estimating Basal Metabolic Rate Based on the World Health
Organization Equation for Children ≥1 Year of Age

Sex	Age			
	1–3 years	3–10 years	10–18 years	18–30 years
Male	60.9W − 54	22.7W + 495	17.5W + 651	15.3W + 679
Female	61W − 51	22.5W + 499	12.2W + 746	14.7W + 496

W = weight in kilograms

BMR = _____
Multiply BMR by an activity/stress factor:
   1.3 for a well-nourished child at bed rest with mild to moderate stress (mild surgery)
   1.5 for a very active child with mild to moderate stress, an inactive child with severe stress (trauma, sepsis, cancer, extensive surgery), or a child with minimal activity who requires catch-up growth
   1.7 for an active child requiring catch-up growth or an active child with severe stress

BMR _____ X Factor _____ = _____ Kcal/day

Source: Data from World Health Organization, 1985, and Nutrition Support Services, 1995.

C. It can be anticipated that treatment (surgery, radiation, chemotherapy, and hematopoietic stem cell transplantation) will cause changes that prevent adequate intake to maintain or restore nutritional status.

III. CRITERIA FOR NUTRITION INTERVENTION

Assess the patient's nutritional status at diagnosis and throughout therapy. Some quick and practical methods that may be used by physicians and nurses are the following:

A. Anthropometric
   1. The current percentile for weight and/or height for age has fallen 2 percentile channels. Complete a growth chart for inpatients and outpatients at diagnosis and throughout therapy.
   2. >5% weight loss from pre-illness weight or >5% weight loss over the last month. Percentage weight loss is derived from the highest previous weight. Weight is inaccurate when a child has edema, large tumor burden, organ congestion, or when excess fluids have been administered (twice maintenance) for chemotherapy.

These guidelines apply to initially obese as well as lean subjects.

3. <10th or >90th percentile weight for age
4. <10th or >90th percentile weight for height
5. <90% ideal body weight for height
    This is calculated as the patient's actual weight divided by the ideal weight for height times 100. Ideal body weight is determined from the appropriate growth curve by first identifying the age for which the measured height is on the 50th percentile, then determining the corresponding 50th percentile weight for that height.
6. <10th percentile height for age
    Height velocity of <5 cm/yr after 2 years of age
7. Degree of malnutrition
    The degree of malnutrition can be determined by assessing wasting—the patient's actual weight divided by the ideal body weight for height—and assessing stunting—the patient's actual height divided by the ideal height for age (see Table 13.3).
8. Other means
    Other, more sophisticated means of evaluating nutritional status can be performed by a registered dietitian including assessment of muscle and subcutaneous fat stores.

Table 13.3.

Anthropometric Criteria for the Diagnosis of Malnutrition and Obesity in Pediatric Cancer Patients

	Degree of Malnutrition			
Criteria	0 (normal)	1 (mild)	2 (moderate)	3 (severe)
Weight-for-height (% expected)	90–110	80–90	70–80	<70
Height-for-age (% expected)	≥95	90–95	85–90	<85

	Degree of Obesity		
	1 (overweight)	2 (obese)	3 (morbid)
Weight-for-height (% expected)	110–120	120–140	>140

Source: Adapted from Motil, 1998; and Walterlow, 1972. Reprinted with permission from Pizzo and Poplack, 2003.

9. BMI <5th or >85th percentile
Body mass index (BMI) is an indirect measure of body fat and controls, to some degree, for the influence of height. BMI is defined as weight in kilograms divided by the square of height in meters (kg/m^2).*

B. Nutrient intake: when intake is <80% estimated needs.

IV. ASSESSMENT OF BIOCHEMICAL DATA

A. Laboratory tests that can be monitored before and during repletion include the following:
1. Obtain laboratory panel to screen for organ function to include: sodium, potassium, chloride, bicarbonate, glucose, creatinine, blood urea nitrogen (BUN), calcium, phosphorus, magnesium, total protein, albumin, triglycerides, cholesterol, alkaline phosphatase, serum aminotransferase, gamma-glutamyltransferase, and total bilirubin.
2. Serum albumin <3.2 mg/dL may indicate decreased protein stores and chronic malnutrition; the level can be affected by hydration and hepatic function.
3. Serum prealbumin level may indicate acute malnutrition; the level can be increased with impaired renal function (normal value varies with age) and decreased with altered hepatic function.

B. Providing nutrition to patients who are depleted can result in abnormalities such as:
1. Refeeding syndrome
This is seen in patients chronically deprived of adequate nutrition and is characterized by metabolic complications, severe fluid shifts, hypokalemia, and hypophosphatemia that occur in patients who are repleted enterally or parenterally. Monitor sodium, potassium, chloride, bicarbonate, BUN, creatinine, calcium, magnesium, and phosphorus.

---

*Please note that the m^2 used in the formula for BMI is not the same as the m^2 used to express body surface area. For example: a patient with weight 82 kg and height 165 cm (1.65 m) would have BMI calculated as follows:

$$BMI = 82/(1.65)^2 = 82/2.72 = 30$$

2. Tube feeding syndrome
    This is characterized by hypertonic dehydration, hypernatremia, and prerenal azotemia in patients receiving highly osmotic enteral feeds.

V. VARIOUS METHODS OF NUTRITIONAL SUPPORT

A. Before determining the most appropriate method of nutritional support, consider the following (see Figure 13.2):
    1. Nutritional assessment/recommendations by registered dietitian
    2. Capabilities of family/patient for learning
    3. Insurance/home care coverage
    4. Ethical issues regarding disease (stage/prognosis).

B. Oral (volitional)
    1. Intervene early by involving a nutritionist at the time of diagnosis or referral for nutritional assessment and counseling.
    2. Provide guidelines for managing complications of treatment (anorexia, alterations in taste, mouth dryness, dysphagia, early satiety, nausea, vomiting, stomatitis, mucositis, diarrhea, or constipation) and for increasing protein or calories. The National Cancer Institute has publications available on nutrition for the child with cancer (1-800-4-CANCER).
    3. Provide oral supplements for trial (e.g., shakes, bars). Review classification of enteral feeding products (see Table 13.4).
    4. Provide specific macronutrients (modulars).
        a. Protein
        b. Carbohydrate
        c. Fat

C. Enteral tube feeding
    If oral feeding is not possible or is inadequate, consider tube feedings. It is important to provide support from registered dietitians, physicians, nurses, and social workers to improve acceptance. (Patients and families need to know that their child can continue to eat with supplemental nutrition.)
    1. Initiate tube feedings:
        a. If mucosal integrity and platelet count permit insertion of tube.

Fig. 13.2.

An Algorithm for Nutritional Support of Children with Cancer

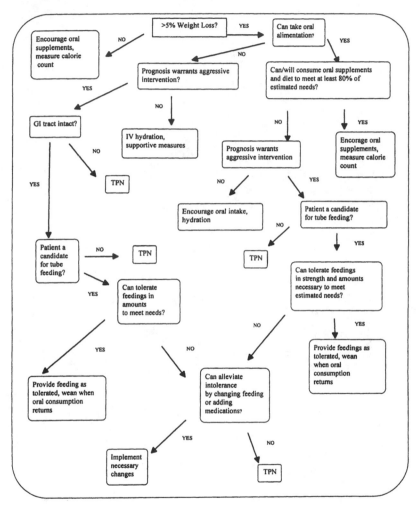

Source: Alexander and Norton, 1993, p. 1026

b. If a patient has a functional gastrointestinal tract along with the ability to tolerate feedings with manageable side effects of nausea, vomiting, and diarrhea.

c. When a patient meets the criteria for nutrition intervention and oral intake is inadequate to meet

Table 13.4.
Characteristics of Enteral Products

Product Description	1–10 Years of Age Tube Feeding and/or Oral	>10 Years of Age Tube Feeding	>10 Years of Age Oral
1. Standard or polymeric Intact macronutrients intended as meal replacements Requires normal digestive and absorptive capacity Usually lactose free unless otherwise indicated	Pediasure Kindercal Nutren Junior Resource Just for Kids TM Compleat Pediatric	Isocal Osmolite Nutren Compleat Modified Promote	Ensure Boost NuBasics Meritene ReSource Fortashake Scandishake Carnation Instant Breakfast
2. High nitrogen Intact macronutrients with >15% total calories as protein Useful in patients with increased protein need (i.e., poor wound healing, radiation)		Isocal HN Osmolite HN Criticare HN	Ensure HN Boost HN TwoCal HN
3. Concentrated or high calorie Contain higher calorie per milliliter than standard formulas May be used with fluid restriction	Nutren 1.5 Nutren 2.0	Nutren 1.5 Nutren 2.0 TwoCal HN Deliver 2.0 Comply Isosource Jevity Plus	NuBasic Plus Ensure Plus Resource Plus Boost Plus TwoCal HN Jevity Plus

Category		Pediatric	Adult	
4. Predigested/elemental	Predigested or partially hydrolyzed peptide-based diet that may be beneficial for child with impaired gastrointestinal function (diarrhea, mucositis, intestinal villous atrophy)	Peptamen Junior Neocate One Plus VivonexPeds TM Pediasure with Fiber EleCare	Peptamen Peptamen VHP Reabilin Tolerex Vivonex TEN	Vital HN
	Many contain medium-chain triglycerides to minimize fat intolerance Can have high osmolality	L-Emental Pediatric	Vivonex Plus Criticare HN Travasorb MCT	
5. Fiber containing	Containing fiber from natural sources or added soy polysaccharides to aid in bowel function	Kindercal Pediasure with fiber Nutren Junior with fiber	Jevity Ultracal Nutren 1.0 with fiber FiberSource	Jevity Ultracal Nutren 1.0 with fiber
6. Disease specific	Macro- and micronutrients modified for disease state		Diabetes: Choice Dm, Glucerna Renal: Nepro, Suplena Pulmonary: Pulmocare, Nutrivent Liver: NutriHep Metabolically stressed: Replete, Impact, Perative	Diabetes: Choice Dm, Glucerna Renal: Nepro, Suplena Pulmonary: Pulmocare, Nutrivent Metabolically stressed: Impact, Replete

cont.

Table 13.4.
continued

Product Description	Cow's Milk	Soy	Predigested
7. Infant formulas (variety of formulas available for premature infants and for infants with poor tolerance). Many infants are lactose intolerant after chemotherapy and benefit from lactose-free formulas. Human breast milk should be used when possible (contains lactose and may not be tolerated well after chemotherapy).	Similac Enfamil Lactofree (lactose free) Gerber Carnation Good Start Similac PM 60/40	Isomil Prosobee	Pregestimil Alimentum Nutramigen
8. Modular components	Protein Casec Pro-mix ProMod NutriSource Protein Elementra	Carbohydrate Polycose Moducal Liquid Carbohydrate (LC) Sumacal NutriSource Carbohydrate NutriSource (long- or medium-chain triglycerides)	Fat Vegetable oil (long-chain triglycerides) Microlipid (long-chain triglycerides) Medium-chain triglycerides
9. Oral electrolyte solutions Provides electrolytes, calories and water during mild to moderate dehydration	Pedialyte Infalyte Equalyte		

estimated needs to provide for normal growth or to provide for repletion of nutritional status.

2. Determine the optimal access route for enteral nutrition based on anticipated duration of tube feeding, risk of pulmonary aspiration, and indications for specific access routes (see Figure 13.3).

   a. Tube selection

      Use the smallest tube possible for greater comfort (6–8-French nasogastric tubes will work in most patients). A larger tube may be needed with fiber-containing formulas or highly viscous formulas. Silicone and polyurethane nasoenteric tubes decrease physical irritation and have less associated risk of pulmonary aspiration. Weighted tubes are designed to assist with postpyloric tube placement and maintenance of tube positions. Placement is assessed by checking pH of aspirated contents or by radiograph.

   b. Nasoenteric: short-term use

      i. Silicone and polyurethane tubes

      ii. Tube lumen size range (6–10 French) based on age/size of child and viscosity of formula.

      iii. Orogastric for infants <34 weeks gestational due to obligatory nose breathers.

      iv. Nasogastric: easy intubation

      v. Nasoduodenal or nasojejunal, which require radiographic proof of placement and can be easily dislodged.

   c. Enterostomy feeding tubes: long-term use

      i. Gastrostomy tubes are made of silicone, polyurethane, rubber, or latex. A Foley catheter may be used for Stamm, Witzel, or Janeway gastrostomies. Surgically or percutaneously placed gastrostomy tubes can be replaced with a button, which is flush with the abdomen once a stoma is formed.

      ii. Jejunostomy tubes are made of rubber, latex, silicone, polyvinyl, silicone rubber, or polyethylene and are surgically placed.

      iii. Complications with enterostomy tubes can include cellulitis and infections (particularly around the time of neutropenia).

Fig. 13.3.
Determining the Optimal Feeding Mode

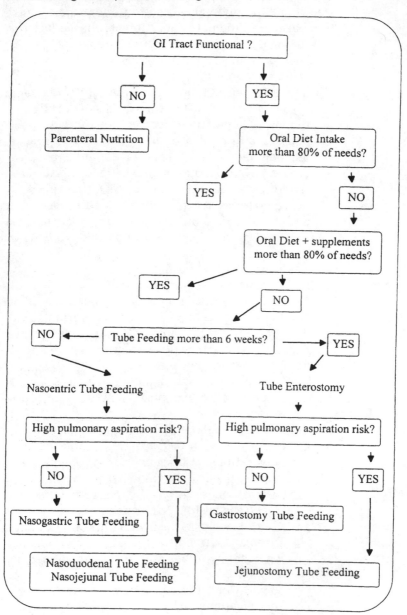

Source: Ideno, 1993, p. 83

3. Determine the method of administration.
   a. An enteral feeding pump provides a reliable, constant infusion rate, decreases the risk of gastric retention, and may prevent gastrointestinal (GI) complications of nausea, vomiting, abdominal cramping/bloating, and diarrhea.
   b. With gravity flow feeding, the flow rate may be adjusted with a clamp that applies pressure on the tubing.
   c. Feeding schedules.
      i. A continuous schedule is more likely to be tolerated than bolus feeds and requires a feeding pump.
      ii. A bolus (intermittent or gravity) schedule more closely mimics normal feeding.
      iii. A combination of continuous nocturnal feeds with daytime boluses could be arranged to meet the patient's nutritional needs.
      iv. The feeding schedule will determine whether a portable or standard pump is required and which pump is reimbursable by insurance.
4. Determine formula based on composition, GI function, age, cost, and resources (e.g., insurance coverage). Use unflavored products for tube feeding. There are many products available for oral use and for tube feedings (see Table 13.4). Children do not generally accept oral products well. In addition, children are usually unable to gain weight with oral products and oral intake and; therefore, usually require supplemental tube feedings.
5. Initiate tube feeding and monitor progression.
   a. If nothing by mouth (NPO) <3 days, begin full strength formula at 1–2 mL/kg/h. Increase by 1–2 mL/kg/h per day as tolerated until the goal is achieved.
   b. If NPO >3 days or if GI problems exist (e.g., mucositis, diarrhea, or gut atrophy), begin half-strength formula at 1–2 mL/kg/h. Advance concentration to full-strength after 12–24 hours, then increase rate by 1–2 mL/kg/h per day to goal.
   c. One option is to provide half estimated needs continuously at night and the remaining half calories in 2–3 boluses during the day. The daily volume can

also be divided into feedings that can be administered every 2–4 hours as desired. Most patients will tolerate continuous feedings better than bolus feedings, particularly if they are nauseated.

d. If fluid needs are not met with oral intake and tube feeding, provide extra free water as flushes or mixed with feeds.

e. Flush tube frequently with water and before/after all medications.

f. Supplementation with potassium, phosphorus, calcium, or magnesium should be divided throughout the day and mixed with feeds for better tolerance. To achieve maximal absorption, do not give calcium and phosphorus at the same time. Medications can be very hyperosmolar and can cause GI irritation. The intravenous form of some medications can be given in tube feedings with less irritation (e.g., magnesium).

6. Watch for mechanical complications of tube feedings.

a. High gastric residual can be caused by delayed gastric emptying. Prokinetic medications (cisapride or metoclopramide) may help as well as elevating the head of the bed at least 30 degrees during and after feeding.

b. Nasopharyngeal and nasolabial irritation can be lessened with small-bore tubes made of silicone or polyurethane and by taping the tube securely to avoid pressure on nares.

c. Skin irritation and excoriation at the ostomy site can be reduced with appropriate enterostomal therapy using topical or oral antibiotics during periods of severe neutropenia.

d. To avoid obstruction of feeding tube lumen, be sure to adequately flush the tube before and after medication and boluses, and every 4 hours during continuous infusion. Use liquid elixirs when possible. If the tube is clogged, mix 1 crushed Viokase enzyme tablet with 1 crushed tablet (324 mg) of sodium bicarbonate and 5 mL of tap water to prepare a pH 7.9 Viokase solution. Inject 5 mL of this enzyme solution through a drum cartridge catheter inserted into the feeding tube. Allow to sit for 5 minutes and reirrigate feeding tube with 20–30 mL water.

   e. Monitor during the administration of tube feeding.

      i. Check body weight, fluid intake/output, and GI function every day when initiating feedings, then 2 times per week when stable.

      ii. Assess biochemical indices (fluid balance, calcium, phosphorus, magnesium, and liver function tests). If refeeding syndrome or depleted stores are suspected, monitor laboratory values daily and increase calories slowly.

      iii. Enteral tubes can stay in place for 4–6 weeks before requiring replacement. Older adolescents may choose to place the tube daily for nocturnal needs.

D. Total parenteral nutrition/hyperalimentation

Total parenteral nutrition (TPN) is indicated for patients when oral and/or tube feedings provide inadequate nutrients or when enteral feeds are contraindicated over a significant period of time. A nutritional assessment should be performed before starting TPN. A central venous catheter is essential if total nutritional requirements are to be met over several weeks or months.

   1. Guidelines for determining TPN requirements

      a. Determine fluid needs.

          <1–10 kg: 100 mL/kg/day

          >10–20 kg: 1,000 mL + 50 mL each kg >10 kg

          >20–30 kg: 1,500 mL + 20 mL each kg >20 kg

          >30 kg: 35 mL/kg/day

      b. Determine calorie needs.

        i. Preterm infant: 90–120 kcal/kg/day

          Full-term infant (0–28 days old): 90–108 kcal/kg/day

          Older infant and child (>28 days old): 60–110 kcal/kg/day

          Older child and adolescent (weight >20 kg): 30–60 kcal/kg/day

        ii. The RDAs may also be used; (see Table 13.1).

        iii. Basal metabolic rate can also be used with appropriate activity/stress factors to determine calorie needs; (see Table 13.2).

    c. Determine protein needs.
      i. Protein provides 4.0 kcal/g.
     ii. Protein requirements are based on age and adjusted for needs. The following assumes normal age-related organ function.
Preterm infant: 2.5–3.5 g/kg/day
Full-term infant (0–28 days old): 2.0–3.0 g/kg/day
Older infant and child (>28 days old): 1.5–3.0 g/kg/day
Older child and adolescent (weight >20 kg): 0.8–2.5 g/kg/day
    iii. Parenteral amino acid products will differ depending on the child's age.
Aminosyn III and Novamine are standard amino acid formulations for children older than 1 year of age. Aminosyn PF and TrophAmine are formulas used for children younger than 1 year of age.
    d. Determine fat/lipid needs.
      i. 20% fat/lipid (Intralipid, Liposyn II) contains 2 kcal/mL and 10% (Liposyn II) contains 1.1 kcal/mL.
     ii. Fat/lipid intake should not exceed 3 g/kg/day, or 60% of total calories. A reasonable goal for fat calories is 30–40% of the daily calories provided.
    iii. Linoleic acid is considered an essential fatty acid. The minimal requirements for linoleic acid are 2–4% of total calories (25–100 mg/kg/day) or 8–10% of the total daily estimated calories as fat.
    e. Determine carbohydrate/glucose needs.
      i. Dextrose provides 3.4 kcal/g.
     ii. Usual rate of glucose administration is:
Preterm infant: 5–7 mg/kg/min with 1–2 mg/kg/min advancement/day, maximum 14–21 mg/kg/min.
Full-term infant (<28 days old): 7–9 mg/kg/min with 1–2 mg/kg/min advancement/day, maximum 14–21 mg/kg/min.

Table 13.5.
Recommended Daily Maintenance Doses of Specific Electrolytes*

	Preterm	Full Term <28 days	Older Infant (>28days) /Child	Older Child/ Adolescent (>20kg)
Amino acids (g)	2.5–3.5	2.0–3.0	1.5–3.0	0.8–2.5
Intravenous fat emulsion (g)	0.5–3	1–3	0.5–3	0.5–2.5
Sodium (mEq)	2–4	2–4	2–4	Individualize 60–150 mEq/day
Potassium (mEq)	1–4	1–4	2–4	Individualize 70–180 mEq/day
Chloride (mEq)	2–3	2–5	2–5	Individualize as needed to maintain acid-base balance
Acetate (mEq) (Use as necessary to maintain acid base balance)				
Calcium (mEq)	1–5	0.5–4	0.5–4	10–40 mEq/day
Phosphorus (mMol)	0.5–2	0.5–2	0.5–2	10–40 mMol/day
Magnesium (mEq)	0.1–0.6	0.25–1	0.25–0.5	8–32 mEq/day

*Values are per kg except as noted for older child/adolescent. Estimated requirements may need to be adjusted for compromised organ function or accompanying medications.

Older infant and child (>28 days old): 5–6 mg/kg/min with 1–2 mg/kg/min advancement/day, maximum 15 mg/kg/min.

Older child and adolescent (>20 kg): 8–14 gm/kg/day, maximum concentration of dextrose solution 25%.

    f.   Determine electrolyte needs.

The appropriate maintenance dose of specific electrolytes is indicated in Table 13.5. Needs may be altered for many causes, which must be considered (e.g., cisplatin causes increased losses of potassium, calcium, magnesium, and phosphorus; amphotericin B causes increased losses of potassium; and renal tubular acidosis requires acetate replacement in TPN).

  2. Guidelines for advancing peripheral line TPN

    a.   Day 1: Start with 10% dextrose protein as required and lipids at 1–2 g/kg/day.

    b.   Day 2: Increase lipids by 1 g/kg/day to goal. Maximum amount of dextrose tolerated is 12.5%.

3.   Guidelines for advancing central line TPN

    a.   Day 1: Give 10% dextrose protein as required and lipids at 1–2 g/kg/day.

    b.   Day 2: Increase dextrose solution and lipids to goal. If the patient is at risk for refeeding syndrome, increase calories more slowly (i.e., 10–15% per day).

4.   Monitoring TPN

    a.   Laboratory
        Obtain baseline-screening panel (see section IVA), then check weekly. Check more frequently with refeeding syndrome.

    b.   Daily weight

    c.   Intake and output daily

5.   Cycling of TPN
Many patients benefit from having TPN cycled over 10–12 hours to allow more time off for normal activity. A portable pump can be used to increase mobility while receiving TPN. The infusion rate of TPN solutions with >10% dextrose should be decreased by 50% during the last hour of the infusion to prevent rebound hypoglycemia.

6.   Complications of TPN

    a.   Hypoglycemia: Avoid abrupt discontinuation of TPN (decrease rate before discontinuation).

    b.   Hyperglycemia: Decrease dextrose concentration or administer insulin with TPN as a separate infusion or provide subcutaneously.

    c.   Fatty liver: Avoid excessive carbohydrate infusion and provide a mix of dextrose, protein, and lipids.

    d.   Cholestatic jaundice: To avoid cholestatic jaundice, cycle TPN as soon as possible and provide enteral feeding.

7.   Weaning
Supplemental nutrition (TPN or tube feeding) can be slowly weaned as oral intake improves.

VI. ETHICAL ISSUES

Each patient/family situation needs to be reviewed concerning the goals, risks, and benefits of nutrition support. The choice to withdraw nutrition by families should be respected. Supplemental nutrition may not benefit patients in the terminal stage of their disease. When goals of the cancer therapy change, the level of nutrition intervention may also change.

Bibliography

Alexander HR, Norton JA. Nutritional supportive care. In Pizzo PA, Poplack DG, eds., *Principles and Practices of Pediatric Oncology*, 2nd ed. Philadelphia: J. B. Lippincott Company, 1993.

Alexander HR, Rickard KA, Godshall B. Nutritional Supportive Care. In Pizzo PA, Poplack DG, eds., *Principles and Practice of Pediatric Oncology.* 3rd ed. Philadelphia: J. B. Lippincott Company, 1997.

Barber JR, Miller SF, Sacks GS. Parenteral feeding formulations. In Gottschlich MM, ed. *The Science and Practice of Nutrition Support.* Dubuque, Iowa: Kendall/Hunt, 2001. Pp. 251–68.

Bechard LJ, Adiv OE, Jaksic T, Duggan C. Nutritional supportive care. In Pizzo PA, Poplack DG, eds., *Principles and Practices of Pediatric Oncology*, 4th ed. Philadelphia: Lippincott Williams & Wilkins, 2003. Pp. 1285–1300.

Bowman L, Hudson M, Gajjar A, Sanders M, Gregornik D, Ringwald-Smith K, Williams R, Thompson K, Lussier, K, Todd J, Howard V, Bagwell, B. *The MISS Handbook. The Metabolic and Infusion Support Policy and Procedure Manual.* St. Jude Children's Research Hospital, 1998.

Hendricks KM, Duggan C, Walker WA, eds. *Manual of Pediatric Nutrition.* Hamilton: B. C. Decker, 2000.

Ideno KT. Enteral nutrition. In Gottschlich MM, Matarese LM, Shroots EP, eds., *Nutrition Support Dietetics Core Curriculum*, 2nd ed. Silver Spring, Md.: American Society for Parenteral and Enteral Nutrition, 1993, p. 83.

Motil KJ. Sensitive measures of nutritional status in children in hospital and in the field. *Int J Cancer* 11(Suppl.) 2, 1998.

Nutrition Support Services, Children's Hospital of Philadelphia. *Nutrition Support Services Policies and Procedures.* Philadelphia: Children's Hospital of Philadelphia, June 1995.

Sacks N. Clinical care guidelines for the pediatric oncology patient. *Nutr Oncol* 2(8&9), 1996.

Schwenk FW, Olson D. Pediatrics. In Gottschlich MM, ed. *The Science and Practice of Nutrition Support.* Dubuque, Iowa: Kendall/Hunt, 2001. pp. 347–72.

Walterlow J. Classification and definition of protein calorie malnutrition. *BMJ* 3:566, 1972.

World Health Organization. *Energy and Protein Requirements.* Tech. Rep. Ser. 724. Geneva: WHO, 1985.

14

Mouth Care

Paula K. Groncy, M.D., and Richard D. Udin, D.D.S.

The oral cavity is a frequent site of therapy-related complications including mucositis, ulcerations, infections, bleeding, and xerostomia. Ulcerated mucosa may provide a pathway for intraoral bacteria to become blood borne. Good oral hygiene, including proper control of plaque to decrease the oral reservoir of microorganisms, plays a major part in the reduction or oral complications of therapy.

I. ORAL PROPHYLAXIS

A. Initial evaluation
   1. Each child should have a thorough medical/dental history with an oral/dental and radiographic examination and a dental deplaquing/scaling before the initiation of therapy.
   2. When this cannot be done, perform an initial screening dental evaluation to rule out any dental conditions that may cause complications during induction therapy or surgery.
   3. Defer any treatment until white blood cell counts recover (absolute neutrophil count [ANC] >1000/µl) after initial chemotherapy.

B. Dental treatment (to eliminate/control the foci of infection)
   1. Before therapy, dental care is indicated in all patients whenever possible. *The treatment of dental problems is mandatory for all patients before radiation therapy that will involve the head and neck.*
      a. Definitive restoration of all carious teeth
      b. Nonsurgical periodontal therapy
      c. Removal of all nonrestorable or exfoliating teeth

    d. Endodontic therapy or pulpal treatment is contraindicated for primary and permanent teeth with periapical pathology

    e. Prosthetic/orthodontic devices should be removed

    f. Prophylactic antibiotics may be considered in patients with a venous access device following the recommendations of the American Heart Association

2. During therapy, use conservative dental therapy as oral and medical conditions permit.

    a. Applications of fluoride gel via custom-fabricated flexible plastic trays are strongly suggested for all patients during radiation therapy to the head and neck (and for selected caries-prone patients during chemotherapy). Alternatively, nightly rinsing with an over-the-counter (0.05% neutral sodium fluoride) fluoride-containing rinse may be as effective (such as ACT or Fluorigard). Commercial mouthwashes are not recommended because they are not bacteriostatic, and many of them have a high alcohol content causing burning, stinging, and desiccation of mucous membranes.

    b. Routine dental examinations with radiographic examination and dental deplaquing/scaling may be performed during treatment only when the ANC is $>1,000/\mu L$ and the platelet count is $>100,000/\mu L$. Prophylactic antibiotics may be considered in patients with a venous access device following the recommendations of the American Heart Association.

    c. When the ANC is expected to fall (e.g., with induction chemotherapy), all elective dental procedures are contraindicated.

    d. *Emergency dental procedures* may be necessary in patients with an ANC $<500–1,000/\mu L$, or falling and expected to reach $<500–1,000/\mu L$.

        i. Consider prophylactic intravenous antibiotics

        ii. Perform extractions 7–10 days before the ANC is expected to fall to $<1,000/\mu L$. Extractions should be performed as atraumatically as possible using primary closure with multiple interrupted sutures. The placement of

intra-alveolar packing agents in extraction sites is not recommended.
   iii. Consider platelet transfusion if the platelet count is <40,000/μL.

II. DAILY REGIMEN OF ORAL HYGIENE

A. Standard regimen (ANC >500/μL, platelets >50,000/μL)
   1. Brush teeth daily with a soft-bristle toothbrush (soak toothbrush in hot water to soften further).
   2. Floss with waxed or unwaxed dental floss depending on the patient's and family's skills.
   3. "Pat and push" a thick paste of sodium bicarbonate (baking soda) and a few drops of warm water into the gingival sulcus and around the teeth using a soft toothbrush or use a fluoride-containing gel toothpaste.
   4. Use mouthwash of mild sodium bicarbonate ($^1/_2$ teaspoon baking soda per cup of water) or 0.12% chlorhexidine gluconate (Peridex, Periogard) b.i.d. or t.i.d.
   5. Use a new toothbrush after any infection.

B. Conservative regimen (ANC <500/μL, platelets <50,000/μL)
   1. Cleanse oral hard and soft tissues with a mild solution of sodium bicarbonate ($^1/_2$ teaspoon baking soda per cup of water) using a 4 × 4 gauze pad or Toothette 2–4 times each day and after each episode of emesis. If unable to tolerate cleansing with a gauze pad or Toothette, use the solution as a mouthwash 2–4 times each day and after each episode of emesis.
   2. Use 0.12% chlorhexidine gluconate mouthwash
      a. Rinse the mouth b.i.d. or t.i.d.
      b. Spit out the mouthwash after rinsing.
      c. Do not eat anything for 30 minutes after rinsing.
   3. For children less than 3 years old, use a gauze pad or Toothette soaked in 0.12% chlorhexidine gluconate.

III. PREVENTION AND TREATMENT OF MUCOSITIS

A. Prevention
   1. The incidence and severity of mucositis have been related to the degree of preexisting mucosal disease, oral hygiene, and the nature of therapy.
   2. Use 0.12% chlorhexidine gluconate rinse (see section IIA4).

3. Maintain daily regimen of oral hygiene (see section IIA, B)

B. Treatment
1. Daily oral hygiene (conservative regimen) (section II B)
2. Sucralfate suspension 1g/10ml (40–80mg/kg/day, max 1g/dose) swish and swallow q.i.d.
3. Topical agents may be tried and continued if they relieve symptoms. Their effectiveness is not proven, but for individual patients, they may bring relief. Use the lowest concentration that provides relief of symptoms (many of the following products are also available as lozenges).
   a. Single agents *Caution:* do not use in infants less than 12 months old.
      i. Amide local anesthetics
         Lidocaine HCl viscous solution, 2%
      ii. Esther local anesthetics
         Benzocaine (Hurricaine spray 20%, Cetacaine spray 14%).
      iii. Miscellaneous
         (1) Dyclonine (Dyclone) solution, 0.5%
         (2) Phenol spray 1.4% (Chloraseptic spray)
         (3) Cocaine applied topically with swab or spray (Cocaine HCl topical solution 4%, 10%; Cocaine HCl Viscous topical solution 4%, 10%)
   b. Combination products
      i. Equal parts by volume of diphenhydramine HCl and kaolin-pectin. *Caution:* some formulations of kaolin-pectin may contain aspirin and should be avoided.
      ii. Equal parts (by volume) of 2% viscous lidocaine, diphenhydramine HCl, and Maalox. Swish and spit, apply with a cotton-tipped applicator, or swish and swallow. *Caution:* if swallowed, do not exceed the standard dose of any component. *Note:* antacids may interact with other oral medications.
4. Dietary changes
   a. Dental/mechanical soft diet
   b. Avoid irritating foods (spicy, acidic, temperature extremes).
5. Systemic analgesics (see Chapter 11, section III)

IV. PREVENTION, DIAGNOSIS, AND TREATMENT OF ORAL INFECTIONS

Mucositis induced by chemotherapy or radiation therapy may be due to reactivation of latent herpes simplex virus (HSV), which occurs in 75% of seropositive patients. Secondary infection, usually with candida, can occur. Marginal gingivitis (recognized by an erythematous periapical line) is presumably caused by anaerobes.

A. Prevention
  1. Good oral hygiene
  2. Use of 0.12% chlorhexidine gluconate (see section IIA4)
  3. Prophylaxis against herpes simplex virus (HSV) (see Chapter 1, section VI C)
     a. Acyclovir 80 mg/kg/day divided into 3–5 doses/day (200 mg/5 ml; 200 mg capsule; 400 and 800 mg tablet)
  4. Prophylaxis against fungal infection (see Chapter 1, section IV)
     a. Fluconazole 3–5 mg/kg/day PO as a single daily dose (suspension 10 mg/ml or 40 mg/ml; tablet 50, 100, 150, or 200 mg)
     b. Ketoconazole 5–10 mg/kg/day PO in 2 divided doses (maximum 800 mg/day); 200 mg scored tablet
     c. Nystatin oral suspension 5 ml q.i.d. swish and swallow (do not use within 30 minutes of 0.12% chlorhexidine gluconate)
     d. Clotrimazole troche 10 mg PO 5 times daily
     e. Oral Amphotericin B solution (0.1 mg/ml) 15 ml q.i.d., swish and spit (for patients refractory to the above).

B. Diagnosis
  1. Direct microscopic examination (wet mount or gram stain)
  2. Cultures
     a. Aerobic and anaerobic bacteria
     b. Fungal
     c. Viral (HSV)

C. Treatment
  1. Candida
     a. Fluconazole 6–10 mg/kg/day PO or IV as a single daily dose

2. Herpes simplex virus
    a. Acyclovir 1,500 mg/m^2/day IV (divided q8h)

V. SALIVARY GLAND DYSFUNCTION

Salivary gland dysfunction includes decreased salivary gland flow, viscous ropy saliva and decreased volume of saliva resulting in a shift to highly cariogenic microorganisms seen with some chemotherapeutic agents (e.g., doxorubicin) and radiation therapy that incorporates the salivary glands in the radiation field.

A. Treatment
    1. Custom gel-applicator trays for self-applied topical neutral sodium fluoride. If the patient cannot use trays (because of pain or gagging), he or she may apply fluoride with a toothbrush, Toothette, or cotton-tipped applicator. Alternatively, nightly rinsing with an over-the-counter (0.05% neutral sodium fluoride) fluoride-containing rinse (such as ACT or Fluorigard) may be used.
    2. Good daily oral hygiene regimen
    3. Helpful aids
        a. Saliva substitutes (Salivart, Xerolube)
        b. Mild sodium bicarbonate rinses ($^1/_2$ teaspoon baking soda per cup of water)
        c. Frequent sips of water (carry plastic squeeze bottle filled with water).
        d. Sugar-free chewing gum and/or sugar-free candy in moderation (effect of protracted use unknown). Excessive use may result in osmotic diarrhea.

VI. ORAL AND/OR GINGIVAL BLEEDING

A. Oral hygiene
    1. Discontinue mechanical hygiene and use good daily oral hygiene (conservative regimen).
    2. A major cause of gingival bleeding is gingivitis, and this must be considered and treated if present.

B. Correct existing platelet and coagulation abnormalities if possible.

C. Topical agents
    1. Thrombin solution: apply with 2 × 2 sterile gauze
    2. Avitene: remove from jar using sterile dry hemostat; press onto bleeding site using 2 × 2 sterile gauze pad.

3. Instat: Cut sheet to size, then press onto gingival tissue using 2 × 2 sterile gauze pad.
4. Aminocaproic Acid (Amicar)
   a. Dosage (PO or IV)
      i. Loading Dose: 100–200 mg/kg (maximum 5,000 mg)
      ii. Subsequent: 100 mg/kg/dose q6hr *or* 30 mg/kg/dose q1hr until bleeding stops (maximum 8 doses) *or* continuous IV infusion at 30 mg/kg/hr
      iii. Maximum 18,000 mg/m^2/24h (30,000 mg/24h)
   b. Preparations
      i. Syrup: 250 mg/mL
      ii. Tablet: 500 mg
      iii. Injectable: 250 mg/ml (20 ml Vial)
5. Tranexamic acid (Cyklokapron)
   a. Dosage
      i. 25 mg/kg/dose PO t.i.d. or q.i.d. for 2–8 days
      ii. 10 mg/kg/dose IV t.i.d. or q.i.d
   b. Preparations
      i. Tablet: 500 mg
      ii. Injectable: 100 mg/ml

Bibliography

American Academy of Pediatric Dentistry. Clinical guideline on the dental management of pediatric patients receiving chemotherapy, bone marrow transplantation, and/or radiation. *Pediatr Dent (Sp Iss)* 23(7):82–84, 2001.

Berg J, Bleyer A. Pediatric dentistry in care of the cancer patient. *Pediatr Dent* 17:257–58, 1995.

da Fonseca MA. Pediatric bone marrow transplantation: Oral complications and recommendations for care. *Pediatr Dent* 20(7):386–94, 1998.

Leggott PJ. Oral complications of cancer therapies: Chronic dental complications. *NCI Monogr* 9:173–78, 1990.

National Institutes of Health, Consensus Development Conference Statement. Oral complications of cancer therapies: Diagnosis, prevention, and treatment. *J Am Dental Assoc* 119:179–83, 1989.

Simon AR, Roberts MW. Management of oral complications associated with cancer therapy in pediatric patients. *ASDC J Dent Child* 58:384–89, 1991.

Taketomo CK, Hodding JH, Kraus DM. *Pediatric Dosage Handbook,* 10th edition. Hudson, Ohio: Lexi-Comp Inc, 2003.

15

Central Venous Access

Connie Goes, R.N., and Joan Ronan, R.N.

Children with a diagnosis of cancer requiring chemotherapy benefit greatly from the placement of a long-term central venous access device (CVAD). Central venous access permits the delivery of chemotherapy, medications, total parenteral nutrition, blood, and blood products. Children on intensive chemotherapy protocols also undergo frequent blood sampling. Placement of a CVAD allows for this easily and painlessly.

Indwelling central venous catheters are available in two main types: external tunneled catheters and implanted subcutaneous ports. Each type comes with its own set of advantages and disadvantages. Several factors to consider when choosing a central venous access device include the age of the child, intensity of therapy, frequency of blood sampling, bathing/activity limitations, and family ability to care for the catheter.

For children who need only short-term central access, a percutaneous intravenous central catheter (PICC) may be a more appropriate choice.

I. VENOUS ACCESS DEVICE: TYPES AND ADVANTAGES/DISADVANTAGES

A. External tunneled catheters
External catheters come in single, double, and triple lumens with the choice depending on the intensity of therapy and the amount of supportive care anticipated.

These catheters are placed surgically by cutdown or percutaneous technique with the tip resting at the superior vena cava/right atrial junction. The catheter is radiopaque allowing for visualization by x-ray and fluoroscopy. The internal jugular, external jugular, and subclavian veins are used most frequently for catheter placement. A Dacron cuff is situated approximately 2 cm proximal to the exit site.

Fibrous tissue secures the catheter in place and prevents microorganisms from migrating up the tunnel.

1. Advantages

   External catheters allow for easy infusion of multiple products and pain-free blood sampling. External catheters also allow for blood samples to be drawn in the home, decreasing visits to the hospital or laboratory. External catheters may be removed in a surgical office under local anesthesia.

2. Disadvantages

   External catheters require daily NS/heparin flushes to maintain patency, periodic dressing changes, occasional cap changes, activity restriction (no swimming), and may negatively impact the child's body image. They may be more easily dislodged in infants and toddlers due to accidental pulling on the line. The risk of infection and thrombus formation is greater than with implanted ports.

3. Contraindications

   The primary contraindication in placing an external tunneled catheter is the inability of the family to properly care for the catheter.

B. Implanted subcutaneous ports

Implanted ports consist of two parts: the reservoir, made of stainless steel or titanium with a self-sealing rubber dome, and a silicon catheter. Double-lumen ports are also available but not generally used in very young children. These devices are placed in the operating room under x-ray or fluoroscopic guidance. The internal jugular, external jugular, subclavian, and facial veins are used most frequently. The reservoir is sutured into an SC pocket and the catheter tip is placed into the superior vena cava/right atrial junction.

Ports are accessed using a noncoring Huber needle using sterile technique.

1. Advantages

   Implanted ports require minimal care. Flushing is recommended monthly and/or after each use. Impact on body image is less than that with external catheters, but scar or keloid formation may be greater. There are no restrictions on bathing/swimming except when accessed.

2. Disadvantages
Accessing a port requires a needle stick. Application of a topical anesthetic cream will decrease anxiety and discomfort during the access procedure. In younger children, anxiety may not be decreased by anesthetic creams due to underlying needle phobia. In an effort to decrease the risk of infection, some institutions do not use the port for routine blood sampling, instead preferring peripheral venipuncture. Many children live a distance from the treating institutions using local laboratories with personnel unqualified to access a port. Implanted port must be removed in the operating room under general anesthesia.

3. Contraindications
Port placement should be avoided in children with extreme obesity and young age as they are more difficult to access and the potential for accidental dislodgment is greater. Children with uncorrectable coagulopathy or prolonged thrombocytopenia are at risk for bleeding during needle placement and removal.

II. IMPACT OF BLOOD COUNTS ON CVAD PLACEMENT

A. Thrombocytopenia
A venous access device can safely be placed in a child with a platelet count >50,000/mm^3. The platelet count should be kept >30,000/mm^3 for up to 72 hours after placement to prevent bleeding at the exit site or port pocket.

B. Neutropenia
An ANC >1,000/mm^3 is preferable at the time of insertion. Unfortunately, many children are neutropenic at the time of diagnosis and initiation of therapy when line placement usually occurs. A one-time dose of a broad-spectrum antibiotic may be given at the time of line placement.

III. INFECTIOUS COMPLICATIONS

A. Catheter-related bacteremia
Device related infections are a major cause of morbidity in children with cancer. Multiple studies have shown the incidence ranging from 2–60%. The most frequent causative organism is coagulase-negative Staphylococcus.

Gram-negative infections are more often seen in children with prolonged neutropenia. With appropriate antibiotic therapy, the infection is generally cleared. However, candida infections are usually resistant to therapy. These infections often require catheter removal and treatment with appropriate antifungal therapy.

1. Definition

   A bloodstream infection in a child with a CVAD who presents with clinical signs of sepsis without an obvious source.

2. Diagnosis

   a. Clinical signs of sepsis (which include fever with or without chills after catheter flush, hypotension, tachycardia, tachypnea), or

   b. Any positive blood culture from the catheter

3. Treatment

   a. Administration of antibiotics to cover gram-positive and gram-negative organisms (neutropenic patients only) seen most commonly in each institution. (See Chapter 3 Section IVB and Table 3.2)

   b. For the clinically stable non-neutropenic child, treatment with a third-generation cephalosporin such as ceftriaxone (50–75 mg/kg/d) may be used alone until blood culture results are known at 72 hours. These children may safely be treated in the outpatient setting. Antibiotic administration should be alternated between lumens per institution policy.

   c. Antibiotic coverage should continue for 7–14 days after blood cultures become negative.

   d. A thrombolytic agent can be used if a catheter thrombus is present. The catheter should be removed if the blood cultures remain positive at 72 hours despite appropriate therapy. Removal is also recommended if the condition of the child deteriorates or with recurrent infections with the same organisms.

B. Tunnel/port pocket infections

   1. Definition

      Erythema, tenderness, and/or swelling along the catheter tunnel or over the port pocket. Drainage may be present at the catheter exit site/port pocket.

2. Diagnosis
   a. Clinical signs (erythema, swelling, tenderness, exudate), or
   b. Positive exudate culture
3. Treatment
   Tunnel/port pocket infections are generally resistant to therapy. IV antibiotics may be given, but removal of the catheter is usually necessary. In neutropenic patients, the classic signs of infection may not be present. As the white blood count recovers, erythema, swelling, tenderness, and/or exudate may develop.

C. Exit site infection
   1. Definition
      Erythema, swelling, tenderness, and exudate at the catheter exit site.
   2. Diagnosis
      Positive exudates culture
   3. Treatment
      Topical antibiotic therapy and frequent dressing changes is generally sufficient. Systemic therapy for neutropenic patients or poor response to local measures may increase the likelihood of salvaging the catheter. Pseudomonas is typically difficult to treat and generally necessitates catheter removal.

D. Catheter replacement
   Replacement of a catheter removed due to infection should not occur until an entire course of antibiotics has been completed and off-treatment blood cultures are documented to be negative.

IV. CATHETER-RELATED THROMBOTIC OCCLUSIONS

A second major complication related to the presence of a venous access device is thrombus formation causing a withdrawal or complete occlusion. A withdrawal occlusion allows infusion of fluids with poor or no blood return. A complete occlusion prevents both fluid infusion and blood return. Risk factors include poor catheter tip placement, placement on the left side of the chest, inadequate flushing, inappropriate catheter size compared to vessel size, and medications causing coagulopathies. Clinical assessment of a poorly functioning catheter includes reaccessing implantable ports, checking for kinks in catheter, changing position, having the child perform a Valsalva maneuver, and infusion of fluid. Imaging assessment for thrombus formation would include an echocardiogram, IV contrast dye study, or a venogram.

A. Types of thrombotic occlusion
   1. Intraluminal: The thrombus is present within a lumen of the catheter, which makes drawing blood and infusing fluids difficult. A total occlusion may occur preventing both infusion of fluids and withdrawal of blood.
   2. Fibrin sleeve: Almost immediately after placing a catheter, fibrin begins collecting along the side of the catheter. The sleeve continues to grow along the catheter and occludes the tip. This type of occlusion acts as a one-way valve allowing fluid to be infused easily, but prevents blood from being drawn.
   3. Portal reservoir obstruction: The thrombus occurs within the reservoir creating a "reverse ball-valve." Blood is drawn without difficulty, but fluids cannot be infused.
   4. Mural thrombus: The vessel becomes thrombosed leading to catheter occlusion.

B. Treatment of withdrawal occlusions (see also Table 5.7)
   1. Tissue plasminogen activator (t-PA) (alteplase) bolus:
      a. t-PA 0.5 or 1 mg/ml concentration.
      b. For external catheters, instill 1 ml (0.5 mg/ml) and allow to dwell for 30–60 minutes.
      c. For implanted ports, instill 2 ml (0.5 mg t-PA/ml) and allow to dwell for 30–60 minutes.
      d. A second bolus dose is indicated if the catheter remains occluded or draws sluggishly.
      e. Once clear, flush the catheter per institution policy.
      f. If the catheter remains occluded after 2 bolus doses, a continuous infusion is indicated.
   2. t-PA infusion
      a. t-PA at a dose 0.01 mg/kg/h is infused over 6–12 hours.
      b. Increase dose to 0.02 mg/kg/h for an additional 6 hours if no improvement.
      c. Increase dose to 0.03 mg/kg/h for an additional 6 hours if line remains occluded.
      d. Monitor fibrinogen (<100 mg/dl) at 6-hour intervals, as it tends to drop rapidly.

e. Monitor for signs of infection or reaction to the t-PA (fever, flushing, chills, bleeding, or oozing).
f. Line removal is indicated if unable to clear after three infusions.

C. Treatment of complete thrombotic occlusion
   1. Negative pressure technique
      a. Attach a 10 ml syringe filled with the appropriate single dose of t-PA to the catheter or Huber needle.
      b. Withdraw as much flush solution as possible and allow the t-PA to be slowly pulled back into the catheter.
      c. Do not permit the plunger to snap back as damage to the catheter may occur.
      d. Repeat this mixing procedure every 5–15 minutes for a half-hour.
      e. After 2–3 mixes, allow the solution to dwell for 60 minutes.
      f. t-PA is slowly dissolving the thrombus if the drawback solution begins to turn red.
      g. If unable to draw blood, give a second dose of t-PA.
      h. Once cleared, flush catheter per institution policy.
      i. Remove the catheter if unable to clear with 2 doses of t-PA.

V. CATHETER-RELATED PRECIPITATE OCCLUSIONS

Total peripheral nutrition (TPN) occlusions are caused by $CaPO_4$ precipitate. Medication precipitates are generally due to inadequate flushing between incompatible medications or infusing drugs at improper dilution. Treatment of these occlusions is geared at changing pH through the use of HCl or $NaHCO_3$ to increase the solubility of the precipitate.

A. Treatment
   1. TPN occlusion
      a. Instill 0.5 ml of 0.1N HCl and allow to dwell for 20 minutes.
      b. Withdraw HCl and assess for patency.
      c. If the catheter is still occluded, attempt HCL dwell for 1–2 additional instillations.
      d. If the catheter clears, flush per institution policy.
      e. If the catheter fails to clear, remove the line.

2. Medication occlusion
   a. Follow same procedure as for TPN occlusion, substituting $NaHCO_3$ (1 meq/ml) for the 0.1N HCl.

VI. MECHANICAL COMPLICATIONS

A. Pinch-off syndrome
   The catheter becomes occluded as the line is compressed between the clavicle and the first rib making sample collection difficult. A chest x-ray may detect compression of the catheter. Blood may be obtained by having the child raise his or her arms or roll his or her shoulders back. A pinched catheter becomes weak and may develop a fracture, permitting fluids to be leaked subcutaneously. The line may break off, resulting in catheter embolism. Serious consideration should be given to removing a catheter with pinch-off syndrome.

B. Malposition
   Malposition may occur as a result of poor placement or by migration of the catheter into a smaller vessel. This may cause difficulty withdrawing blood, pain on infusion, or complaint of an audible sound in the ipsilateral ear when flushed. A lateral chest x-ray will demonstrate tip location. In general, if the line is not functioning properly, it will need to be replaced.

C. Extravasation
   1. External tunneled catheter
      Extravasation results from two complications. The presence of a large sleeve thrombus may cause the infused solution to backtrack between the catheter and sleeve. If the thrombus extends up to the vessel insertion site, the fluid may leak through the venotomy site. The second cause of extravasation is due to catheter fractures within the tunnel, most commonly due to the pinch-off syndrome.
   2. Implanted port
      Improper insertion of the Huber needle will result in extravasation. Dislodgement of the Huber needle due to an inappropriate size needle, poor stabilization of the needle, obesity, and accidental tugging on the IV lines can be another cause of extravasation. Mechanical causes include separation of the catheter from the

reservoir, fracture of the catheter distal to the cannu-
lated vein, and failure of the reservoir.
3. Treatment
    a. For extravasation of a vesicant, (see Chapter 8).
    b. For extravasation of a nonvesicant solution, use
        warm packs to enhance resorption of fluid and pain
        medications as needed.

D. Fracture
    A fracture is a break in the external or internal portion of the
    catheter. Fractures of the catheter within the tunnel or port
    reservoir can be diagnosed by either clinical symptoms of
    difficulty with infusion, pain on infusion, swelling in the
    area, or by an IV contrast study. Catheter embolization, a
    complete break of the internal portion of the catheter, may
    occur as a result of the pinch-off syndrome. The catheter
    is squeezed between the clavicle, breaks off, and travels to
    the right ventricle or pulmonary artery.
    1. External fracture
        Manufacture repair kits are available for the external
        portion of tunneled catheters. The repair is performed
        under sterile conditions by a nurse or physician. The
        catheter may be used immediately if necessary, but it
        may be prudent to wait 24 hours if possible. A tem-
        porary repair may be performed, also under sterile
        conditions, by use of a Jelco needle. The catheter is
        cleansed with Betadine, then cut between the fracture
        and the exit site. A Jelco needle with the stylet pulled
        back slightly to prevent puncture is inserted into the
        lumen. The stylet is removed and an empty syringe is
        attached. A permanent repair is performed as soon as
        possible.
    2. Internal fracture
        These lines are not reparable and must be removed. It
        may be possible to preserve the port pocket for inser-
        tion of another device.
            An embolized catheter is removed in the cardiac
        catheterization lab.

Bibliography

Andris D, Krzywda, E. Central venous access. *Nursing Clinics of North America* 32:719–37, 1997.

Bagnall-Reeb H, Perry S. Surgery. In *Nursing Care of Children and Adolescents with Cancer,* 3rd edition. Philadelphia: W. B. Saunders Company, 2002, pp. 101–8.

DiCarlo I, Fisichella P, Russello D, et al. Catheter fracture and cardiac migration: A rare complication of totally implantable venous devices. *J Surgical Oncology* 73:172–73, 2000.

Duffy L, Kerzner B, Gebus V, Dice J. Treatment of central venous catheter occlusions with hydrochloric acid. *Journal of Pediatrics* 114:1002–4, 1989.

Hastings C. Central venous catheters. In *The Children's Hospital Oakland Hematology/Oncology Handbook*. St. Louis: Mosby, 2002.

Hooke C. Recombinant tissue plasminogen activator for central venous device occlusion. *J Pediatric Oncology Nursing* 17:174–78, 2000.

Hoope B. Central venous catheter-related infections: Pathogenesis, predictors, and prevention. *Heart and Lung* 24:333–37, 1995.

Keung Y, Watkins K, Chen S, et al. Comparative study of infectious complications of different types of chronic central venous access devices. *Cancer* 73:2832–37, 1994.

Rackhoff W, Ge J, Harland N, et al. Central venous catheter use and the risk of infection in children with acute lymphoblastic leukemia: A report from the Children's Cancer Group. *J Pediatric Hematology/Oncology* 21:260–67, 1999.

Ross V, Orr P. Prevention of infections related to central venous catheters. *Critical Care Nursing Quarterly* 20:79–88, 1997.

16

The Sexually Mature Young Adult Patient with Cancer

Paula K. Groncy, M.D., and Melissa E. Huggins, M.D.

The sexually mature teenager with cancer presents a special challenge to the pediatric oncologist. This chapter touches briefly on ways the pediatric oncologist and co-professionals may assist these young people as they assume their new responsibilities in the transition to adulthood while facing the additional burdens of cancer treatment.

I. **PRETREATMENT RECOMMENDATIONS**

    A. At the onset of treatment, a relationship based on respect, trust, and confidentiality between the patient, the physician, and other health care providers must be established. The physician must set the model for open, honest, and trustworthy communication. It must be clear to the young patient that he or she has a personal physician who will represent his or her interests and concerns.

    B. Discussions about sexuality with the teenage patient must take place privately and may include the patient's parents when the patient gives permission.

    C. In addition to educating the patient about the cause, treatment, and prognosis of the cancer, the impact of the disease on school, normal activities, friendship, and sexuality should also be discussed. Because of changes in physical and psychosocial status before, during, and after treatment, these topics should be reviewed with the patient at corresponding intervals.

    D. Before induction of chemotherapy, the female patient should have a complete gynecologic history. A negative pregnancy test should be documented.

E.   For the sexually active patient, birth control options should be encouraged and initiated. Options that decrease menstrual frequency or induce amenorrhea should be encouraged. These include the oral contraceptive pill (OCP), and depo-medroxyprogesterone acetate (DMPA).

F.   The possibility of current and future pregnancy should be addressed with the female patient. The potential physical stress of pregnancy on the patient's disease and treatment course should be discussed. Additionally, the patient's future fertility related to the disease and treatment must be addressed. If future fertility is threatened, discuss indications for cryopreserved oocytes or cryopreserved embryos before treatment.

G.   The difference between fertility and virility should be explained to the male patient. Sperm banking should be recommended before initiation of chemotherapy if there is a risk of potential oligospermia and aspermia with treatment.

II. PREVENTION AND MANAGEMENT OF INFECTION

A.   Abrasions
1.   Vaginal abrasions and mucosal abnormalities have been associated with the use of tampons. The immunocompetent person is at an increased risk of infection with superabsorbency tampons or when a tampon is left in place longer than recommended. Therefore, immunodeficient patients should use sanitary napkins for menstrual bleeding to decrease infection risk.
2.   To decrease mucosal injury and infection, the diaphragm, vaginal contraceptive sponge, cervical cap, intrauterine device, and contraceptive vaginal ring should be avoided birth control options.
3.   Over-the-counter water-based lubricants (e.g., Astroglide) may be used to limit mucosal abrasions during intercourse.

B.   Intercourse
1.   Sexually active female patients with an absolute neutrophil count (ANC) <500/mm^3 have an increased risk of vaginal mucosa disruption and bacterial shower with subsequent infection. Therefore, abstinence is recommended.

2. Both male and female patients must be informed that infection risk is increased with any episode of intercourse despite the ANC level.
3. Condoms should be recommended to decrease infection risk. Vaginal spermicides (e.g., nonoxynol-9) are not effective in preventing sexually transmitted disease and increase risks of vaginal irritation and urinary tract infection. Condoms should be used in addition to a more efficacious method of birth control (e.g., OCP or DMPA) in the female patient.

C. Sexually transmitted diseases
   1. Human papillomavirus (HPV) infection can manifest as visible genital warts or as a subclinical infection without a visible lesion. Certain strains of HPV are associated with a greater risk of developing cervical, vulvar, and vaginal cancer, especially in the immunodeficient patient. A definitive diagnosis of high-risk HPV is achieved by detecting the viral nucleic acid (DNA or RNA) or capsid protein. This test is not indicated as a screening test, even in the immunodeficient patient. It is, however, recommended when a PAP smear result demonstrates atypical cells of undetermined significance (ASCUS).
   2. Rates of chlamydia and gonorrhea are highest in females 15–19 years old. Asymptomatic females should undergo screening. All male patients with urethritis should undergo screening. Advancement of untreated disease can result in pelvic inflammatory disease in females and epididymitis in males.
   3. Genital herpes simplex is more likely to be acquired and to recur in immunodeficient states. To decrease outbreaks, daily suppressive therapy may be required with antiviral medications (e.g., acyclovir, valacyclovir, and famciclovir).
   4. Testing for HIV, hepatitis, and syphilis should be offered to the sexually active patient.

III. PREVENTION AND MANAGEMENT OF EXCESSIVE MENSTRUAL BLEEDING

A. Prevention
   Consider menstrual suppression to decrease the risk of associated hemorrhage and anemia before induction of

chemotherapy. The goal of prophylactic therapy is to decrease menstrual frequency or induce endometrial atrophy.

1. Menstrual frequency can be decreased with daily administration of a low-dose, monophasic, combined oral contraceptive pill. This regimen can be continued for up to 4 months without withdrawal bleeding. The patient should be instructed to remove the 7 placebo pills in each pack. When the platelet count is $>50,000/mm^3$ and expected to remain stable, a withdrawal bleed can occur by stopping the oral contraceptive pill for 1 week.

   a. To minimize breakthrough bleeding risk, prescribe a monophasic OCP containing 30 or 35 ug ethinyl estradiol with norgestrel (e.g., Lo/Ovral), norgestimate (e.g., Ortho-Cyclen), or levonorgestrel (e.g., Nordette).

   b. Daily dosing of oral contraceptive pills requires patient compliance. Unfortunately, monthly injectable combined contraception with medroxyprogesterone/estradiol cypionate (e.g., Lunelle) is not an appropriate alternative because it is associated with increased bleeding irregularities compared to OCPs, and withdrawal bleeding cannot be suppressed under the recommended dosing guidelines.

   c. The World Health Organization guidelines for OCP use include the contraindications of a history of deep vein thrombosis or pulmonary embolism, liver cancer, breast cancer, surgery of the lower extremities, and/or prolonged immobilization. These guidelines should be referred to for other comorbid conditions that may be contraindicated.

2. Endometrial atrophy and amenorrhea can be achieved with depo-medroxyprogesterone acetate (DMPA) 150 mg IM every 12 weeks. It is a superior alternative to OCPs for increased compliance, avoidance of estrogen side effects, and negligible medication interaction.

   a. Irritability, depression, and anxiety have been associated with DMPA use.

   b. Because DMPA has been shown to induce decreased bone mineral density, *it should be avoided in the adolescent at risk for osteoporosis.* This includes patients with significant steroid exposure, chronic renal disease, chronic amenorrhea, eating disorders, or those who are nonambulatory.

B. Management
Pregnancy, thrombocytopenia, and coagulopathy must be ruled out when excessive bleeding occurs. Once these are excluded from the differential diagnosis, the most likely cause is dysfunctional uterine bleeding. After assessing hemodynamic stability, the clinician should perform a pelvic exam to determine the origin of the bleeding.
1. Normal hemoglobin
   a. Monitor with frequent hemoglobin levels during heavy bleeding episode.
   b. If the patient is currently taking an OCP, confirm compliance. Breakthrough bleeding can occur in the first months of OCP use, but is minimized with pills containing norgestrel, norgestimate, or levonorgestrel. Increase dose to 2 pills a day until bleeding resolves or add 20 ug of ethinyl estradiol for 7–10 days.
   c. DMPA is associated with initial irregular bleeding. Simultaneous estrogen administration for the first 3 weeks of the first 2 injections can decrease this undesirable effect. Amenorrhea is achieved in 3 months in 30% of the patients, and in 12 months by more than 50% of the patients.
   d. If the patient is not on prophylaxis with OCP or DMPA, begin therapy with OPCs as described above. Administering DMPA with active bleeding during chemotherapy may initially worsen the bleeding profile.
   e. Begin iron supplementation.
2. Hemoglobin 8–12 g/dL
   a. Patients can often be managed in the outpatient setting if hemodynamically stable.
   b. Start a taper regimen with a combined, monophasic oral contraceptive pill containing 35 ug of estrogen (e.g., Lo/Ovral). Administer one pill every 6–8 hours for 24–48 hours. If bleeding continues, increase the estrogen dose to 50 ug (e.g., Ovral) every 6 hours. With cessation of bleeding, increase the dosing interval over 1 week until patient is taking

1 pill per day. Continue with the 35 ug estrogen dose for up to 3 months with a scheduled withdrawal bleed as described above. An antiemetic is recommended approximately 30 minutes before each dose of the oral contraceptive pill during the multiple dose taper.

   c. Begin recombinant human erythropoietin (e.g., Epogen, Procrit) with iron supplementation.

3. Hemoglobin <8 g/dL

   a. Hospitalization with IV hydration and prompt hormonal therapy is required. First administer a 50 ug combined oral contraceptive (e.g., Ovral) every 6 hours to stabilize the endometrium. If bleeding doesn't respond after 1 or 2 doses, add IV conjugated estrogen (e.g., Premarin) 25 mg every 6 hours to the existing regimen. Discontinue the Premarin as soon as the bleeding has stopped, not to exceed 6 doses. Taper the oral contraceptive to 1 pill per over one week. Continue with the 35 ug estrogen dose for up to 3 months with a scheduled withdrawal bleed as described above. An antiemetic is recommended approximately 30 minutes before each dose of the oral contraceptive pill during the multidose taper.

   b. Dilation and curettage is rarely required in the adolescent population.

   c. RBC transfusion may be necessary.

IV. SEXUALITY AND CONTRACEPTION

A. Communication

Every young man and woman needs the opportunity to discuss the developmental issues of sexuality that encompass more than sexual function. The combined experience of the physiologic changes of sexual development in the period of adolescence with physical alterations from cancer and its treatment will affect patients' perception of themselves and their body. Counseling should be available to address the physical issues of decision-making, family conflicts, peer pressure, and physical alterations from cancer treatment.

B. Contraception
   1. Discuss the need for contraception with every sexually active teenage patient.
   2. Emphasize that contraception dose not eliminate the spread of HIV/AIDS.
   3. Both male and female patients should be counseled that if a woman is using OCPs or DMPA to prevent pregnancy, condoms must also be used to prevent infection.
   4. Discuss emergency contraception with the patient and a parent. Plan B is a commonly used regimen consisting of 2 doses of levonorgestrel 0.75 mg at 12-hour intervals. Emergency contraception should be administered as soon as possible after unprotected intercourse, not to exceed 72 hours.

Bibliography

Centers for Disease Control and Prevention. Guidelines for treatment of sexually transmitted diseases. *Morb Mortal Wkly Rep* 47(RR-1):4–6, 1998.

Greydanus DE, Patel DR, Rimso ME. Contraception in the adolescent: An update. *Pediatrics* 107(3):562–73, 2001.

Kaunitz AM. Long-acting injectable contraception with depot medroxyprogesterone acetate. *Am J Obstet Gynecol* 170:1543, 1994.

Kaunitz AM. Injectable contraception: New and existing options. *Obstet Gynecol Clin North Am* 27(4):741–80, 2000.

Mitan LA, Slap GB. Adolescent menstrual disorders. *Med Clin North Am* 84(4):851–68, 2000.

Munro MG. Contemporary management of abnormal uterine bleeding. *Obstet Gynecol Clin North Am* 27(2):287–304, 2000.

Workowski KA. Sexually transmitted diseases treatment guidelines, 2002. *Morb Mortal Wkly Rep* 51(RR-6): 1, 2002.

World Health Organization. *Improving Access to Quality Care in Family Planning: Medical Eligibility Criteria for Contraceptive Use.* Geneva: World Health Organization, 1996.

17

Care of the Hematopoietic Stem Cell Transplant Patient after Leaving the Transplant Center

Kenneth De Santes, M.D., and Adrianna Vlachos, M.D.

Hematopoietic stem cell transplantation (HSCT) is an established treatment for a variety of malignant, hematologic, and immunologic disorders. The stem cells used for transplant may be obtained from the patient (autologous transplant), or from a related or unrelated donor who is human leukocyte antigen (HLA) compatible with the patient (allogeneic transplant). Stem cells are currently derived from three different sources: bone marrow, peripheral blood, and umbilical cord blood. There are potential advantages and drawbacks associated with each stem cell product (see Table 17.1). Many other factors influence the nature and severity of various post-transplant complications including the pretransplant conditioning regimen, HLA compatibility of the donor, graft manipulation (e.g., T cell depletion, tumor purging), as well as the patient's age, underlying disease, and prior therapy.

The conditioning regimen is used to prepare patients for the stem cell infusion and generally consists of high-dose chemotherapy, with or without regional or total body irradiation (TBI). The goals of the conditioning regimen may include the eradication of malignant cells, creation of "space" in the marrow by destroying host stem cells, and/or induction of immunosuppression to facilitate engraftment of allogeneic donor cells. After the transplant, there is an obligatory period of pancytopenia, which has been shortened, to some extent, by the use of peripheral blood stem

Table 17.1.
Characteristics of Different Hematopoietic Stem Cell Grafts

Stem Cell Source	Risk of Graft Failure	Tempo of Engraftment	Risk of Acute GVHD	Risk of Chronic GVHD
Autologous donor				
Bone marrow	Low	Moderate	None	None
Peripheral blood	Low	Fast	None	None
Matched related donor				
Bone marrow	Low	Moderate	Moderate	Moderate
Peripheral blood	Low	Fast	Moderate	High
Umbilical cord blood	Low	Slow	Low	Low
Unrelated donor				
Bone marrow	Low	Moderate	High	High
Peripheral blood	Low	Fast	High	High
Umbilical cord blood	Moderate	Slow	Moderate	Low
T-cell depleted bone marrow or blood	Moderate	Variable	Low	Moderate

cells (PBSC) and hematopoietic growth factors. Discharge from the transplant center usually occurs when the patient achieves a stable ANC $>500–1000/mm^3$, resolves any acute infectious or other transplant-related complications, and is obtaining adequate nutritional support. At the time of discharge, all HSCT patients remain profoundly immunocompromised, especially those who develop graft versus host disease (GVHD), and many still require platelet and red blood cell transfusion support.

Economic pressures and the increased use of mobilized PBSC have resulted in earlier discharge from the HSCT unit. Consequently, general pediatricians and pediatric oncologists who may have limited transplant experience are assuming greater responsibility for the care of these children. Management of the HSCT patient requires knowledge of the complications that can arise at different times after transplant, recognition of these problems, and the early implementation of appropriate therapy.

I.   HEMATOLOGIC SUPPORT

A. Background
1. HSCT patients are generally not discharged from the transplant unit until they have achieved stable neutrophil engraftment (ANC $\geq 500/mm^3$). However, it is not unusual for patients to require red blood

cell and/or platelet transfusion support after leaving the hospital. Generally, transfusion independence is achieved 1–2 months after transplant. A prolonged delay in hematopoietic reconstitution, or the development of late cytopenias after initial recovery, mandates further evaluation. Hematologic deficiencies may be due to poor graft function, peripheral destruction of blood cells, or a combination of these events. Possible causes include infections, drugs, GVHD, autoimmune disease, late graft failure, relapse of the underlying malignancy, or the development of secondary leukemia or myelodysplasia.

2. Management of cytopenias involves:
   a. Identifying and treating possible causes
   b. Providing red blood cell and/or platelet transfusions
   c. Use of hematopoietic growth factors

3. Blood products should *always* be irradiated before administration to eliminate the risk of transfusion-associated GVHD.

4. If both patient and donor are CMV-negative, then CMV-negative products should be provided whenever possible. If CMV-negative products are unavailable, then a leukocyte filter should be used to reduce the risk of CMV transmission. Leukocyte filters may also reduce the risk of alloimmunization.

5. If patient and/or donor are CMV-positive, most blood banks will not release CMV-negative products and leukocyte-filtered blood products should be used.

B. Anemia

Most patients do not attain a normal hemoglobin level for several months after HSCT. However, the persistence of severe anemia requiring transfusion support beyond 2–3 months, or the development of anemia after achieving normal erythropoiesis requires investigation.

1. Possible causes, diagnostic procedures and treatment options are listed in Table 17.2.

2. Transfusion with irradiated, CMV-negative and/or leukocyte-filtered packed red blood cells should be considered if:
   a. The hemoglobin falls below 7.0–8.0 gm/dl, or
   b. Symptoms develop (e.g., fatigue, dizziness)

Table 17.2.

Hematologic Problems after HSCT

Problem	Etiology	Diagnostic Studies	Treatment Options
Anemia	Drugs	(e.g., CSA)	Consider EPO if level <500 U/L
	HUS	RBC morphology, LDH, creatinine, platelet count	Consider stopping CSA; plasmapheresis
	Autoimmune hemolytic	Coombs test, reticulocyte count, bilirubin	Steroids, CSA, IVIG, other immuno-suppressive agents, rituximab, splenectomy
	Parvovirus	PCR for parvovirus	IVIG
	Graft failure	Engraftment studies	Second transplant
	Relapse	Bone marrow aspirate	Consider stopping CSA; donor leukocyte infusion; second transplant
	Unknown	EPO level, bone marrow aspirate	Consider EPO if level <500 U/L
Thrombocytopenia	GVHD	Biopsy, bilirubin, GGT	Steroids, CSA, ATG, other immuno-suppressive agents
	Infection	Cultures	Antibiotics
	Relapse	Bone marrow aspirate	Consider stopping CSA; donor leukocyte infusion; second transplant
	Drugs	(e.g., azathioprine)	Consider alternative agent
	ITP	Platelet-associated Ig, bone marrow aspirate	IVIG, WinRho, steroids, splenectomy
	Graft failure	Engraftment studies	Second transplant
	Unknown	Bone marrow aspirate	Platelet transfusion
Neutropenia	Drugs	(e.g., ganciclovir, TMP/SMX, azathioprine)	Consider alternative agent, G or GM-CSF
	GVHD	Biopsy, bilirubin, GGT	Steroids, CSA, ATG, other immuno-suppressive agents
	CMV infection	CMV DNA or antigen detection	Ganciclovir, IVIG, foscarnet
	Graft failure	Engraftment studies	Second transplant
	Unknown	Bone marrow aspirate	Consider G or GM-CSF if ANC <500/mm^3

Note: HSCT, hematopoietic stem cell transplant; IVIG, intravenous immunoglobulin; HUS, hemolytic uremic syndrome; TTP, thrombotic thrombocytopenic purpura; CSA, cyclosporin; PCR, polymerase chain reaction; EPO, erythropoietin; GVHD, graft versus host disease; ATG, antithymocyte globulin; ITP, immune thrombocytopenic purpura; CMV, cytomegalovirus.

3. Erythropoietin (EPO) therapy may be considered for the patient with low EPO levels. The patient will generally convert to the donor's blood type. During this period, which occurs 2–4 months after transplant, patients may require more transfusion support. EPO may be effective at this time to decrease the number of transfusions.

C. Thrombocytopenia
Most children become independent of platelet transfusions within 2 months of their transplant. The persistence of a transfusion requirement beyond 2–3 months, in the absence of an obvious cause (e.g., severe GVHD), requires investigation. Similarly, the development of thrombocytopenia after attaining a normal platelet count mandates further evaluation.
1. Possible etiologies, suggested evaluations, and treatment options are listed in Table 17.2.
2. Transfusion with CMV-negative and/or leukocyte-filtered platelets should be considered if:
    a. The platelet count falls below 10–$15,000/mm^3$, or
    b. Bleeding occurs
3. If a patient experiences significant bleeding (e.g., gross hematuria) the platelet count should be maintained $50,000/mm^3$.
4. Apheresis units should be used, if possible, to reduce donor exposures.
5. Minimal data are currently available regarding the use of thrombopoietic growth factors (e.g., thrombopoietin, IL-11) in stem cell transplant recipients.

D. Neutropenia
Patients are generally not discharged from the HSCT unit until they have recovered from the obligatory period of neutropenia early after transplant.
1. The ANC may fluctuate for several months after transplantation but does not usually fall below $500/mm^3$.
2. Persistent severe neutropenia after discharge requires further evaluation and treatment (see Table 17.2).
3. Some patients may benefit from intermittent doses of G-CSF or GM-CSF (3–7 days/wk) to maintain an ANC $>500/mm^3$.

II. NUTRITIONAL CONSIDERATIONS

A. Nutritional support and monitoring
    Nearly all children require nutritional support at the time
    of HSCT and for several weeks to months thereafter. Caloric
    supplementation may be provided by intravenous hyperal-
    imentation or nasogastric feeds, depending on the child's
    clinical status and preferences of the transplant team. Sup-
    port is gradually weaned over 2–4 weeks as the patient
    resumes normal dietary habits. Close monitoring of nutri-
    tional status is an important component of post-transplant
    care.
    1. Reasons for poor dietary caloric intake early after
        transplant may include:
        a. Anorexia, nausea, and mucositis consequent to the
            conditioning regimen
        b. Psychological food aversions
        c. Depression
        d. Gastrointestinal GVHD, oral GVHD
        e. Xerostomia and/or damaged taste buds
        f. Infection or other complications that cause general
            malaise
        g. Dietary restrictions placed on patients because of
            iatrogenic immunodeficiency (see IIB)
    2. Weight and dietary history should be obtained weekly
        after discharge until all significant nutritional problems
        have resolved.
    3. Parents should be instructed to keep a log of their
        child's oral intake.
    4. Once a child is taking ~75% of his or her caloric re-
        quirements by mouth, consideration should be given
        to stopping supplemental enteral/parenteral support.
    5. Consultation with a nutritionist may be quite helpful,
        especially for patients who require prolonged nutri-
        tional support.
    6. Special attention should be given to new or worsening
        nausea, anorexia, vomiting, or diarrhea since this may
        be indicative of:
        a. Infection
        b. Gastrointestinal GVHD
    7. Common dietary problems and suggested solutions are
        shown in Table 17.3.

Table 17.3.
Common Dietary Problems after HSCT and Suggested Solutions

Problem	Suggestions	Comment
Nausea and vomiting	Eat small, frequent meals Avoid foods with strong odors Avoid fatty or spicy foods Drink clear cool liquids Drink liquids slowly Consider use of antiemetics	Very common If persistent or worsening, consider evaluation for GVHD, gastritis, sinusitis, or association with a specific drug.
Anorexia	Eat small frequent meals Consume high-calorie foods, such as milkshakes, nutritional formulas (e.g., Ensure), peanut butter Try to make mealtime fun and relaxed Praise good eating; avoid arguing or nagging	Very common If persistent or worsening, consider evaluation for upper GI GVHD, oral infection, depression.
Diarrhea	Avoid fatty/greasy foods Limit intake of dairy products or consider use of lactase or low-lactose milk products Consume easy-to-digest carbohydrates, such as rice, white bread, potatoes Drink fluids frequently between meals to avoid dehydration Avoid caffeinated soft drinks	Consider evaluation for infection (e.g., CMV, Cryptosporidium), and GI GVHD
Xerostomia	Add sauces or broths to food Drink liquids with meals (citrus juices may stimulate saliva production) Keep mouth moist with rinsing, ice chips, sugarless hard candy or gum Consider use of an over-the-counter saliva substitute	Consider evaluation for oral chronic GVHD
Change in taste	Select foods with strong flavors; try tart foods Select foods that smell appetizing Use plastic utensils if foods taste metallic Add sauces to foods, try marinades on meats Try eating meat with something sweet such as cranberry sauce or applesauce	

B. Dietary restrictions and recommendations

The CDC, Infectious Diseases Society of America, and American Society of Blood and Marrow Transplantation have recently published guidelines for food and beverage safety after HSCT. The recommendations resulting from this collaborative effort are summarized in IIB.1–3 and in Table 17.4. In general, these precautions should be observed for 3 months after autologous HSCT, and until all immunosuppressive medications have been discontinued after allogeneic HSCT and immune reconstitution has been achieved. Individual transplant centers may also have policies regarding dietary precautions, which address concerns specific to that geographic region. The transplant center should have final responsibility to determine when dietary restrictions can be eliminated for a particular patient. Any questions regarding food and beverage safety should be discussed with the transplant physician.

1. Water safety
   a. Private well water should not be used.
   b. Public well water may be used if tested for bacterial contamination ≥ 2 times/day.
   c. Tap water may be treated to further reduce risk of Cryptosporidium by:
      i. Boiling water for ≥ 1 minute.
      ii. Use of a filter (must be able to remove particles ≥ 1 μm diameter), home distiller, or reverse osmosis unit.
   d. Bottled water may be used if it has been processed to remove Cryptosporidium by one of the methods listed above. This information can be obtained by contacting the bottler directly or by contacting the International Bottled Water Association at (703) 683-5213 or *http://www.bottledwater.org*.

2. Other beverage safety
   a. Avoid fountain beverages and ice made from tap water at restaurants, theaters, etc.
   b. Do not drink unpasteurized milk or juice.
   c. The following beverages are generally considered safe:
      i. National brands of carbonated soft drinks
      ii. Commercially packaged noncarbonated drinks that contain fruit juice (e.g., juice boxes)

Table 17.4.
Foods That Pose a High-Risk for HSCT Recipients
and Safer Substitutions

Food That Poses a High-Risk	Safer Substitution
Raw and undercooked egg* and food containing it (e.g., french toast, omelette, salad dressing, egg nog, and puddings)	Pasteurized or hard-boiled egg
Unpasteurized dairy products (e.g., milk, cheese, cream, butter, and yogurt)	Pasteurized dairy products
Fresh-squeezed, unpasteurized fruit and vegetable juices	Pasteurized juices
Unpasteurized cheeses or cheeses containing molds	Pasteurized cheeses
Undercooked or raw poultry, meats, fish, and seafood	Cooked poultry, well-done meats, fish, and seafood
Vegetable sprouts (e.g., alfalfa, bean, and other seed sprouts)[†]	Should be avoided
Raw fruits with a rough texture (e.g., raspberries)[‡]	Should be avoided
Smooth raw fruits	Should be washed under running water, peeled, or cooked
Unwashed raw vegetables[§]	Should be washed under running water, peeled, or cooked
Undercooked or raw tofu	Cooked tofu (i.e., cut into ≤1-inch cubes and boiled for ≥5 minutes in water or broth before eating or using in recipes)
Raw or unpasteurized honey	Should be avoided
Deli meats, hot dogs, and processed meats[‖]	Should be avoided unless further cooked
Raw, uncooked grain products	Cooked grain products, including bread, cooked, and ready-to-eat cold cereal, pretzels, popcorn, potato chips, corn chips, tortilla chips, cooked pasta, and rice
Maté tea[#]	Should be avoided
Moldy and outdated food products	Should be avoided
Unpasteurized beer (e.g., home-brewed and certain bottled or canned, or draft beer that has been pasteurized after fermentation)	Pasteurized beer (i.e., retail microbrewery beer)
Raw, uncooked brewers yeast	Should be avoided: HSCT recipients should avoid any contact with raw yeast (e.g., they should not make bread products themselves)
Unroasted raw nuts	Cooked nuts
Roasted nuts in the shell	Canned or bottled roasted nuts or nuts in baked products

Source: Morbidity and Mortality Weekly Report 49 (RR-10):1–125, CEI-7, 2000.
* Centers for Disease Control, 1996.
† Taormina, Beuchat, and Slutsker, 1999.
‡ Herwaldt and Ackers, 1997.
§ Centers for Disease Control, 1998.
‖ Centers for Disease Control, 1999.
Kusminsky et al., 1996.

iii. Pasteurized juices

iv. National brands of fruit juice concentrates that are reconstituted with water from a safe source

3. Food safety

Recommendations regarding safe food preparation are generally applicable to all persons, regardless of their immune status. However, HSCT patients should observe special precautions regarding food consumption.

a. Recommendations applicable to all persons include:

i. Wash hands thoroughly before handling/preparing foods and before eating.

ii. Raw meat/fish/poultry/seafood should be handled on a separate surface than other food items, and the surface should be thoroughly washed with warm soapy water after use.

iii. After handling raw meat/fish/poultry/seafood, individuals should wash their hands and cooking utensils thoroughly with warm soapy water.

iv. Refrigerate leftovers within 2 hours of cooking.

v. Reheat leftovers to $\geq 165°F$ before serving.

vi. Bring leftover soups, sauces, or gravies to a rolling boil before serving.

b. Recommendations especially important for HSCT patients include:

i. Consume a low-microbial diet (see Table 17.4).

ii. Do not share eating or drinking utensils.

iii. Avoid unpasteurized dairy products.

iv. Avoid raw or undercooked eggs, meat, fish, seafood, or poultry (use of a cooking thermometer to monitor the internal temperature of food is recommended).

III. INFECTION

A. Background

The risk of infection after HSCT is largely determined by the rapidity of myeloid recovery and the rate of T and B cell immune reconstitution. While the vast majority of HSCT patients will have achieved a normal neutrophil count by 3–4 weeks after transplant, restoration of adequate immunologic function is highly variable and dependent on many factors including the stem cell source, HLA compatibility of the donor, graft manipulation (e.g., T cell depletion), and the presence or absence of GVHD. In general, recipients of unrelated donor or mismatched related grafts have slower immune recovery compared with patients receiving HLA-matched sibling grafts. The former group is also at greater risk for developing GVHD, which results in further immune dysregulation and the initiation or extended use of immunosuppressive therapy. However, all HSCT patients should be considered severely immunocompromised early after transplant (i.e., between days +30 and +100). Measures to reduce infection risk during this time include the use of prophylactic antibiotics, minimizing environmental exposures, and possibly, the administration of intravenous immunoglobulin (IVIG).

After day +100, severe infections are more commonly seen in patients diagnosed with GVHD. Children who develop chronic GVHD incur significant deficits of humoral immunity, cell mediated immunity, and reticuloendothelial cell function. Consequently, they remain at increased risk for viral, fungal, and bacterial infections (especially with encapsulated organisms). Constant vigilance, with early recognition and treatment of infection, is crucial to optimize the probability of a successful outcome. Each transplant center has its own policies to safeguard patients against infection. Some general guidelines will be discussed below.

B. General precautions
    1. Prophylactic antibiotics
        a. *Pneumocystis carinii* prophylaxis
            i. Trimethoprim/sulfamethoxazole (TMP/SMX) 2.5 mg/kg/dose (max dose = 160 mg) TMP PO b.i.d. on 3 consecutive days each week is usually administered for prophylaxis against *Pneumocystis carinii* pneumonia (PCP) for at least 6 months after transplant, or until immunosuppressive medications have been discontinued and T cell function has significantly improved. TMP/SMX is started only after engraftment has occurred to avoid delays in neutrophil recovery.

      ii. Dapsone 2 mg/kg (maximum dose = 100 mg) PO q day is a suitable alternate for patients unable to tolerate TMP/SMX.

     iii. Aerosolized pentamidine given by Respirgard II™ inhaler 300 mg (for children ≥5 years old) or 8 mg/kg (for children <5 years old) q 21–28 days, or IV pentamidine 4 mg/kg q 14–28 days has also been used for patients intolerant of TMP/SMX.

  b. Candida species prophylaxis

      i. Fluconazole 3–6 mg/kg (for children ≤13 years old) or 400 mg (for children >13 years old) IV or PO QD is frequently administered for prophylaxis against invasive fungal disease at the start of conditioning and early after transplant, but is often discontinued once stable engraftment has occurred (~ day +30). Some institutions continue fluconazole treatment while patients are receiving immunosuppressive medications.

     ii. Certain Candida species (e.g., *C. krusei, C. glabrata*) are resistant to fluconazole and breakthrough infections with these organisms have been reported.

     iii. Clotrimazole troches and nystatin suspension are useful in preventing oral candidiasis, are not protective against invasive fungal disease.

  c. Herpes simplex virus (HSV) prophylaxis

      i. Acyclovir 250 mg/m^2/dose IV q8h is often administered to HSV seropositive patients during the peritransplant period.

     ii. Acyclovir should be continued at least until engraftment occurs and mucositis has resolved.

     iii. Some centers continue prophylaxis with oral acyclovir for a longer period of time. The recommended oral dose is 600–1,000 mg/day in 3–5 divided doses (maximum pediatric dose = 80 mg/kg/day in 3–5 divided doses).

  d. CMV prophylaxis

      i. All HSCT patients at risk for CMV disease (CMV-seropositive patients or seronegative patients who have seropositive donors) should be closely monitored for evidence of infection until 100 days after transplant, or longer if there is continued use of immunosuppressive therapy for treatment of GVHD.

ii. Prevention of CMV disease is accomplished by prophylaxis or pre-emptive therapy with antiviral drugs and by providing CMV-negative blood products for CMV-seronegative patients who have seronegative donors.

iii. Ganciclovir is the most common agent used for the prevention and treatment of CMV infection. However, ganciclovir is myelosuppressive, and its use early after transplant may interfere with engraftment.

iv. Acyclovir 500 mg/m²/dose IV q8h is often administered to patients at risk for CMV until engraftment has occurred.

v. Pre-emptive therapy with ganciclovir is implemented if patients develop CMV infection detected by screening blood ≥1 time/week for viral antigen or DNA.

vi. Some centers use prophylactic ganciclovir for all allogeneic CMV-seropositive patients. This approach has, perhaps, been more commonly employed for HSCT recipients who are at especially high-risk for CMV reactivation. High-risk patients include those seropositive patients receiving unrelated donor, mismatched related, or T cell depleted grafts.

vii. Various ganciclovir dosing regimens have been used for pre-emptive therapy. For allogeneic HSCT recipients <100 days after transplant, ganciclovir may be administered at a dose of 5 mg/kg/dose IV b.i.d. for 7–14 days, then 6 mg/kg/day IV 5 days/week for at least 3 weeks or until day 100, whichever is longer, and CMV viremia or antigenemia has cleared. For allogeneic HSCT recipients >100 days after transplant or autologous graft recipients, ganciclovir may be administered at a dose of 5 mg/kg/dose IV b.i.d. for 7 days, then 6 mg/kg/day IV 5 days/week for 2 weeks.

      viii. Patients receiving ganciclovir should be clo-
sely monitored (e.g., twice a week) for renal
and hematologic toxicity. Dose adjustment is
required for renal impairment. Discontinuation
of ganciclovir should be considered if the ANC
falls below 1000/mm^3. Administration of G-CSF
or GM-CSF may be helpful in maintaining the
ANC >1000/mm^3.

      ix. Foscarnet may be used for pre-emptive ther-
apy if patients are unable to tolerate ganciclovir. Different dosing regimens have been
used. Foscarnet may be administered at a dose
of 90 mg/kg/dose IV (infused over 1$\frac{1}{2}$–2 hours)
q12h or 60 mg/kg/dose IV (infused over a minimum of 1 hour) q8h for 14 days, then 90–
120 mg/kg IV q day until day +100.

  e. Antibiotic prophylaxis for patients with GVHD
Children being treated for acute or chronic GVHD
require prolonged antibiotic prophylaxis (see section IV).

2. Intravenous immunoglobulin
The use of IVIG after transplant varies depending on
the preferences of each transplant center.

  a. Many centers administer IVIG 250–500 mg/kg
weekly, or 500 mg/kg every 2 weeks, to allogeneic
HSCT patients until 3 months after transplant.

  b. Routine use of IVIG in autologous HSCT recipients
is not recommended.

  c. Patients transplanted for severe combined immunodeficiency syndrome should continue to receive
IVIG until they demonstrate adequate antibody
production.

  d. Prolonged use of IVIG should be considered for
other allogeneic HSCT recipients who are experiencing frequent sinopulmonary infections and
have low serum IgG levels or a documented IgG
subclass deficiency (e.g., IgG2a). The dose of IVIG
is 400–500 mg/kg every 4 weeks; however, dosing
should be adjusted to maintain serum trough levels
>400 mg/dl.

3. Environmental precautions
After discharge from the HSCT unit, patients should

minimize environmental exposures that increase their risk of infection. These precautions are generally maintained until 6 months after transplant, or longer for those patients still receiving immunosuppressive therapy for GVHD prophylaxis or treatment. Any questions regarding environmental restrictions should be discussed with the HSCT center since policies often vary among different transplant programs.

a. HSCT recipients should wash hands thoroughly with antimicrobial soap:
    i. Before eating
    ii. After handling pets
    iii. After returning from outdoors
    iv. After playing with friends
    v. After touching sand or dirt (playing with sand or dirt is discouraged)

b. Many centers require patients to wear masks when traveling outside their home.

c. If possible, patients should avoid exposure to:
    i. Crowds
    ii. Ill friends and family members (if contact with an ill caregiver is unavoidable, the caregiver is encouraged to wash hands frequently and thoroughly and to wear a surgical mask for respiratory illnesses)
    iii. Construction sites
    iv. Moldy or dusty environments
    v. Environmental tobacco or marijuana smoke

d. In general, pets do not need to be removed from the home, although contact with animals should be minimized early after transplant. Obtaining new pets early after transplant is discouraged.

e. Direct contact with ill pets should be avoided and prompt veterinary care obtained.

f. Cat litter boxes should be changed daily (not by the patient) and kept in rooms where eating or food preparation does not occur.

g. HSCT recipients should not:
    i. Clean animal cages or fish tanks
    ii. Change cat litter boxes
    iii. Handle reptiles, ducklings, or chicks

h. Dietary modifications are discussed in section II.

C. Recognition and management of specific infections
1. Bacterial infections
   Bacterial infections with either gram-positive or gram-negative organisms are relatively common within the first year after HSCT. Patients at highest risk include those with active GVHD and recipients of unrelated donor or mismatched related grafts. Infections occurring after 1 year after HSCT are generally limited to patients diagnosed with chronic GVHD. This latter group is particularly susceptible to illness caused by encapsulated organisms, especially *Streptococcus pneumoniae, Hemophilus influenzae,* and *Neisseria meningitides.* These pathogens may result in otitis media, pneumonia, sinusitis, meningitis, and septicemia. Many centers institute penicillin prophylaxis for patients with chronic GVHD (125 mg PO b.i.d. for children <5 years old, 250 mg PO b.i.d. for children 5 and older).

   Any transplant patient experiencing fever, especially within the first 6 months after HSCT, should be promptly evaluated for infection. Empiric therapy with broad-spectrum antibiotics should be considered pending blood culture results. This should always be done for patients who have an indwelling catheter device. Persistent unexplained fever should prompt radiographic evaluation of the sinuses. Other studies may be required, as clinically indicated. Patients experiencing frequent sinopulmonary infections should have an IgG level measured and, if normal, be tested for an IgG subclass deficiency. Children with low IgG levels, or an IgG subclass deficiency, may benefit from IVIG replacement therapy (section IIIA2).

2. Viral infections
   a. Cytomegalovirus
      i. Diagnostic considerations
         CMV is the most common, virus causing, life-threatening infection after HSCT. Risk factors for late CMV infection include chronic GVHD, use of unrelated donor or T cell depleted grafts, and persistently low CD4 counts. CMV disease usually manifests as pneumonitis or gastroenteritis, though hepatitis and retinitis can also occur. The diagnosis of CMV

pneumonia is usually made by culturing the virus (or detecting CMV by other means) in bronchial fluid obtained from a bronchoalveolar lavage (BAL). Early recognition and treatment of pulmonary disease is critical for averting a fatal outcome. CMV gastroenteritis is diagnosed by performing endoscopy and obtaining biopsies of involved mucosal tissue.

Another important diagnostic tool for CMV is the detection of viral pp65 antigen in peripheral blood leukocytes by immunofluorescence or viral DNA in the blood by PCR. These techniques are highly sensitive and can aid in the diagnosis of CMV disease. The virus may also be cultured using standard techniques or a rapid shell-vial culture system. However, cultures require a minimum of 48 hours to complete and are not as sensitive as antigen detection or PCR.

ii. Treatment

Treatment of life-threatening CMV disease usually involves a combination of drug therapy and IVIG (or cytomegalovirus immune globulin, Cytogam). Ganciclovir is started at an induction dose of 5 mg/kg/dose IV b.i.d. for 14–21 days, and then continued at a maintenance dose of 5 mg/kg IV q day. IVIG is given at an induction dose of 500 mg/kg IV q.o.d. for 2 weeks, and then at a maintenance dose of 500 mg/kg IV q week. Treatment should continue until symptoms have resolved and the virus has been cleared from the blood. Patients treated with ganciclovir should be closely monitored for hematologic and renal toxicity. Therapy with foscarnet or cidofovir should be considered for patients unable to tolerate ganciclovir or when ganciclovir-resistance is suspected.

b. Varicella-Zoster virus (VZV)

i. Diagnostic considerations

VZV is one of the most common viral infections encountered after HSCT with an incidence as high as 50% at 5 years. Risk factors for VZV infection include pretransplant seropositivity,

use of TBI in the conditioning regimen and age
≥ 10 years. Although most infections are dermatomal, systemic dissemination can occur,
especially within the first year after transplant.
The diagnosis of VZV is made by recognition of
the characteristic vesicular rash, which classically follows a dermatomal distribution and
may be pruritic or painful. Lesions appearing
outside the primary sensory dermatomes may
be observed in immunocompromised patients.
The diagnosis can be confirmed by scraping a
lesion for a Tzanck preparation or direct fluo-
rescent antigen testing.

   ii. Treatment

HSCT recipients <24 months after transplant,
who are exposed to VZV, should receive Varicella Zoster immune globulin (VZIG). Any
HSCT recipient who is ≥ 24 months after transplant, but still receiving immunosuppressive
therapy, should also receive VZIG if exposed to
VZV. Ideally, VZIG should be administered as
soon as possible after VZV exposure and certainly within 96 hours. The recommended dose
is 1 vial (125 Units) per 10 kg body weight IM
with a maximum dose of 5 vials. The minimum
dose is 1 vial.

       Patients with an established VZV in-
fection should be treated with acyclovir
500 mg/m^2/dose IV q8h. Treatment with oral
acyclovir is not recommended in immunocompromised patients.

  c. Adenovirus

    i. Diagnostic considerations

Adenovirus is increasingly being recognized
as an important pathogen in HSCT recipients.
The virus can cause enteritis, upper respiratory infection, pneumonia, hepatitis, hemorrhagic cystitis, and encephalitis. Dissemination can occur rapidly with a mortality rate
of approximately 60%. Patients at greatest risk
are those most profoundly immunocompromised including recipients of unrelated donor
or T cell depleted transplants. The diagnosis of

adenovirus infection is typically made by culturing the virus from stool, urine, CSF, nasal secretions or bronchial fluid, or by identifying viral DNA in the blood or bodily secretions using PCR. Characteristic morphologic features can also be seen on tissue biopsy and the diagnosis confirmed by immunoassay.

ii. Treatment

Several antiviral agents have been used to treat adenovirus infections including ribavirin, ganciclovir, vidarabine, and cidofovir. Limited data suggest that cidofovir may be the most effective agent and should be considered for initial therapy. Cidofovir has been administered at a dose of 5 mg/kg IV q week for 3 weeks followed by 5 mg/kg IV every 10–14 days. Treatment should continue until symptoms resolve and the virus is no longer detectable. The drug is nephrotoxic and IV fluid hydration with normal saline should be provided before and after cidofovir infusion. Co-administration of probenecid may reduce renal toxicity. The dose of probenecid is 2 g per 1.73 m^2 PO, 3 hours before cidofovir, and 1 g per 1.73 m^2, 2 and 8 hours after cidofovir infusion. Prolonged treatment with cidofovir may be required to prevent reactivation of the virus.

Donor leukocyte infusions (DLIs) have also been used to treat severe adenoviral infections. Although this approach may be efficacious, data are quite limited.

d. Respiratory syncytial virus (RSV)

i. Diagnostic considerations

Any HSCT recipient demonstrating URI symptoms before transplant, or early after transplant, should be tested for RSV. The virus can be isolated by nasopharyngeal culture, though rapid diagnostic tests are readily available. RSV can cause severe pneumonia in immunocompromised patients with a fatality rate of ~70%. Early diagnosis and treatment of an RSV URI may prevent dissemination to the lower respiratory tract and facilitate eradication of the virus.

ii. Treatment

While there is no uniformly accepted treatment of RSV infections in HSCT patients, many transplant centers employ a combination of ribavirin and IVIG or RSV immune globulin. Ribavirin (6 gm) has been administered at a concentration of 20 mg/ml for 18 hours/day q day using a small particle aerosol generator (SPAG-2). IVIG is given concomitantly at a dose of 500 mg/kg q.o.d. Alternatively, RSV immune globulin has been used in lieu of IVIG, given as a single dose of 1,500 mg/kg.

e. Influenza

i. Preventative strategies

Influenza can cause severe illness in immunocompromised patients. It is; therefore, recommended that family members and household contacts of HSCT recipients be vaccinated against influenza during each flu season starting before transplant, and continuing for 2 years after transplant, to minimize patient exposure risk. If vaccination is administered during an influenza A outbreak, it is recommended that family members and household contacts also receive 2 weeks of chemoprophylaxis with amantadine or rimantadine. Zanamivir or oseltamivir may be substituted for amantadine/rimantadine if the latter drugs cannot be tolerated, the influenza A strain is amantidine/rimantidine resistant, or the outbreak strain is influenza B.

These policies should be continued >2 years after transplant if the HSCT recipient remains significantly immunocompromised (e.g., is being treated for chronic GVHD), until immunocompetence is restored.

HSCT recipients who are ≥6 months after transplant should receive seasonal vaccinations against influenza. HSCT recipients who are <6 months after transplant should receive

chemoprophylaxis with amantadine or rimantadine during influenza A outbreaks.

ii. Treatment
HSCT recipients who develop influenza A infections should be treated with amantadine. The
recommended dose is 5 mg/kg/day PO in 1 or
2 divided doses. The maximum daily dose is
150 mg for children 1–9 years old and 200 mg
for children ≥10 years old. Amantadine is not
FDA approved for use in children <1 year old.

f. Parainfluenza virus
i. Diagnostic considerations
Parainfluenza virus can cause both upper and
lower respiratory tract disease in HSCT recipients. Pulmonary involvement portends a poor
prognosis with a mortality rate ≥30%. The diagnosis of parainfluenza virus infection is made
by culturing the virus from nasopharyngeal secretions or bronchial fluid. Rapid antigen detection assays are also available.

ii. Treatment
Ribavirin has been used to treat parainfluenza
virus infections in HSCT recipients but efficacy
has not been clearly established.

g. Epstein-Barr virus
i. Diagnostic considerations
Epstein-Barr virus (EBV) infection or reactivation in HSCT recipients can cause a clonal
B cell proliferation resulting in a complication termed post-transplant lymphoproliferative disorder (PTLD). Risk factors for the development of PTLD include T cell depletion
(including in vivo T cell depletion with anti-
T cell antibodies), use of unrelated donor or
HLA-mismatched grafts, and increased donor
age. The presenting symptoms are variable,
but often include fever and lymphadenopa-
thy, especially in the tonsillar and cervical
regions. Hepatomegaly, splenomegaly, and GI
tract involvement may be evident. Patients
presenting early after transplant often experience a particularly fulminant course with

multiple-organ infiltration and overwhelming sepsis.

The diagnosis of PTLD is made by biopsy of affected tissue, which is analyzed for clonality, immunophenotype, and for the presence of EBV. The detection of EBV DNA in the blood by quantitative PCR may also be helpful. Although PTLD is a relatively uncommon complication of HSCT, it is associated with a very poor prognosis. Recent therapeutic advances may improve outcome, especially if the diagnosis is promptly established allowing for early intervention.

ii. Treatment

The first approach taken in the management of PTLD is usually a reduction of immunosuppressive therapy. This may suffice for patients with minimal disease; however, most HSCT recipients will require more aggressive interventions. Many different agents have been used to treat PTLD including antiviral drugs (e.g., acyclovir, ganciclovir), IVIG or CMV immune globulin, a-interferon, anthracycline-based chemotherapy regimens (e.g., CHOP), and anti-B cell monoclonal antibodies (e.g., rituximab). More recently, EBV-specific cytotoxic T lymphocytes derived from the stem cell donor have been used for prophylaxis and treatment with encouraging results.

The regimen used to treat PTLD will ultimately depend on the patients' clinical circumstances and the expertise and preferences of each transplant center.

3. Fungal infections

Candida and aspergillus species account for the majority of fungal infections in HSCT recipients. Most infections occur early after transplant as a consequence of prolonged neutropenia, mucosal breakdown, and the use of broad-spectrum antibiotics. Late fungal disease is primarily seen in patients who experience engraftment failure or prolonged immunosuppressive therapy for treatment of GVHD.

a. Candida species
   i. Diagnostic consideration
      Candida albicans, C. tropicalis, C. krusei, and
      C. glabrata are the most common pathogens
      isolated from HSCT recipients. Superficial in-
      fections involving the skin and oral mucosa
      are quite common and usually can be diag-
      nosed based on their characteristic clinical
      appearance. Invasive disease can manifest as
      esophagitis, pneumonia, hepatosplenic can-
      didiasis, endocarditis, osteomyelitis, endoph-
      thalmitis, meningitis, and urinary tract infec-
      tion. The diagnosis is made by culturing the
      organism from infected tissue or blood or by
      the identification of yeast and/or pseudohy-
      phae on histochemical stains.
   ii. Treatment
      Superficial infections can generally be treated
      topically with nystatin or clotrimazole prepa-
      rations. Oral infections and skin infections also
      may be treated with oral fluconazole at a dose
      of 6 mg/kg/day.
      Treatment of invasive disease requires
      Amphotericin B 0.5–1 mg/kg/day given for 4–6
      weeks. Certain infections such as esophagitis
      may only require 10–14 days of therapy.
b. Aspergillus species
   i. Diagnostic considerations
      Measures should be taken to reduce exposure
      of HSCT recipients to aspergillus and other
      molds, as discussed above. Aspergillus infec-
      tion most commonly manifests as pneumonia
      and/or sinusitis. However, other sites of dis-
      ease may include the brain, skin, kidneys, gas-
      trointestinal tract, heart, and bones. The diag-
      nosis of aspergillosis is made by culturing the
      organism from infected tissue. Pulmonary in-
      fections may be difficult to diagnose because
      aspergillus is only sporadically recovered from
      bronchial fluid. Fine needle aspiration, trans-
      bronchial, or open lung biopsy may be re-
      quired to establish a microbiologic diagnosis.
      However, because of the morbidity of these

procedures, presumptive therapy is sometimes initiated based on characteristic radiographic features seen on CT scanning.

ii. Treatment

Aspergillus infections have been associated with a very high mortality rate and aggressive treatment is required. Amphotericin B 1–1.5 mg/kg/day IV for a minimum of 4–6 weeks is often used for initial therapy. Liposomal amphotericin preparations have also been employed and generally cause less nephrotoxicity than conventional amphotericin. Liposomal amphotericin has also been used as salvage therapy for patients not responding, or intolerant of, conventional amphotericin (see Table 3.1 for dosages). Itraconazole (and more recently Voriconazole) has also been used to treat Aspergillus infections, although data regarding efficacy in children are limited.

In addition to aggressive antifungal therapy, surgical resection or debridement of infected tissue is sometimes required to facilitate eradication of the organism.

4. Protozoal infections

a. *Pneumocystis carinii*

Although the incidence of PCP has decreased dramatically due to widespread use of antibiotic prophylaxis, infections still occur as a consequence of noncompliance or antibiotic resistance. The diagnosis of PCP should be entertained in any HSCT recipient who develops a diffuse interstitial pneumonitis. Diagnosis is made by identification of the organism in bronchial fluid. Treatment should be initiated with TMP/SMX (20 mg/kg/day TMP) IV divided every 6 hours.

b. *Toxoplasma gondii*

Toxoplasmosis is an uncommon infection in HSCT recipients that results from reactivation in seropositive patients who are receiving aggressive immunosuppressive therapy. The infection most commonly involves the central nervous system, although pneumonia and myocarditis can also occur.

It has been recommended that HSCT candidates with a prior history of chorioretinitis due to Toxoplasma, or seropositive patients undergoing treatment for GVHD, should receive prophylaxis with TMP/SMX 150 mg/m^2/day TMP PO in 2 divided doses on 3 consecutive days each week. However, few data are available regarding the efficacy of this regimen, and breakthrough infections have been reported.

IV. GRAFT VERSUS HOST DISEASE

A. Background

GVHD occurs when donor T lymphocytes recognize histocompatibility antigens expressed on host tissue as "nonself" and mount an immunologic response. The process may begin while the patient is hospitalized or can develop subsequently, after discharge. It can be subdivided into two phases:

1. Acute GVHD (aGVHD) develops during the first 100 days after transplant.

2. Chronic GVHD (cGVHD) either persists beyond or first manifests after 100 days following HSCT. It may occur in decreasing order of frequency:

   a. Evolve directly from acute GVHD (persistent cGVHD),

   b. Redevelop after resolution of the acute phase (quiescent cGVHD), or

   c. Be the first manifestation of GVHD (de novo cGVHD).

B. Acute GVHD (aGVHD)

1. The primary target organs of aGVHD in decreasing order of frequency are skin, GI tract, and liver (see Table 17.5). Most patients have skin involvement, which often begins on the palms and soles, soon thereafter spreads to face, scalp, nape of neck and ears, and then involves the rest of the body. This often occurs in a step-wise fashion, "marching down" a patient's body. Skin GVHD presents as a maculopapular rash, which can become confluent and may be pruritic.

2. Isolated GI or hepatic involvement is uncommon, although a subset of patients may present with only upper GI disease manifesting as anorexia, nausea and

Table 17.5.
Clinical Classification of Acute Graft versus Host Disease According
to Organ Injury

	Skin	Liver (Bilirubin)	Gut
Stage			
1	Maculopapular rash on <25% of body surface	2–3 mg/dl*	300–600 ml/m² stool/day or nausea*†
2	Maculopapular rash on 25–50% of body surface	>3–6 mg/dl	>600–900 ml/m² stool/day
3	Maculopapular rash on >50% of body surface	>6–15 mg/dl	>900 ml/m² stool/day
4	Maculopapular rash on >50% of body surface with bullae and desquamation	>15 mg/dl	severe abdominal pain with or without ileus
Clinical Grade		*Stage*	
I (mild)	1 or 2	0	0
II (moderate)	3 or	1 or	1
III (severe)	—	2–3 or	2–4
IV (life threatening)	4 or	4	—

Source: Modified from a consensus conference on aGVHD grading (*BMT* 15:825–28,1995)
*Downgrade one stage if additional cause for elevated bilirubin or diarrhea is documented
†Persistent nausea with histologic evidence of GVHD in the stomach or duodenum

vomiting. In general, gut GVHD manifests as watery diarrhea, often with cramping. Persistence of gut GVHD
can lead to bloody diarrhea. Liver GVHD most commonly manifests with hyperbilirubinemia, but also can
present with elevated transaminases.

3. Diagnosis of aGVHD usually can be made by skin biopsy
    and involvement of the other organs inferred in the
    appropriate clinical context. For those uncommon pa-
    tients whose skin is spared, endoscopic biopsy of an
    involved portion of the GI tract or liver biopsy may
    be necessary to establish a diagnosis. A biopsy also
    may be required to exclude other causes of GI or hep-
    atic dysfunction. Viral and opportunistic infectious eti-
    ologies should be thoroughly pursued via culture, and
    PCR testing, along with histochemical and pathological
    methods, if possible.

4. The prophylactic regimen used to prevent GVHD
    depends on the type of transplant (related vs.

unrelated) and individual preferences of the transplant center. Cyclosporine (CSA) or tacrolimus is commonly used, often in combination with other agents such as methotrexate (MTX) and/or methylprednisolone (MP).

a. Cyclosporine (CSA) is usually started intravenously at a dose of 3 mg/kg/day ÷ Q12 hrs. More frequent administration (e.g., Q6–8 hrs or continuous infusion) may be required to achieve a therapeutic serum level, especially in very young children. Once the patient is able to tolerate oral medications, the IV CSA can be converted to an equivalent oral dose. There are currently two oral preparations available, Neoral® and Sandimmune®. If Neoral® is used, then the conversion factor from IV to PO is 3:1 (i.e., the oral dose is 3 times the intravenous dose). A higher conversion factor (e.g., 4:1) may be required for Sandimmune®, since its' bioavailability is lower than Neoral's®'. After converting from IV to oral CSA, trough serum levels should be monitored to ensure a therapeutic serum concentration is attained.

b. Pharmacological monitoring of CSA levels may be performed by high pressure liquid chromatography (HPLC) or by immunoassay. The methodology utilized will influence the therapeutic range reported by the laboratory. The patient's clinical circumstance may also have some bearing on the desired CSA level. For example, some transplant centers may target a higher CSA serum concentration for recipients of unrelated donor grafts because of the increased risk of GVHD. Hence, interpretation of CSA levels should be made in conjunction with the transplant center.

c. The CSA dose may need to be modified for renal insufficiency (see Table 17.6).

d. If GVHD does not develop, then the CSA is usually tapered by 5% per week starting 2–4 months after transplant.

e. A slower taper regimen is sometimes used for patients receiving unrelated donor grafts because of the increased risk of GVHD.

Table 17.6.
CSA Dosing for Renal Insufficiency

Serum Creatinine	CSA Dose
<1.5 x baseline	Full dose
1.5–1.9 x baseline	50% dose
2.0 x baseline	Hold dose

f. The most commonly used MTX schedule is the "short-course" regimen, which includes 15 mg/m^2 on day +1, then 10 mg/m^2/day on days +3, +6, and +11 after transplants.

g. Many different MP dosing schedules exist. Most regimens require an increase in dosing at the time of highest risk of GVHD, usually day +7 or day +15. Tapering of MP is begun on day +28 if no signs of GVHD are present. MP is used most often with cord blood transplants, usually in place of MTX, as well as in mismatched and unrelated HSCT recipients in addition to MTX.

5. Treatment of newly diagnosed aGVHD, or a flare of aGVHD, will depend on which medications the patient received for GVHD prophylaxis or for prior therapy. Initiation or change of therapy should be done in consultation with the transplant center.

a. Steroids are the treatment of choice for aGVHD. If the patient has not been on steroids, then prednisone or methylprednisolone, 2 mg/kg/day in divided doses, should be started.

b. Once there has been a satisfactory response, an initial taper of 0.5 mg/kg every 7–14 days can be instituted.

c. Patients who fail to respond to standard dose steroids and CSA may be treated with high-dose "pulse" methylprednisolone (10–30 mg/kg/day), or horse antithymocyte globulin (20 mg/kg QD or QOD × 7 doses). Other treatment modalities that have been used are listed in Table 17.7.

d. CSA has also been used to treat acute GVHD at the same dose used for GVHD prophylaxis. Recently, tacrolimus has been used in lieu of CSA at a dose of 0.03–0.05 mg/kg/day IV usually as a continuous

Table 17.7.
Alternative Therapies for Acute Graft versus Host Disease

Agent	Example
Newer immunosuppressive drugs	rapamycin, tacrolimus, mycophenolate mofetil, pentastatin
Anti–T cell monoclonal antibodies	anti-CD3 (e.g., visilizumab)
Antibodies that block cytokines	anti-TNF (e.g., infliximab)
Antibodies that block cytokine receptors	anti-IL-2R (e.g., daclizumab)

infusion. This can be converted to an oral dose of 0.15–0.20 mg/kg/day in 2 divided doses. The level of tacrolimus is determined by one of two assays, a microparticle enzyme immunoassay (MEIA) and an ELISA. Both methods use the same monoclonal antibody for tacrolimus. Usually whole blood concentrations are maintained between 5 and 20 ng/mL.

   e. Patients can be changed from CSA to tacrolimus, or vice versa, if acute GVHD is not controlled with initial management or if chronic GVHD develops and persists despite alternative treatments.

   f. If there is GI involvement causing significant diarrhea, the patient may need to be made NPO and begin parenteral nutrition. It is often also necessary to resume intravenous CSA and MP because of the decreased absorption of oral medications in this setting. If the diarrhea is secretory, octreotide therapy may be beneficial (1 mcg/kg/dose q12h; may slowly increase dose up to 10 mcg/kg as needed). As the disease comes under control, enteral feeding should be gradually reintroduced.

6. The immunosuppressive agents used for prophylaxis or to treat GVHD can cause numerous complications. The side effects of steroids are well known to most medical personnel and will not be reviewed here. CSA commonly causes neurologic symptoms and renal dysfunction (see Table 17.8). Serum CSA levels, creatinine, electrolytes, and magnesium should be monitored on a regular basis, usually every 1–2 weeks, or more often

Table 17.8.
Cyclosporine Toxicity

Neurotoxicity
  Common
    Tremor
    Headache
    Dysesthesia
  Uncommon
    Seizures
    Ataxia
    Somnolence
    Leukoencephalopathy
Renal toxicity
  Common
    Elevated creatinine
    Hypomagnesemia
    Hyperkalemia
    Hypertension
  Uncommon
    Acute renal failure
    Hemolytic uremic syndrome with:
      renal insufficiency
      microangiopathic hemolytic anemia
      thrombocytopenia
Hirsutism
Hepatic insufficiency

as necessary. The most frequent toxicities requiring intervention are:

a. Hypomagnesemia
   i.   Potentiates the neurotoxicity of CSA
   ii. Often requires treatment with IV or oral magnesium
b. Hypertension
   i.   Especially common in patients on concomitant steroids
   ii. Often responds well to vasodilating calcium channel blockers (e.g., nifedipine, isradipine)
   iii. Additional antihypertensive agents may be required (e.g., enalapril, labetalol, clonidine)
c. Renal insufficiency
   i.   Increased hydration will decrease the risk of nephrotoxicity.

Table 17.9.
Clinical Grading of Chronic Graft versus Host Disease

Limited (better prognosis)
  Localized skin involvement or hepatic dysfunction
Extensive (worse prognosis)
  Generalized skin involvement or localized skin involvement plus any of
  the following:
    chronic hepatitis or cirrhosis
    keratoconjunctivitis
    oral mucosal involvement (xerostomia, lichen planus)
    involvement of any other organ (e.g., lung, gastrointestinal tract)

     ii.   To ensure good renal function, an oral intake of $1{,}500\text{--}2{,}000\ cc/m^2/day$ should be maintained.
    iii. The side effects of tacrolimus are similar to those of CSA, although decreased nephrotoxicity and neurotoxicity have been reported with tacrolimus.
   7. Early recognition and prompt treatment of complicating bacterial, fungal, and viral infections are essential, as patients are severely immunocompromised. Maintain prophylaxis against *Pneumocystis carinii* prophylaxis, fungus, and herpes viruses (see section IIIB).
 C. Chronic GVHD
   1. cGVHD can be classified as limited or extensive (see Table 17.9). It may affect the same target organs as the acute form, but may also involve the mouth (xerostomia, lichen planus), eyes (keratoconjunctivitis sicca), and lungs (bronchiolitis obliterans) as well as other organ systems (see Table 17.10). The clinical manifestations often resemble those of a persistent autoimmune disease.
   2. Screening tests for cGVHD include biopsy of involved organs, assessment of pulmonary and hepatic function, CBC, and Schirmer's test (see Table 17.10).
   3. Immunodeficiency persists with propensity to opportunistic infections and infections with encapsulated bacteria. Infection is often the cause of death in these patients.
   4. If there is progressive bronchiolitis obliterans, death may be due to respiratory failure.

Table 17.10.
Chronic Graft versus Host Disease: Clinical Features
and Screening Studies

Organ/System	Clinical Features	Screening Study
Skin	Lichenoid or sclerodermatous changes, xeroderma, desquamation, erythema, dyspigmentation, alopecia, onychodystrophy	Punch biopsy of skin
Oral cavity	Lichen planus, xerostomia	Lower lip biopsy
Ocular	Sicca, keratitis	Schirmer's test
Liver	Icterus	Bilirubin, alkaline phosphatase, GGT
GI tract	Dysphagia, malabsorption, diarrhea, anorexia, weight loss	Endoscopy with biopsies
Pulmonary	Bronchiolitis obliterans producing obstructive lung disease, cough, dyspnea, exercise intolerance	Pulmonary function tests, CT scan of lungs
Immunologic	Opportunistic infections, encapsulated bacterial infections, frequent sinopulmonary infections	T cell function and subsets, quantitative immunoglobulins, IgG subclasses
Hematologic	Thrombocytopenia, eosinophilia	CBC

5. Treatment of cGVHD is most efficacious when administered early in its course. Screening tests help identify patients in need of therapy. For those patients whose cGVHD is not a direct progression from unresolved aGVHD, clinical manifestations of cGVHD may become apparent as post-transplant immunosuppressive therapy is tapered.

6. Patients who develop cGVHD during a CSA taper should, at a minimum, stop the taper and have their dose increased to the amount prescribed before the development of GVHD. It may be necessary to return to full therapeutic dosing (12 mg/kg/day PO in 2 or 3 divided doses). If this fails to produce resolution, then the first line of therapy for cGVHD, as for aGVHD, is corticosteroid administration. To minimize the long-term side effects of steroid therapy, patients eventually may be placed on an alternate day dosing schedule.

Table 17.11.
Alternative Therapies for Chronic Graft versus Host Disease

Agent	Toxicity	Comment
Azathioprine	Bone marrow suppression Thrombocytopenia is a relative contraindication	Monitor CBC regularly
Psoralen and ultraviolet A therapy (PUVA)	Erythroderma, xeroderma, hyperpigmentation, pruritis, nausea	Used for cutaneous cGVHD Psoralen may be given orally or in bath Extracorporeal PUVA has also been effective and may provide systemic benefit Avoid concomitant photosensitizing drugs
Thalidomide	Somnolence, dizziness, rash, constipation, headache, xerostomia, xeroderma, peripheral neuropathy	Drowsiness abates after a few weeks Discontinue drug if patient develops evidence of peripheral neuropathy May be helpful to monitor plasma levels
Etretinate	Scaling of skin, chelitis, xerosis, eye irritation	Has been used for sclerodermatous cGVHD
Hydroxychloroquine	Retinopathy, keratopathy, nausea, diarrhea	Regular eye exams required
Mycophenolate mofetil	Nausea, diarrhea, leukopenia	Monitor CBC regularly
Clofazimine	Nausea, constipation, diarrhea, hyperpigmentation	Experience with this modality is very limited
Total lymphoid irradiation	Leukopenia	Experience with this modality is very limited

a. A commonly employed regimen consists of prednisone 1 mg/kg/day PO and cyclosporine 12 mg/kg/day PO in 2 divided doses.

b. Patients who fail to respond to the above regimen may be tried on alternative therapies (see Table 17.11). Alternative agents such as mycophenolate mofetil (CellCept) are often added in an attempt to wean the patient off steroids.

c. Patients with refractory oral disease may respond to steroid rinses or photochemotherapy to the oral cavity. Photochemotherapy, in the form of Psoralen with ultraviolet A radiation (PUVA) therapy, also has been effective for isolated chronic skin GVHD. Extracorporeal PUVA has been used to treat GVHD involving multiple organ systems.

   d. If possible, patients should be enrolled in open clinical trials to evaluate the efficacy of different cGVHD therapeutic regimens.

7. Additional supportive care measures are critical and include:

   a. Prophylaxis against *Pneumocystis carinii,* fungal infection, and infection with encapsulated bacteria (see section III B)

   b. Protection from sun exposure by covering commonly exposed areas and use of sunscreen

   c. Artificial tears for patients with eye involvement

   d. Monthly IVIG at a dose of 400–500 mg/kg may be beneficial, especially in patients with hypogamma-globulinemia or IgG subclass deficiencies

   e. Hypervigilance for viral, fungal, and bacterial infections

V. ENDOCRINE CONSIDERATIONS

A. Background

Abnormalities of linear growth, sexual maturation, and thyroid function may be encountered after HSCT and are related to the transplant conditioning regimen, age at transplant, development of cGVHD, the patient's underlying disease, and prior therapy.

B. Growth

Many children who undergo HSCT subsequently experience impaired growth, especially at the time of puberty. The most important factors associated with diminished growth include use of TBI for conditioning and younger age at the time of transplant. In addition, boys tend to experience a greater loss of height than girls. However, despite iatrogenic disturbances in growth, most pediatric transplant recipients will ultimately reach a final stature that is within the normal range for adults.

1. Use of TBI as part of the transplant conditioning regimen consistently has been associated with impaired growth. TBI may directly damage growth plates and cause gonadal injury and hormonal deficiencies, all

of which impede normal growth. The effect is particularly prominent among children who have received prior cranial or craniospinal irradiation. Fractionated TBI protocols cause less growth retardation compared to single-dose regimens.

2. Conditioning regimens that use chemotherapy alone, including busulfan, appear to cause significantly less growth impairment than TBI-based regimens.

3. After HSCT, children should have their height measured every 6–12 months until they attain final adult stature.

   a. Children experiencing subnormal growth velocity should be evaluated by a pediatric endocrinologist.

   b. The administration of exogenous growth hormone to HSCT patients may improve growth velocity in select cases; however, final adult stature may not be altered by this approach.

C. Sexual development

1. The use of TBI has been associated with a significant risk of gonadal failure resulting in:

   a. Delayed pubertal development

   b. Amenorrhea

   c. Infertility

2. Data regarding the effect of busulfan on gonadal function are more limited; however, use of this agent has been associated with a significant risk of gonadal failure, primarily in girls.

3. Most children treated with cyclophosphamide alone appear to regain normal gonadal function 6–12 months after transplant and fertility is usually unimpaired.

4. Tanner scores should be determined yearly after transplant until pubertal development is complete. Patients manifesting delayed puberty, or showing other signs of gonadal dysfunction (such as hot flashes), should be evaluated by a pediatric endocrinologist. Girls appear to be at greater risk of gonadal failure than boys (except those boys treated with prior testicular irradiation), and are more likely to require sex hormone replacement therapy.

5. Both busulfan and TBI-based transplant regimens carry a very high-risk of infertility among male and female HSCT recipients. Nonetheless, pregnancies have been

reported among female patients or female partners of male patients. Pregnancies among female patients have been associated with an increased risk of spontaneous abortion and premature delivery. There does not appear to be an increased risk of congenital anomalies in children born to HSCT recipients.

D. Thyroid function
1. Hypothyroidism develops in approximately 10–30% of patients exposed to fractionated TBI and can occur many years after the HSCT.
2. In most cases, compensated hypothyroidism is diagnosed (elevated TSH with normal T4 index), but occasionally overt hypothyroidism occurs (low T4 index).
3. Rarely, hypothyroidism has been reported in patients conditioned with chemotherapy alone.
4. Thyroid studies (TSH and T4 index) should be obtained yearly for patients exposed to TBI, and the neck should be palpated to detect any nodules suggestive of a secondary malignancy.
5. The management of compensated hypothyroidism is controversial, but hormone replacement therapy should be considered for patients manifesting a significant and persistent elevation of TSH.
6. Overt hypothyroidism requires treatment with thyroid hormone, which should be administered after consultation with a pediatric endocrinologist.

VI. DELAYED ORGAN TOXICITY

A. Background
Delayed organ toxicity (see Table 17.12) in the HSCT patient is often multifactorial.
1. Previous chemotherapy and radiation therapy may have already produced toxicity or increased the risk of toxicity from the conditioning regimen.
2. Doses of radiation and chemotherapy used for conditioning often approach the tolerance limits of non-hematopoietic tissues.
3. Toxicity also may result from, or be exacerbated by, drugs used for the prevention and treatment of infection or GVHD.

Table 17.12.
Delayed Complications after HSCT

Organ	Process	Onset after HSCT	Diagnostic Test	Risk Factor
Kidney	HUS	months	CBC, LDH creatinine	TBI, CSA
Bladder	Hemorrhagic cystitis	weeks-months	Urinalysis, viral culture	Cyclophosphamide, busulfan
Eye	Sicca syndrome	months-years	Schirmer's test	cGVHD
	Cataracts	months-years	Slit lamp exam	TBI, steroids
	Retinopathy	months	Fundus exam	CSA
Heart	Myocardial failure	years	Echocardiogram, MUGA scan	Anthracyclines, chest radio-therapy
Liver	Cholestasis	months-years	Liver function tests	cGVHD
	Hepatitis	months-years	Liver function tests, Hepatitis C PCR, HBSAg	Infection with: Hepatitis C or Hepatitis B
Lung	Restrictive changes	months-years	Pulmonary function tests	Bleomycin, BCNU, chest radio-therapy or thoracotomy, conditioning with busulfan or BCNU
	Obstructive changes	months-years	Pulmonary function tests, chest CT, lung biopsy	cGVHD

Note: HUS, hemolytic uremic syndrome; TBI, total body irradiation; CSA, cyclosporine; cGVHD, chronic graft versus host disease; PCR, polymerase chain reaction; HBSAg, hepatitis B surface antigen.

B. Renal and bladder toxicity
1. Renal toxicity can be a consequence of administering any of the following drugs singly or in combination:
   a. Aminoglycoside antibiotics
   b. Amphotericin B
   c. Ganciclovir and acyclovir
   d. Foscarnet
   e. Pentamidine
   f. Cyclosporine and tacrolimus
2. Whenever possible, minimize the number of potentially nephrotoxic drugs.
3. Renal toxicity also can result from endothelial cell damage produced by the conditioning regimen (TBI)

or cyclosporine/tacrolimus or both. Pediatric patients seem to be particularly prone to a hemolytic uremic-like syndrome, which develops after transplant and is characterized by renal insufficiency, microangiopathic hemolytic anemia, and thrombocytopenia.

a. Patients at highest risk include:

    i. Recipients of TBI (especially when the dose exceeds 1,200 cGy)

    ii. Infants and young children

    iii. Allogeneic HSCT recipients receiving cyclosporine/tacrolimus

b. Treatment is primarily supportive care:

    i. Transfuse with packed red blood cells if Hgb <7–8 gm/dl or if patient is clinically unstable

    ii. Transfuse with platelets as clinically indicated

    iii. Discontinue cyclosporine/tacrolimus

    iv. Plasmapheresis has been advocated by some centers

4. Bladder toxicity is most often due to hemorrhagic cystitis.

a. Early onset (days to weeks after transplant) hemorrhagic cystitis usually results from cyclophosphamide administration but can occasionally occur following busulfan (i.e., even in patients who do not receive cyclophosphamide).

b. Late-onset hemorrhagic cystitis (weeks to months) may be due to infection with adenovirus, BK papovavirus, or CMV.

c. Management is largely symptomatic and involves:

    i. Adequate hydration to maintain a good urine output

    ii. Bladder irrigation if blood clots develop

    iii. Smooth muscle relaxants to alleviate bladder spasm

    iv. Platelet transfusions for thrombocytopenic patients

d. Other therapeutic options may include:

    i. Antiviral therapy for patients with CMV or adenovirus

    ii. Aminocaproic acid (cystoscopy required to remove all clots within the bladder before administration)

   iii. Intravesicular instillation of various prosta-
        glandins (PGE_1, PGE_2, PGF_2 alpha)
   iv. Intravesicular instillation of formalin (ureteral
        reflux is a contraindication)
C. Ocular toxicity
   1. Anterior segment pathology includes:
      a. Conjunctival involvement in acute and chronic
         GVHD. Patients with keratoconjunctivitis sicca
         may have:
         i.   Burning
         ii. Irritation
         iii. Photophobia
         iv. Painful punctate erosions
      b. Posterior subcapsular cataracts usually develop 2–
         6 years after transplant. Patients at risk are those
         who received TBI (especially ≥1,200 cGy) and/or
         required prolonged systemic corticosteroid ther-
         apy.
   2. Posterior segment pathology consists primarily of an
      ischemic retinopathy characterized by cotton wool ex-
      udates and occasionally by disc edema.
      a. It occurs in patients treated with cyclosporine.
      b. It develops within the first 6 months after trans-
         plant.
      c. If cyclosporine can be discontinued, the retinopa-
         thy is usually reversible.
D. Cardiac complications
   1. Therapies received before HSCT are the most impor-
      tant determinants of late cardiac complications. The
      cumulative anthracycline dose and mediastinal irradi-
      ation both individually and collectively determine the
      risk for cardiac complications. HSCT patients who have
      these risk factors should be monitored closely for late
      cardiac dysfunction.
   2. TBI can further increase the risk of late cardiac compli-
      cations.
   3. Patients may remain asymptomatic or present with any
      of the following symptoms:
      a. Fatigue
      b. Shortness of breath
      c. Poor exercise tolerance
      d. Palpitations with or without chest pain

4. Children demonstrating poor cardiac function or arrhythmia should be referred to a pediatric cardiologist for further evaluation and management.

E. Hepatic complications
   1. Allogeneic HSCT patients with acute or chronic GVHD often have liver involvement.
      a. Patients are usually asymptomatic but may have the following biochemical abnormalities:
         i. Hyperbilirubinemia
         ii. Elevated gamma-glutamyl transpeptidase (GGT)
         iii. Elevated serum alkaline phosphatase
         iv. Modest elevation of transaminases
      b. Most cases respond to immunosuppressive therapy
      c. Occasionally patients develop progressive cholestasis and ultimately biliary cirrhosis
         i. Histologically this entity can be difficult to distinguish from chronic active hepatitis.
         ii. Ursodeoxycholic acid may lower bilirubin levels and alleviate pruritis.
   2. Autologous and allogeneic HSCT recipients also may develop chronic active hepatitis. They may have:
      a. Fluctuating transaminase levels
      b. Evidence of hepatitis C virus infection (positive antibody titers in patients not receiving IVIG and/or detection of hepatitis C virus RNA by PCR in serum or liver)
      c. Evidence of hepatitis B virus infection (positivity for HBsAg, IgM anti-HBc)
   3. In allogeneic HSCT patients, chronic active hepatitis may be difficult to distinguish clinically from chronic hepatic GVHD. A liver biopsy sometimes may be helpful in arriving at a definitive diagnosis. Patients with progressive hepatitis may be candidates for clinical trials of antiviral therapy.

F. Pulmonary complications
   1. Pulmonary complications may result from prior lung infections or from therapies received before transplantation such as:
      a. Chemotherapy with BCNU, bleomycin, or busulfan

      b. Radiation therapy to the mediastinum, the lungs, or both

      c. Thoracotomies to remove pulmonary metastases

2. Mild restrictive abnormalities in pulmonary function that do not produce any clinical symptoms have been reported in the following patients:

      a. Recipients of autologous HSCTs conditioned with high-dose chemotherapy only:

          i. In most cases, therapies administered before HSCT were thought to be responsible for the abnormalities in pulmonary function.

         ii. In other cases, BCNU or busulfan administered as part of the conditioning regimen may have contributed to the abnormalities.

      b. Recipients of autologous or allogeneic HSCTs who have received TBI or busulfan

3. Obstructive abnormalities, varying from mild to severe, occur primarily in recipients of allogeneic HSCTs as a manifestation of cGVHD.

      a. Patients at greatest risk are those with cGVHD who:

          i. Received allografts from mismatched related or unrelated donors

         ii. Have hepatic involvement

      b. Chest x-ray often either is normal or demonstrates mild hyperinflation unless there is:

          i. Intercurrent infection

         ii. Extensive interstitial involvement

        iii. Pneumothorax/pneumomediastinum

      c. More severely affected patients may have:

          i. Cough

         ii. Dyspnea

        iii. Wheezing

        iv. Pneumothorax/pneumomediastinum

         v. Propensity to recurrent bronchopulmonary infections

      d. Diagnosis can be made by:

          i. Pulmonary function tests demonstrating obstruction (FEV1 is usually decreased, FVC is usually normal, and FEV1/FVC is decreased)

         ii. Chest CT scans demonstrating bronchiolitis obliterans or bronchiolitis obliterans organizing pneumonia

      iii. Bronchoalveolar lavage and/or lung biopsy may be needed to exclude infection as the primary cause of the pulmonary process

  e. Therapy

      i. Immunosuppression is the primary mode of treatment.

      ii. Treatment of intercurrent sinopulmonary infection is essential.

      iii. Symptoms may be worsened by coexistent gastroesophageal reflux. Thus, if demonstrated by endoscopy or pH probe, the patient should commence treatment for this problem as well.

VII. IMMUNIZATIONS

A. Background

  1. Patients undergoing autologous or allogeneic HSCT sometimes have immunologic reconstitution with cells that retain immunologic memory for antigens to which they had previously been exposed. However, this is far from certain. Furthermore, infants and young children who serve as their own stem cell donors, or as stem cell donors for allogeneic HSCT, will have received few, if any, immunizations before the transplant.

  2. Recipients of cord blood transplants and T cell depleted transplants receive stem cell products largely devoid of memory cells.

  3. Most HSCT patients will require a complete set of immunizations after the transplant.

  4. Immunizations will not be effective until immune reconstitution has occurred. As a rule, recipients of allogeneic transplants have slower return of immunologic function than recipients of autografts. Immune function may be impaired for prolonged periods of time (24 months or more) after T cell depleted or partially HLA-matched HSCT, and may never return to normal in patients with cGVHD.

B. Immunization guidelines

  1. General recommendations for post-transplant immunizations are summarized in Table 17.13.

Table 17.13.
Recommended Immunizations after HSCT

Vaccine	Time after HSCT	Comment
DT or DTP	12, 14, and 24 months	For children <7 years old
Td	12, 14, and 24 months	For children ≥7 years old
IPV	12, 14, and 24 months	Use for all patients
Hib	12, 14, and 24 months	Use for all patients
Hep B	12, 14, and 24 months	Use for all patients
Pneumococcal	12 and 24 months	Use 23-valent pneumococcal polysaccharide vaccine
Influenza A	Yearly beginning at 6 months	
MMR	24 months	Do not administer to patients still receiving immunosuppressive therapy or patients with cGVHD
Varicella	Do not administer to patient	Should administer to susceptible household contacts

Note: DT, diphtheria toxoid-tetanus toxoid; DTP, diphtheria toxoid-tetanus toxoid-pertussis; Td, tetanus-diptheria toxoid; IPV, inactivated polio vaccine; Hib, Haemophilus influenzae b conjugate vaccine; Hep B, Hepatitis B; MMR, measles-mumps-rubella.

2. Children receiving IVIG should not begin immunizations until 3 months after the last dose is given to avoid interference by passive antibody.

3. Postimmunization antibody titers should be obtained to ensure the patient is adequately protected.

4. It may be prudent to document responses to killed vaccines (e.g., DTP, IPV) before immunizing with a live virus (e.g., MMR).

5. For patients with cGVHD or patients on immunosuppressive therapy:
    a. Do not administer any live virus vaccines such as MMR.
    b. Immunization with killed vaccines is safe; however, efficacy is uncertain.
    c. Alternatively, the patient can be maintained on monthly IVIG.

VIII. NEUROPSYCHOLOGICAL FUNCTIONING

A. Background
    Many children undergoing HSCT will show minimal, if any, cognitive impairment. However, some patients may

demonstrate a decline in global measures of intelligence or develop deficits in specific areas of neuropsychological functioning. In practical terms, this can result in learning disabilities and a deterioration of academic performance. Many factors contribute to intellectual impairment after HSCT including exposure to neurotoxic drugs (e.g., busulfan, cyclosporine) or radiation (e.g., TBI), protracted absences from school, social isolation imposed because of immunodeficiency, and poor overall health caused by late transplant sequelae. In addition, prior therapy directed at the CNS such as prophylactic or therapeutic cranial irradiation may have a significant impact on post-transplant cognitive development.

The identification of patients at risk for cognitive problems should allow for early assessment with appropriate neuropsychological tools and the accession of supportive services to help maximize academic potential.

B. Risk factors
Several studies have identified variables that appear to place patients at higher risk for developing significant cognitive deficits.
1. Age at time of HSCT
Younger children, especially those ≤3 years old, have shown significant declines in IQ testing at 1 year after transplant, which may further deteriorate over time. Children between 3 and 6 years of age also appear to be at higher risk for intellectual impairment. Older, school-aged children are less likely to demonstrate a significant decrease in IQ after HSCT.
2. Prior therapy and conditioning regimen
Interestingly, most studies have not shown a correlation between the type of conditioning regimen administered at the time of transplant (i.e., TBI versus chemotherapy only) and post-transplant neuropsychological testing. However, patients exposed to prior cranial irradiation, who then receive TBI, are at higher risk for cognitive impairment.
3. Type of transplant
While there are few data correlating type of transplant with probability of neuropsychological dysfunction, it is likely that recipients of allogeneic transplants are at greater risk than those receiving autologous transplants. Children transplanted with allografts are more

likely to be exposed to neurotoxic drugs such as cyclosporine or tacrolimus, endure a longer period of social isolation, and are more likely to experience late transplant complications (e.g., chronic GVHD), which may adversely affect their cognitive development.

C. Nature of cognitive deficits
1. In many cases, cognitive deficits are identified only at the time of specialized neuropsychological testing. However, some children will manifest significant learning disabilities and/or behavioral problems.
2. Investigators have identified several areas of cognitive impairment including deficits in:
    a. Global intelligence (IQ)
    b. Perceptual-motor skills
    c. Memory
    d. Attention
    e. Academic achievement

D. Recommendations
By 1 year after HSCT, most school-aged children have returned to the classroom. Health care personnel and teachers should be vigilant of potential learning difficulties experienced by HSCT patients, especially those identified as high-risk. All patients may benefit from age-appropriate developmental testing, conducted by a child psychologist, one year after HSCT in order to ascertain any learning disabilities that may impede scholastic performance. Additional yearly testing may be useful, especially for younger children, since new problems may become evident over time.

E. Acute neurologic toxicity
Occasionally, children experience acute neurologic toxicity after discharge from the HSCT unit. Causes for neurologic dysfunction include infection, drug toxicity, and treatment-related leukoencephalopathy.
1. CNS infections are relatively uncommon after transplant and are:
    a. Usually caused by aspergillus or candida species
    b. Occasionally caused by other fungal species (e.g., cryptococcus), *Toxoplasma gondii,* bacterial, or viral pathogens
    c. Usually seen in patients being treated for GVHD

2. Cyclosporine may cause a variety of neurologic symptoms (see Table 17.8).
   a. The diagnosis is typically made by ruling out other causes of neurologic dysfunction (e.g., infection) and demonstration of characteristic abnormalities on brain MRI (relatively symmetric high T2-weighted signal changes in the cerebral hemispheres, cerebellum, and/or corpus callosum).
   b. CSA should be discontinued, if possible, for patients experiencing significant neurotoxicity.
   c. Tacrolimus has sometimes been used in lieu of CSA for patients experiencing CSA neurotoxicity, though neurologic dysfunction has also been associated with this drug.
   d. CSA levels should be monitored on a regular basis to reduce the risk of severe neurotoxicity.
3. Severe leukoencephalopathy is occasionally seen in patients who have received extensive prior CNS therapy.
   a. The risk may be increased by administering post-transplant intrathecal chemotherapy.
   b. Symptoms (e.g., lethargy, confusion, dysarthria, ataxia, seizures) usually develop within a few months after TBI.
   c. Patients should be evaluated by MRI, which shows white matter destruction and ventricular dilatation.
   d. A lumbar puncture may be helpful to confirm the diagnosis by demonstrating an elevated myelin basic protein and to rule out a CNS infection.

IX. SURVEILLANCE FOR RELAPSE

A. Leukemias
   The risk of relapse after transplant depends on the type of leukemia, disease status before transplant, the marrow donor (autologous versus allogeneic, related versus unrelated), and other factors.
   1. A CBC and physical exam should be performed monthly during the first year after transplant. Confirmation of engraftment by FISH (for sex-mismatched transplants) or by VNTR also can be helpful in detecting a leukemic relapse. This should be done at the initial time of

Table 17.14.
Relapse Surveillance after HSCT

Years after HSCT	Time Interval between Studies (Months)	
	Leukemias*	Solid Tumors[†]
1	1	3
2	3	4
3	4	6
4	6–12	12
5	6–12	12

*CBC, physical exam
†Radiological studies, biochemical markers, physical exam

engraftment, repeated at 6 months, and then every 6–12 months thereafter. More frequent testing may be indicated for patients at high risk of relapse.

2. Stable patients could then be followed every 3 months during the second year, every 4 months during the third year, and every 6–12 months thereafter until 5 years after transplant (see Table 17.14).

3. Performing routine surveillance bone marrow exams is of questionable benefit unless required for research purposes. One exception may be CML patients in whom the detection of persistent Ph+ cells after transplant has prognostic significance and may alter patient care. This same rationale could be applied to other leukemias when a molecular marker has been identified that could be detected by surveillance marrow exams. Patients thought to be experiencing an early relapse might benefit from a rapid taper of immunosuppressive therapy or the initiation of DLIs.

B. Solid tumors
Children with high-risk or recurrent solid tumors may be candidates for HSCT. The risk of relapse after transplant depends on the patients' disease, disease status at time of transplant, conditioning regimen, and biologic characteristics of the tumor. The frequency of disease evaluations after transplant is usually dictated by protocol. Guidelines are presented in Table 17.14.

X. SECONDARY MALIGNANCIES

A. Background

The lifetime risk of a secondary malignancy occurring in a HSCT patient appears to be 7–11 times greater than that observed in the general population. Secondary malignancies can be broken down into the following categories:

1. EBV-related lymphomas
2. Myelodysplasia (MDS) / acute nonlymphoblastic leukemia (ANLL)
3. Solid tumors

B. EBV-related lymphomas

1. EBV can cause a post-transplant lymphoproliferative disorder (PTLD), which is the most common secondary malignancy among allogeneic HSCT recipients.
2. The tumors are large cell lymphomas and have identical features to those developing after solid organ transplants. They are EBV-driven proliferations of donor B cells and can be either polyclonal or monoclonal.
3. Risk factors, clinical features, and management are discussed in section III C.

C. MDS/ANLL

MDS or leukemia usually develops at a later time than PTLD but invariably within the first decade after HSCT; it occurs in recipients of autologous as well as allogeneic grafts.

1. Patients whose conditioning included radiation appear to be at higher risk than those conditioned with chemotherapy alone.
2. In allogeneic HSCT recipients, the malignant cells may be of donor origin.
3. In autologous HSCT patients, prior treatment with agents known to induce secondary MDS/ANLL appears to be a risk factor.
4. A therapeutic option for autologous HSCT patients with secondary MDS/ANLL is an allogeneic HSCT. A second allogeneic HSCT for those allogeneic patients is possible but fraught with many potential complications. The outcome is generally poor.

D. Solid tumors
Various solid tumors of epithelial origin can occur many
years after HSCT. Exposure to TBI or ATG appears to be
risk factors in their development.
1. Most common are various skin cancers including basal
cell carcinoma, squamous cell carcinoma, and malignant melanoma. Patients at greatest risk are those who
develop cGVHD.
2. Brain tumors may develop (e.g., meningioma, glioblas-
toma multiforme).
3. Bone tumors may occur including osteosarcoma and
malignant fibrous histiocytoma.

XI. WHEN TO REFER A PATIENT BACK
TO THE TRANSPLANT CENTER

A. Many problems that develop after HSCT do not require return of the patient to the transplant center. However, it
may be useful to have select biopsy specimens reviewed
by pathologists versed in HSCT pathology. Their consultation can be particularly valuable when a diagnosis of GVHD
is being entertained.

B. Patients who should be referred back to the transplant center include those with:
1. Newly diagnosed acute or chronic GVHD.
2. Severe aGVHD patients who are refractory to conventional therapy and are candidates for experimental
therapy administered at the transplant center.
3. Severe cGVHD patients who are refractory to conventional therapy and are candidates for experimental
therapy that must be initiated at the transplant center.
4. Graft failure.
5. Life-threatening viral infections that require adoptive
immunotherapy with donor lymphocytes.
6. Relapsed leukemia patients who are candidates for immunotherapy with DLI.
7. PTLD patients who are candidates for adoptive immunotherapy with donor-derived T cells.
8. A relapsed malignancy patient who is a candidate for a
second transplant.
a. Any regimen-related toxicity from the first transplant should have resolved.

b. If TBI was used for conditioning before the first transplant, sufficient time (often up to 12 months) must have elapsed to permit recovery from radiation injury to normal tissues and allow the patient to undergo conditioning with a non-TBI based regimen without excessive regimen-related toxicity.

c. If TBI was not used for the first transplant, the time interval before a second transplant can be performed may be considerably shorter.

d. Ideally, patients who receive second transplants for disease recurrence should be in remission or, alternatively, be in early relapse at the time of the second HSCT.

Bibliography

Bhatia S, Ramsay N, et al. Malignant neoplasms following bone marrow transplantation. *Blood* 87:3633–39, 1996.

Boulad F, Sands S, and Sklar C. Late complications after bone marrow transplantation in children and adolescents. *Current Problems in Pediatrics* 28:273–97, 1998.

Centers for Disease Control. Outbreaks of *Salmonella* serotype enteritidis infection associated with consumption of raw shell eggs, United States, 1994–1995. *MMWR* 45(34):737–42, 1996.

Centers for Disease Control. Foodborne outbreak of cryptosporidiosis, Spokane, Washington, 1997. *MMWR* 47(27):535–37, 1998.

Centers for Disease Control. Update: multistate outbreak of listeriosis, United States, 1998–1999. *MMWR* 47(51):1117–18, 1999.

Cohen A, Rovelli R, et al. Endocrine late effects in children who underwent bone marrow transplantation: Review. *Bone Marrow Transplantation* 21, Suppl. 2:S64–67, 1998.

Cohen A, Rovelli A, et al: Final height of patients who underwent bone marrow transplantation for hematological disorders during childhood: A study by the working party for late effects—EBMT. *Blood* 93:4109–15, 1999.

Dini G, Castagnola E, et al. Infections after stem cell transplantation in children: state of the art and recommendations. *Bone Marrow Transplantation* 28, Suppl. 1:S18–21, 2001.

Ferrara J, Deeg H. Graft-versus-host disease. *N Engl J Med* 324:667–74, 1991.

Giorgiani G, Bozzola M, et al. Role of busulfan and total body irradiation on growth of prepubertal children receiving bone marrow transplantation and results of treatment with recombinant human growth hormone. *Blood* 86:825–31, 1995.

Gross TG, Steinbuch M, et al. B cell lymphoproliferative disorders following hematopoietic stem cell transplantation: risk factors, treatment, and outcome. *Bone Marrow Transplantation* 23:251–58, 1999.

Guidelines for preventing opportunistic infections among hematopoietic stem cell transplant recipients. *Morbidity and Mortality Weekly Report* 49 (RR-10):1–125, CEI-7, 2000.

Herwaldt BL, Ackers ML. Outbreak in 1996 of cyclosporiasis associated with imported raspberries. *New Engl J Med* 336(22):1548–56, 1997.

Hoyle C, Goldman JM. Life-threatening infections occurring more than 3 months after BMT. *Bone Marrow Transplant* 14: 247–52, 1994.

Kusminsky G, Dictar M, Arduino S, Zylberman M, Sanchez Avalos JC. Do not drink Maté: an additional source of infection in South American neutropenic patients. *Bone Marrow Transplant* 17(1):127, 1996.

Moe GL. Low-microbial diets for patients with granulocytopenia. In Bloch AS, ed., *Nutrition Management of the Cancer Patient*. Rockville, Aspen Publishing, Inc., 1990, pp. 125–34.

Phipps S, Dunavant M, et al. Cognitive and academic functioning in survivors of pediatric bone marrow transplantation. *J Clin Oncol* 18:1004–11, 2000.

Schultz K, Green G, et al. Obstructive lung disease in children after allogeneic bone marrow transplantation. *Blood* 84:3212–20, 1994.

Somani J, Larson R. Review: reimmunization after allogeneic bone marrow transplantation. *Am J Med* 98:389, 1995.

Sullivan K, Witherspoon R, et al. Alternating-day cyclosporin and prednisone for treatment of high-risk chronic graft-v-host disease. *Blood* 72:555–561, 1988.

Taormina PJ, Beuchat LR, Slutsker L. Infections associated with eating seed sprouts: an international concern. *Emerg Infect Dis* 5(5):626–34, 1999.

18

Psychosocial Care

Robert B. Noll, Ph.D., and Anne E. Kazak, Ph.D.

As the prognosis for children with cancer improves due to more aggressive treatments, more attention must be placed on the social, emotional, and behavioral quality of life for them and their families. These children, their families (siblings, parents, grandparents), friends, and the professionals (teachers, nurses, physicians, psychosocial providers, etc.) who care for them are placed in numerous stressful situations. These challenging life events can be overwhelming, but they also can be managed in positive ways that encourage families to continue to function in the best possible fashion and facilitate personal growth.

Although most pediatric cancer centers provide psychosocial care (e.g., psychology, social work, Child Life, psychiatry), the amount and structure of these services vary widely. The current challenge is to provide services that are accessible to families, effective and cost efficient, while also addressing the multiple and ongoing needs of children with cancer and their families, and ensuring that psychosocial care is integrated with medical care. At a minimum, psychosocial expertise is necessary in the following general areas: (1) knowledge of childhood cancer and the impact of serious illness on children and families; (2) clinical interviewing of children and families; (3) behavioral and cognitive behavioral approaches to pain and distress management; (4) consultation skills for working with complex medical teams and families; (5) psychodiagnostic skills; (6) neuropsychological and psychoeducational screening and evaluation; (7) school intervention; (8) psychotherapy; (9) ability to identify resources to assist families in addressing financial and social concerns; (10) strong skills in teaching medical and nursing staff; and (11) collaborative styles for working with multidisciplinary teams. Each pediatric cancer center must determine the optimal manner for their center to provide this broad array of essential psychosocial services to every child with cancer and their families.

I.   ESTABLISHING OPEN COMMUNICATION AT DIAGNOSIS

A.   The multidisciplinary treatment team should introduce psychosocial team members as integral to care. Psychosocial concerns should be acknowledged as "normal" responses to extraordinary circumstances. It is essential to avoid suggesting that psychosocial care is reserved for families having problems.

B.   It is helpful to have a psychosocial team member present at the initial informing meeting with the family and at other meetings where critical medical information is provided to the family. The psychosocial team member can:
1.   Support the family during this meeting.
2.   Note familial reactions to information and the family's style of responding and mobilizing to care for their child.
3.   Facilitate the family's understanding by asking questions during the meeting.
4.   Provide additional assistance in clarifying details of treatment protocols and informed consent.

C.   It is unlikely that all necessary information can be obtained during one interview with the newly diagnosed child and family. Follow-up interviews should:
1.   Include parents, siblings, ill child, grandparents, etc.
2.   Model communication for discussing difficult health care issues with children.
3.   Include consideration of the following topics:
a.   Disease, treatment, prognosis, side effects, invasive medical procedures (to ensure clarity of communication and re-education as needed)
b.   Insurance, financial concerns, social support resources (e.g., baby sitting for siblings), transportation to the medical center, religious/spiritual needs, any special social or economic issues
c.   Identification of risk factors that are antecedent to the diagnosis of cancer and which may interfere with the child's care:
i.   Marital difficulties
ii.   Parental emotional problems or existing mental health histories
iii.   Children's behavioral/emotional/academic problems
iv.   Other stressors that the family is experiencing

4. Psychosocial professionals should have diagnostic skills to identify difficulties in the above domains.

5. Impressions from family meetings must be reviewed with the child's health care team to facilitate the development of a comprehensive care plan.

6. Several follow-up interviews during the first week or two are almost always required.

D. Follow-up interviews are recommended again about 1–2 months after diagnosis and regularly thereafter (every 4–6 months) to review issues again and evaluate the child's and family's adjustment to cancer.

1. After the shock of the initial diagnosis and treatment have subsided.

2. Consider including siblings, grandparents, and other meaningful supportive individuals in these meetings.

3. The frequency of these follow-up meetings will depend on the needs of the family. Some families need standard follow-up; others require consistent and frequent meetings.

E. Parental reluctance (or refusal) to meet with psychosocial professionals is unusual. When encountered-

1. Reasons should be explored:
   a. Cultural issues (race, ethnicity, language)
   b. Timing
   c. Manner of contacting family (e.g., fit with the style of the psychosocial team member, miscommunication about purpose of meeting)
   d. Other reasons

2. Difficulties in establishing communication with the family about psychosocial concerns should be discussed as a multidisciplinary team in order to develop alternate plans to ensure that the family's needs are met while their concerns are also respected.

II. ADAPTATION OF CHILDREN

A. Distinct social, emotional, and behavioral challenges are associated with the specific developmental phase of the child, but considerable data strongly suggest that the social, emotional, and behavioral functioning of children with cancer is quite robust.

1. Infants, toddlers, and preschoolers are sensitive to separations from caregivers and prone to angry outbursts (tantrums). Babies are often cranky when hospitalized and/or receiving either inpatient or outpatient care.

2. Preschoolers often have a difficult time with medical procedures and may demonstrate regressive or aggressive behavior (tantrums).

3. It is common for school-aged children to have anticipatory worries about medical procedures, separation anxieties, and school re-entry, but these should not interfere with treatment.

4. If problems emerge with pill swallowing, procedural anxiety, etc., a referral should be make as soon as possible to a mental health professional with special training in these areas.

5. Adolescent issues of eating, pill swallowing, procedural anxiety, and adherence are reviewed below.

B. Depression and/or anxiety are the most common reasons for psychological/psychiatric referral during treatment. However, there are minimal data supporting the presence of these problems in children receiving treatment for cancer except brain tumors (see section VII.D). While many children have symptoms of depression or anxiety, these are often understandable reactions to their disease and treatment rather than symptoms that met criteria for a psychiatric diagnosis. Approaches include:

1. Finding out what has been helpful in the past if there is a history of being anxious and depressed when placed in stressful situations.

2. The majority of instances where the youngster appears excessively depressed or anxious, these responses are normal reactions to feeling bad physically or acute life circumstances such as:
   a. Reactions to hospitalizations
   b. Side effects of therapy
   c. Missing meaningful activities

3. When evaluation indicates the presence of clinical depression, suicidality should be explored. More intensive treatment options should be considered with the family or the child alone. Consultation with a mental

health professional who specializes in childhood psychopathology or family problems should be sought.

4. Successful use of antidepressant medications in children/adolescents with cancer has *not* been reported in the research literature.
   a. Medication use should be limited to the following instances:
      i. Strong family history of problems with depression.
      ii. Premorbid difficulties were present.
      iii. Current problems are chronic, unremitting, and interfere with day to day functioning.
      iv. Psychotherapeutic interventions have not been successful.
   b. Antidepressant medications are less effective for adjustment reactions.
   c. If antidepressant medications are used, an awareness of interactions with chemotherapeutic agents should be reviewed with a child psychiatrist.

III. ADAPTATION OF ADOLESCENTS

A. Special attention is required for adolescents because of the documented difficulties they encounter with adverse reactions to chemotherapy and well-substantiated nonadherence to treatment recommendations.

B. Significant changes in the demeanor of the adolescent such as excessive anxiety, moodiness, undue passivity, undesirable changes in behavior, academic difficulty, or more conflict at home require attention.

C. The adolescent who is nonadherent with treatment is a significant challenge.
   1. Nonadherence with oral medications is high, up to 60%.
   2. Psychosocial management of the teenager might include:
      a. Preventively, parents can work with teens to ensure that medications are taken. It is helpful to have parents anticipate nonadherence in teens and, if needed, to monitor medication taken.
      b. Providing regular psychosocial interventions with a focus on adherence.

    c. A team approach that integrates information from the medical team along with input from parents, grandparents, teachers, peers, and other outside resources that are meaningful to the teenager.

    d. Use of positive interventions such as developing routines, parental monitoring, and reinforcement for adherence to encourage and motivate teens to take medications, despite their side effects, are strongly recommended. Scare tactics are typically not effective. Unfortunately, education is also typically not effective.

  D. Fostering connections between adolescent patients can be very beneficial, especially when they have opportunities to participate in non-oncology-related activities such as camps, special activities (e.g., trips to amusement parks, pizza parties).

  E. Teen patients may need additional resources when a friend with cancer relapses or dies. Team members with expertise in mental health and available community resources must make contact with the adolescent and their family to determine what might be helpful.

IV. SIBLINGS

  A. Understanding siblings' reactions to the diagnosis and making certain that parents are able to deal with their reactions are essential to family centered care.

    1. If concerns are raised, additional information should be obtained from the sibling, family, and teachers to ascertain the full extent of difficulties.

    2. Sibling reactions that are troublesome for parents may be manifest by:

      a. Extreme anxiety

      b. Apparent unconcern and unusual apathy

  B. Siblings of children with cancer commonly have immediate concerns about changes to family routines, the health of their ill sibling, etc. There has been little research on siblings and their long-term adjustment.

  C. Common sibling concerns include:

    1. The desire for more information about their siblings' illness.

2. Jealousy about the extra attention their ill sibling is receiving.
3. Fears that their sibling is dying.
4. Being left behind
5. Donor issues
6. Contagion effects
7. Guilt related to the patient's diagnosis (children can believe that they caused the cancer).

D. Visits to the hospital and outpatient clinic are strongly recommended but can be stressful. Care must be taken to prepare healthy siblings before visits.
   1. The initial visit should occur as soon as possible after diagnosis.
   2. The staff should make certain visits are not overwhelming.
      a. Preparation about technical medical equipment is helpful.
      b. Preparation about how ill their sibling looks is helpful.
         i. Verbal descriptions
         ii. Photographs

E. Although siblings of children with cancer commonly do *not* have social or academic difficulties at school, parents should routinely be asked about sibling functioning at school so problems can be addressed immediately.
   1. School-focused interventions with collaboration from the medical treatment team.
   2. Education of teachers and peers regarding what is occurring for the ill sibling are often useful.

F. Major worries of many siblings are related to the illness and not having accurate information. Misinformation is a common problem as siblings talk to teachers, peers, neighbors, etc. With increasing age, siblings will benefit from knowing greater details about:
   1. The specific illness (e.g., leukemia)
   2. A description of the illness (cancer of the blood)
   3. Side effects of treatment (especially those that can be observed)
   4. Length of treatment
   5. Ill child's prognosis

   a. Many siblings are specifically concerned about
      whether their ill brother or sister will die, but are
      afraid to ask adults.
   b. Psychosocial professionals need to take a leader-
      ship role for the family.

V. PARENT AND FAMILY COPING AND ADJUSTMENT

A. The diagnosis of cancer in a child is one of the most distressing experiences for families. In the short-term, mothers and fathers of children with cancer may have difficulties
   with anxiety, depressed mood, sleep, somatic complaints,
   and interpersonal relationships.
   1. Most research has been conducted on mothers. It is
      essential to include fathers in clinical care and in re-
      search. Mothers and fathers have many similar reac-
      tions but may express distress differently.
   2. Cognitive-behavioral problem solving interventions
      are effective to reduce distress for parents at diagnosis
      and are highly recommended. They can reduce distress
      and have the potential to improve problem-solving abil-
      ities.
   3. Careful monitoring of parental mental health is a nec-
      essary component of cancer care for children. Knowl-
      edge of premorbid adjustment and previous reactions
      to stress are helpful in predicting how parents will cope.
   4. Over the first year from diagnosis, parental and fam-
      ily adaptation improves. Careful assessment at diag-
      nosis may reveal risk factors to identify those families
      who will experience more difficulty coping with the de-
      mands of treatment.

B. Parents will profit from contact with psychosocial professionals during routine patient visits. These meetings
   should focus on coping with stress with special attention
   to:
   1. Family functioning
   2. Parental distress
   3. Siblings
   4. Grandparents
   5. Problems with misinformation from outside sources
      a. Many people know about cancer in adults but not
         in children.

      b. Experience with adult cancers are often presumed to hold true for childhood cancers.

      c. When parents use an open communication model, problems in this area are less frequent and less burdensome.

C. Most parents will report having symptoms of anxiety, depression, and feeling overwhelmed; however, problems with day to day functioning are not typical. If difficulties with day to day functioning occur, immediate referral should be made for regular psychotherapy, or community support groups, or community agencies that specialize in providing support to families when a family member has cancer.

    1. Psychotropic medications for dealing with the stress of childhood cancer and its treatment should be limited to parents who do not respond to psychotherapy or parents with pre-existing psychiatric difficulties.

    2. Psychotropic medications are less effective for adjustment reactions.

    3. It is strongly recommended that pediatric oncologists do not prescribe psychotropic medications to parents but rather refer parents to their internist, family physician, or to a psychiatrist.

D. Family coping needs to be monitored during treatment.

    1. The stress associated with childhood cancer can be especially challenging when parents have different styles of coping.

    2. Treatment of childhood cancer demands considerable parental time, and parents often must re-allocate available resources and redefine roles within the family. Assistance with these processes can be very helpful.

E. Despite the many strains that childhood cancer places on the marriage, cancer in a child is *not* associated with long-term marital conflicts or increased divorce rates when compared with families not affected by childhood cancer. Serious marital problems should be referred to psychotherapy.

F. Chronic distressing symptoms related to their child's cancer such as unexpected intrusive thoughts about cancer, difficulties making hospital visits, heightened concerns over minor health problems (i.e., colds, flu) for all of their children, or recurrent dreams are commonly experienced by parents.

1. Post-traumatic stress symptoms are common but typically do not interfere with daily activity.
2. When symptoms are so severe that they adversely affect day to day functioning, interventions must be initiated. These might include:
   a. Mental health professionals on the team assisting with coping strategies, helping parents to stay focused, or accept their distress
   b. A referral for outside assistance from cancer-related agencies or professional therapist with post-traumatic stress disorder experience
   c. A referral for medications from a psychiatrist with experience with post-traumatic stress disorder

VI. GRANDPARENTS

A. Grandparents often play a key role with child care, daily living tasks, and care of the child with cancer.
B. While little research has been done examining the reactions of grandparents to the diagnosis of childhood cancer, clinical observations suggest that they may be at risk for excessive worry, depressed mood, and somatic complaints.
C. Some grandparents are in double jeopardy as they observe the pain of their adult child coping with their grandchild's cancer, and they observe the difficulties for their grandchild.
D. Help for grandparents can be accomplished by specifically including them in family meetings to provide accurate information about disease, prognosis, and treatment plans.

VII. SCHOOL RE-ENTRY

A. After parental permission is obtained, school personnel should be contacted as soon as possible to let them know about the child's disease. The child's peers should be informed about what is happening to preclude misinformation.
   1. Contacting the school with specific medical information helps school personnel feel more in control and facilitates dissemination of accurate information about the child's illness and treatment.

2. Children, teachers, and principals may associate childhood cancer with death. Knowledge of the child's disease; treatment, side effects, anticipated days of school to be missed, and duration of treatment; prognosis; and special issues (e.g., emergency catheter care).
3. Information should be obtained about how the child has performed (academically and socially) in the past.
4. When school nurses are available, they can be an excellent conduit for information between the hospital staff and school personnel.

B. If an extended absence from school is inevitable, school personnel should be encouraged to maintain contact with the patient and family via homebound teachers, letters, tapes, etc.
   1. Video tapes from classmates are especially helpful for morale.
   2. Peers should be encouraged to sustain contact during hospitalizations.
   3. Homework should be completed insofar as it is medically feasible.

C. As soon as possible after initial diagnosis and treatment, within the limits of medical care, children should be encouraged to return to school.
   1. Before the child returns to school, the psychosocial professional or an educational liaison specialist should talk with the child and parents about concerns they have about the child's return to school. Common concerns are:
      a. Changes in the child's physical characteristics
      b. Ways the child can talk with peers about their illness
      c. Childhood cancer is not contagious
   2. School attendance signals the return to normal routines and provides parents and children reassurance regarding improving health and the need to re-establish normal expectations and routines for the child.
   3. Maintaining friendships and routine interactions with peers are essential to normal psychological development and are as, or more, important than academic issues.

4. Homebound teaching should be considered when the option to attend school does not exist.

5. Attending school even for short periods of time is important as social interactions with schoolmates are extremely important.
   a. Combinations of homebound instruction along with limited school attendance when feeling better are common solutions
   b. Flexibility based on the child's changing health status is critical

6. Peer relationships of children with cancer should not be adversely affected by their disease and its treatment (except brain tumors).

D. Children with brain tumors or malignancies that can compromise central nervous system (CNS) integrity through their therapies (ALL with CNS disease; whole-brain radiation therapy) can have special problems related to school. These patients commonly experience difficulties with intellectual abilities, academics, and socialization that are not always obvious unless explored.

1. Neuropsychological evaluations should be completed by a professional with experience working with children with malignancies and the cognitive sequelae of their diseases.
   a. Facilitate appropriate classroom placements and the development of appropriate education programs.
   b. Results must be carefully reviewed with parents and school professionals to guarantee understanding of the child's cognitive abilities. Attendance at the Individual Education Plan by the testing neuropsychologist is encouraged.

2. Recommended scheduling of neuropsychological evaluations:
   a. Before school re-entry: neuropsychological screening (e.g., WISC-III subtests, individual achievement tests)
   b. Within 6 months of diagnosis: comprehensive neuropsychological assessment
   c. 1–2 years after diagnosis: comprehensive neuropsychological assessment (earlier if problems are being reported)

    d. 3–5 years after diagnosis: comprehensive neuro-psychological assessment. These tests are needed to:

       i. Fully appreciate the extent and nature of late effects

      ii. Direct comparisons with earlier test results are critical to understanding the neuropsychological impact of the disease and treatment

   3. Children with brain tumors are at high risk for problems fitting in with peers. They can become socially isolated and experience less social acceptance.

  E. School intervention programs are exceptionally valuable at maintaining liaison between the family, medical staff, and school professionals. Their routine use is strongly encouraged.

  F. When families have a difficult relationship with schools before a child is diagnosed, school intervention staff can be especially helpful.

  G. Remember, school personnel do not always understand issues related to confidentiality and HIPAA. Discussions should be held about appropriate use of health-related information and confidentiality.

VIII. RELAPSE, DEATH, AND DYING

  A. Relapse is a time of great stress for families and is often more devastating than the initial diagnosis. Psychosocial attention at this point is essential. Continuity of care and the opportunity to work with known staff members is particularly helpful at this point.

  B. After a relapse, the psychosocial provider must meet with the entire family, including healthy siblings and grandparents, to ensure understanding of what occurred and what will happen. Parents are generally overwhelmed by the relapse, so professional guidance is typically necessary.

  C. Assistance with anticipatory grieving before the loss of the child should be accomplished whenever possible. Some believe that long-term coping is enhanced when this has been explored.

   1. Fear of death becomes more prominent and should be explored.

2. Professional guidance should be offered as the majority of parents are not able to lead these discussions with their children or extended family.
3. Parents and children should be able to share concerns about death, and affirm their relationships with one another-to say goodbye to the dying child. Children who are terminally ill frequently know what is happening to them.
4. Particular attention should be paid to siblings and grandparents, to ensure they have an opportunity to say goodbye and understand what has occurred.
5. Silence can result in unnecessary suffering and diffuse fears about what is happening.

D. Sustained contact should be maintained during terminal phases of treatment by the psychosocial provider and local health professionals.

IX. BEREAVEMENT AND FAMILIES

A. Many believe that parents, siblings, grandparents, and close friends of a child who dies from cancer are at increased risk for psychosocial morbidity.
1. Grieving typically takes many years, and moderate to severe psychological distress is not uncommon.
2. We recommend discussion with the family about continued contact with the treatment team. Many families welcome phone calls over the first year after the child's death. The circumstances of the death and the family's relationship with the treatment team may determine the nature of ongoing contact.
3. As a part of formal/planned bereavement follow-up, one focus of the call should be to ascertain whether excessive psychosocial morbidity is present so that an appropriate referral can be made.

B. Styles of successful coping with loss are diverse.
1. Some individuals try to remember as much as possible while others try to forget-both can be successful.
2. Help families to appreciate diversity in styles of coping with loss.

C. Recommendations for follow-up are as follows:
  1. Key members of the primary treatment team (attending, fellow, nursing, psychosocial) should meet shortly after the death of a child to develop a follow-up plan. This plan should review plans for attendance at funerals and visitations and follow-up phone contact.
  2. Team members are encouraged to attend visitations and funerals in pairs.
  3. Decisions regarding attendance must be based on the needs of the family.
      a. Visitations are typically more lengthy visits at which more support can be provided.
      b. Funerals are typically more formal events at which the presence of hospital staff is important to families, but less specific support can be provided.
  4. We recommend calling families 2–4 weeks after the death of a child. This call should focus on psychological issues related to grieving and determining how the treatment team can be helpful.

X. STRESSES ON HEALTH PROFESSIONALS

A. Professionals who work with children with cancer are often in the midst of human tragedy that results in personal emotional pain.
  1. Common immediate reactions to this type of stress are anxiety, frustration, irritability, helplessness, and anger.
  2. Delayed stress reactions are lingering sadness, grief, or guilt.

B. Numerous strategies exist for professionals to lessen the burden of distressing events and accelerate recovery including:
  1. Psychosocial debriefings with the oncology team members to discuss critical incidents.
  2. Informal or formal support groups that meet regularly to focus on these complex issues.
  3. Regular physical exercise to reduce stress reactions.
  4. Use of relaxation techniques, imagery, or self-hypnosis.

XI. LONG-TERM SURVIVORS

A. The majority of children diagnosed with cancer will become long-term survivors. Cancer and its treatments can result in numerous late effects (e.g., risk for second malignancies, learning disabilities, reproductive failure, growth problems, organ toxicity) that can be distressing to long-term survivors and their families.

B. Even many years after treatment ends, upsetting memories of their child's treatment can continue to cause distress to the patient, parents, and family. However, most survivors and their families do well psychologically after cancer and are able to integrate their memories adaptively.

C. It is strongly recommended that a psychosocial professional be integrated into long-term follow-up visits to monitor adverse reactions by survivors and their families so appropriate interventions can be initiated with maximal ease. Psychological distress can become more prominent in young adulthood, and survivorship programs should attend to the psychosocial needs of survivors as they transition into adulthood.

Bibliography

Butler RW, Hill JM, Steinherz PG, et al. The neuropsychological effects of cranial irradiation, intrathecal methotrexate and systemic methotrexate in childhood cancer. *J Clin Oncol* 12:2621–29, 1994.

Hobbie, W, Stuber, M, Meeske, K, et al. Symptoms of posttraumatic stress in young adult survivors of cancer. *J Clin Oncol* 18:4060–66, 2000.

Kazak A, Simms S, Rourke M. Family systems practice in pediatric psychology. *J Pediatr Psychol* 27:133–43, 2002.

Lemanek K, Kamps J, Chung N. Empirically supported treatment in pediatric psychology: Regimen adherence. *J Pediatr Psychol* 26:253–75, 2001.

Mulhern RK, Wasserman AL, Friedman AG, et al. Social competence and behavioral adjustment of children who are long-term survivors of cancer. *Pediatr* 83:18–25, 1989.

Noll RB, Gartstein MA, Vannatta K, et al. Social, emotional, and behavioral functioning of children with cancer. *Pediatr* 103:71–78, 1999.

Riddle MA, Kastelic EA, Frosch E. Pediatric pharmacology. *J Child Psychol Psychiat* 42:73–90, 2001.

Ris MD, Noll RB. Long-term neurobehavioral outcome in pediatric brain tumor patients: Review and methodological critique. *J Clin Exp Neuropsychol* 16:21–42, 1994.

Sahler OJZ, Varni JW, Fairclough DL, et al. Problem-solving skills training for mothers of children with newly diagnosed cancer: A randomized trial. *J Dev Beh Pediatr* 23:77–86, 2002.

Seravalli EP. The dying patient, the physician, and the fear of death. *NEJM* 319:1728–30, 1988.

Stuber M, Kazak A, Meeske K, et al. Predictors of posttraumatic stress in childhood cancer survivors. *Pediatr* 100:958–64, 1997.

19

Recognition, Prevention, and Remediation of Burnout in Pediatric Oncology Staff

Corin M. Greenberg, Ph.D., Maru Barrera, Ph.D., Elizabeth Nichol, R.N., Linda Waterhouse, M.S.W., R.S.W., and Mark L. Greenberg, O.C., M.B., Ch.B., FRCPC, FAAP

Stress and burnout in health practitioners are of increasing concern in the field of pediatric oncology. The nature of the practice encompasses many risk factors for professional caregivers where unmanaged stress has enormous potential to disrupt the delivery of optimal care. The cohesive operation of the multidisciplinary team and the careers of professionals are at their peak or at the point of entry. More than a decade ago, a U.S. study reported that burnout affected 47% of university-linked oncologists and 39% of pediatric oncologists (Whippen and Canellos, 1991). A more recent study of Canadian cancer clinicians documented emotional exhaustion in oncology physicians and other health staff members (53.3% and 37.1%, respectively), a feeling of low accomplishment (48.4% and 54.0%), and evidence of depersonalization (21.1% and 4.3%). The prevalence of psychological morbidity among physicians was 25.4%.

As in other "people-oriented" professionals, staff are vulnerable to burnout because of: (1) work environments with high demands and low resources; (2) implicit standards/expectations and social norms for putting the needs of others first, working long hours, and going to any length to help patients; and (3) the pivotal place in their work of significant relationships with patients and their families. Unlike other disciplines, however, pediatric oncology practice involves a roller coaster course of treatment, uncertain outcomes, frequent revisions and reversal of care plans, and there is a substantial demand for effective communication and third-party problem-solving by professionals, teams, and families during a chronic course of illness that includes multiple acute episodes. These characteristics create an environment with unusual interpersonal and team challenges. Durable, long-term, high levels of collaboration with colleagues and families, predicated on excellent, nuanced, partner-sensitive communication are central to the provision of care.

I. WHAT IS BURNOUT?

A. Burnout is the inability to cope with the demands of the workplace—a cumulative and fairly stable stress reaction occurring in individuals chronically exposed to occupational stressors. Burnout is thought to be progressive. It has been described as a slowly advancing, multiple-step process arising from persistent exposure to problems at work characterized by, and sometimes progressing through, recognizable stages such as mental and physical exhaustion; indifference and cynicism; a sense of failure as a professional; a sense of failure as a person; and emotional numbness, which may be accompanied by exiting the profession or suicidal intent.

B. Burnout can be conceptualized as a mismatch between individual and workplace occurring in one or several of six areas of work life, namely:
1. Overload
2. Degree of control
3. Community
4. Personal-organizational values
5. Fairness
6. Reward/recognition.

C. Burned-out staff members are chronically exhausted, cynical, and disengaged. They feel ineffective and their work and working relationships decline. In contrast, engaged staff members are energetic, strongly involved and effective, and exhibit a high level of ability to adapt to change, creativity, and work quality.

II. RELATED AND CONTRASTING CONCEPTS

A. "Stress" and "failures of coping" are broad concepts that encompass physiologic, psychological, and social dimensions of poor adaptive functioning. Burnout is a distinct subset of stress/failure of coping, distinguishable by its chronicity, intensity, and occurrence in the context of work.

B. Post-traumatic stress disorders (PTSDs) are acute stress reactions that develop in response to a single, identifiable critical incident. In contrast, burnout evolves slowly and incrementally in response to multiple workplace experiences.

C. "Compassion fatigue," which is described increasingly frequently among health care workers, is best understood as vicarious traumatization prompted by listening to the accounts of fear, pain, and suffering of others—a secondary PTSD. Compassion fatigue is characterized by the re-experiencing of traumatic events, persistent arousal, and reduced social engagement with patients or colleagues. It can be a component of, or precursor to, burnout and an early indicator of dysfunction requiring intervention in its own right.

III. INDICATORS AND MANIFESTATIONS OF BURNOUT

A. Strong indicators of burnout are:
1. Overwhelming exhaustion
2. Cynicism
3. Frustration
4. Anger
5. A sense of failure

B. Additional indicators, particularly when these are associated with personal dysfunction and deterioration in physical and mental health, are:
1. Decreased commitment to work
2. Job dissatisfaction
3. Staff turnover and absenteeism

C. Indicators may be subjective or objective.
1. Principal subjective indicators are: a general state of severe fatigue accompanied by a loss of self-esteem, resulting from a feeling of professional incompetence; reduced job satisfaction; multiple physical symptoms of distress in the absence of organic illness; problems with concentration; irritability; and negativism.
2. The main objective indicator is a significant decrease in work performance over a period of several months—observable by patients as a deteriorated level of

service received; by colleagues as a general loss of interest in work; and by supervisors as decreased effectiveness and increased absenteeism.

D. Several researchers caution that a diagnosis of burnout should not be made in the presence of major psychopathology; major family problems; continuing and unchanged low level of competence on the job; or severe fatigue resulting from high and/or monotonous workload in the absence of feelings of incompetence.

E. Symptom profiles of burnout may vary across professional disciplines. Among nurses in a number of different specialties, physical symptoms and irritability are frequently reported, as are feelings of isolation and lack of support; symptoms of depression; and diminished general physical health. In contrast, among physicians, the most common symptoms of burnout are high levels of physical fatigue and emotional exhaustion, low levels of personal accomplishment and work dissatisfaction.

F. Indicators are grouped here in three categories to pave the way for a later discussion of choosing appropriate interventions with reference to specific symptom manifestations and the history of their development. These categories are: individual—personal; interpersonal—community; and organizational.
   1. Individual indicators
      Individual indicators typically include:
      a. Extreme fatigue and emotional exhaustion, a predictor of various physical symptoms reported by a majority (53.3%) of oncologists.
      b. Loss of confidence and a diminished sense of self-worth and personal accomplishment escalating to a sense of failure, isolation, and even self-hatred. Low accomplishment was reported in 48.4% of oncology clinicians in Ontario, Canada, and is strongly associated with workplace indicators such as low morale, poor performance, low productivity, and high staff turnover.
      c. Physical symptoms such as headaches; tiredness; neck, back, and shoulder pain; gastrointestinal disorders; muscle tension; hypertension; cold/flu episodes; and sleep disturbances.

      d. Psychological morbidity: health professionals working in oncology units exhibited levels of psychological morbidity often comparable to that of their patients. Physicians and nurses seem equally susceptible to social dysfunction, somatic, and anxiety disorders.

      e. Difficulty in balancing work and private life; and difficulties with personal relationships.

2. Interpersonal indicators

      a. A cluster of important symptoms of burnout are interpersonal in nature and can be detected by:

         i. Monitoring the work environment for high-risk conditions

         ii. Close observation of team function

         iii. Tracking the nature and frequency of staff—patient conflict, and

         iv. Attending to individuals' reflections on their own well being.

      b. Interpersonal symptoms of burnout include:

         i. Unresolved conflict among members of the health team and signs of low team cohesiveness. Nurses report conflict among medical staff to be particularly stressful.

         ii. Cynicism and depersonalization (i.e., negative, excessively, and chronically detached interactions with patients and/or colleagues). These are associated with a loss of idealism and thought to be symptomatic of more advanced "second stage" burnout. Staff members exhibiting depersonalization symptoms are typically in work overload and exhibit high levels of emotional exhaustion.

         iii. Feelings of emotional over involvement and an inability to maintain professional boundaries.

         iv. Persistent staff difficulty in bonding with new employees often observed in the restructured hospital environment.

3. Organizational indicators

From the perspective of the organization, the following indicators of burnout have been documented across the developed world:

      a. Staff absenteeism

      b. Low productivity

c. Decreased morale
d. Job dissatisfaction
e. Perceived organizational unfairness
f. Staff distress arising from work overload
g. Staff expressions of loss of control over the work environment
h. Major organizational change (e.g., restructuring, downsizing, turnover in leadership)

IV. RISK FACTORS ASSOCIATED WITH BURNOUT

A. Research and anecdotal accounts of health professionals concur that age, experience, coping style, constant exposure to serious illness, and the following workplace conditions are risk factors for burnout:
1. Work overload
2. Personal conflict
3. Limited autonomy and involvement in decision-making
4. Disruption of the social substrate of the team
5. Lingering shadows cast by questionable fairness
6. Replacement or removal of leaders and mentors
7. The absence or disruption of mechanisms of reward and recognition, and
8. Conflict of values

B. These factors are reported to be more potent stressors than patient suffering including death.

C. The literature points to different risk factors and appropriate interventions with various subpopulations of staff. In anticipation of the later discussion of appropriate interventions, risk factors for poor coping and burnout are grouped as: personal, interpersonal, and organizational.
1. Personal risk factors
Personal risk factors include:
a. A limited ability to manage conflicting demands on time.
b. Difficulty maintaining personal boundaries.
c. Persistent carryover of work stress to the home environment, which can undermine two critical protective factors; family support and a balance between work and home life.
d. Age and experience: younger cancer clinicians are reported to suffer more stress and burnout than

their older colleagues. Less experienced staff members may perceive patients and/or families as more needy than they are. This can lead, potentially, to a disruption of the optimal balance between professional and personal involvement. Younger (surgical) nurses exhibited more stress, lower self-esteem, and a lesser capability for social intimacy than older nurses during hospital downsizing.

e. Coping style: emotion-focused coping (observed in student nurses) has been associated with depersonalization, a common antecedent of burnout. In contrast, effective coping styles, which are correlated with greater experience, with a higher sense of personal accomplishment, and higher levels of work satisfaction are problem-focused coping (making a plan of action); existential coping (finding a sense of meaning and coherence); and preventive coping (trying to reduce anticipated problems).

2. Interpersonal risk factors
  a. Examples of interpersonal risk factors include:
    i.   Interactions with patients and families who are highly stressed, fearful, and/or angry.
    ii.   Having to suppress legitimate anger toward patients and families in their time of suffering.
    iii. Needing to maintain professional boundaries to ensure that caregivers support, but do not undertake, the emotional burdens of patients and families.
    iv.   Difficulty with setting boundaries: boundary setting appears to be a particular issue for pediatric oncology nurses who report that:
      (1) Without great involvement with patients, their nursing care would be incomplete;
      (2) Patient and family contact is a key source of their job satisfaction; and
      (3) Patients are extremely needy.
    v.   Having to constantly support, and provide hope for, fragile families, even when the outlook is grim.
    vi.   Dealing on a daily basis with life-threatening illness and limited therapeutic success.

      vii. Having repeatedly to break bad news.

     viii. Experiencing feelings of guilt after unexpected adverse events.

      ix. Shifting goals of patient care when resistant disease is encountered.

       x. Grief saturation.

      xi. Conflicting opinions among staff and parents in the context of third-party decision-making.

     xii. The attendant necessity for close, frequent, and complex communication leading to group consensus about the best interests of the child.

  b. The necessarily different perspectives of each child's caregivers (health care staff, parents, and guardians), in addition to the need for prolonged association through the difficult times and fluctuating disease status, make conflicts of opinion about the appropriate and ethical course of action unavoidable and superior problem-solving strategies an essential skill. Additional risk-loading characteristics of today's pediatric oncology units/ professional communities are the increased numbers and complexity of cases and increased clinical and academic demands arising from rapid advances in cancer treatment.

3. Organizational risk factors

  a. Health care work environments contain many risk factors for burnout. Characteristically, these workplaces:

       i. Have limited resources.

      ii. Hold to social norms of selflessness.

     iii. Require the development of multiple, sustained relationships to mediate their success.

     iv. Contain significant potential for a clash of values regarding patient care among professional colleagues; between professionals and parents; and/or between professionals and the organization.

      v. May set professional and organizational values on a collision course (e.g., when fiscal objectives cannot be reconciled with the caregiver prioritization of optimal resources for patient care). Early discharge policies and special permission processes required to carry out certain treatment procedures such as bone marrow transplantation further exemplify organizational stressors.

b. Organizational factors that may result in positive engagement include:

i. Sufficient recognition of staff.

ii. Perceived fairness regarding promotions and dismissals.

iii. Opportunities to develop professionally, which may include mentorship and management positions that constitute accessible sources of knowledge and problem-solving and can assist staff with workload management, rebuilding of the team, and valuable leadership. In this regard, the retention of a hierarchy of unit managers and experienced nurse educators seems to have a significant impact on nurses.

c. Many of these organizational issues are exacerbated in a health care environment characterized by budget cuts and funding reductions, and are more damaging when they occur concurrently with an increased service demand per patient, coupled with stable or shrinking staffing complements in the pediatric oncology setting—conditions that pertain to many pediatric oncology practice contexts over the past decade.

d. Low control in the work environment coincides with stress intrinsic to a high morbidity, relatively high mortality discipline with persistently increasing work loads.

e. The following events should trigger increased vigilance for symptoms of stress and burnout:

i. Expressed concern about limited/lost control over the work.

ii. A number of patient deaths in a short period of time.

iii. Unexpected or adverse outcomes, particularly in the context of significant organizational change as detailed in the next section.

iv. Elimination of middle management.

     v. Changes in departmental or nursing leader-
ship.

    vi. Threats to the integrity of the team (e.g., after
radical restructuring and loss of staff).

   vii. Persistence of identified risk factors or evidence of their intensification.

f. Recognizing these causes and risk factors for
burnout enables staff and leaders to intervene pre-
ventatively to augment the enormous sense of grat-
ification that can accrue to staff from this discipline
and remedially to re-establish a positive work experience.

V. INTERVENTIONS

A. Individual, interpersonal, and organizational-level interventions have emerged from a burgeoning 30-year literature on strategies to address burnout and promote workplace coping.

B. The timing of interventions falls into three categories:
1. Preventive interventions involve the pre-emptive management of predictable high-risk stressors. Such interventions aim to achieve a work environment that
fosters staff energy, involvement, effectiveness, and
satisfaction.
2. Secondary level interventions more effectively address
established, moderate levels of stress, and optimally
include one or more interventions selected to match
the type of symptom and its antecedents.
3. Remedial work is called for when health care providers
are evidently suffering severe psychological or physical effects of burnout. Effective intervention at this late
stage should include individual counseling and is likely
to require multilevel strategies to address the multiple
dimensions of established burnout.

C. Principles and guidelines for the selection of effective
interventions
1. Preventive interventions
    a. Intervening pre-emptively may include:
       i. The creation of opportunities for staff mem-
bers to develop selected skill sets that directly

address identified stressors (e.g., communication skills training). These have substantial potential to foster a professional community, positive staff—patient interaction, and problem-solving strategies.

ii. Maintaining the distinctive and especially fitting culture of pediatric oncology care (i.e., family-centered care with a developmental perspective); a culture of collaboration; and team-based delivery enriched by the different literatures and skills sets of multiple disciplines.

iii. Modification of the environment within the hematology-oncology program (institution-wide, where possible), for example, through:

(1) Effective reduction of escalating workloads including increasing human resources.

(2) Conscientious recognition of staff contributions.

(3) Inclusion of confidential employee assistance programs.

(4) Introduction of principles of program operation that include fairness and due process.

(5) Realistic expectations (including the inevitability of some interpersonal stress).

(6) Policies that help staff members to balance academic, teaching, and clinical responsibilities.

(7) Rotation of staff between the oncology inpatient unit and clinics where positive outcomes are more evident.

(8) Participatory decision-making. Active staff involvement in decision-making facilitates the sharing of staff knowledge and experience within the collegial group and has been shown to promote a sense of control and engender commitment. It is consistently associated with higher levels of personal accomplishment and lower levels of staff exhaustion.

(9) Creation of a culture of consultation and mentorship in which informal contacts

with senior staff are encouraged within and across disciplines, and knowledge transfer formats such as tumor boards and multidisciplinary rounds are promoted.

   iv. Monitoring at-risk staff populations for personal, interpersonal, and discipline-related symptoms (e.g., young nurses who have been shown to suffer more stress than experienced nurses).

2. Secondary and remedial interventions

   a. In planning secondary and remedial interventions, it is important to:

      i. Explore the etiology of presenting problems; classify sources of stress as individual, interpersonal and/or organizational, and expect to find multiple antecedents and expressions of burnout.

      ii. Match the intervention to the problem profile. For example, in addressing "interpersonal" and nature-of-practice problems, communication training and support groups may be more effective. Optimal interventions for severe individual burnout include psychological counseling and cognitive therapy. Stress and burnout related to organizational stressors may be best addressed by strategies such as advocacy for better patient-to-staff ratios, exposure to appropriate role models, allowing time off on short notice, participation in education programs, and increased vacation time (69% of U.S. oncologists proposed the latter as an antidote for burnout [Whippen and Canellos, 1991]).

      iii. Consider multilevel interventions. Since burnout is typically the result of chronic exposure to multilevel stressors, some combination of individual, team, and organizational programs or strategies will often be most effective.

      iv. Choose or construct interventions that offer longer contact times, since these achieve more sustained changes in psychological well being. The following formats have proven effective: a total of nine hours of weekly, one-hour sessions, and six 90-minute sessions, held weekly, followed by refresher sessions over the next 18 months (Rowe, 1999).

v. Where team morale, cohesiveness, and productivity are of concern, consider hiring team assessment and team-building experts (e.g., Myers-Briggs Type Indicator and True Colors team building, communication, and life skills workshops *[www.career-lifeskills.com/ products_services]*).

vi. Match the intervention to proven staff receptivity. For example, nurses respond to ongoing staff support groups with increased job satisfaction and self-esteem, reduced toxicity errors, and are more affected by groups conducted by an external facilitator. Nurses also benefit from methodical problem-solving skills training and the use of humor. Physicians are reported to gain from interactive communications training. Which promotes step-by-step techniques for difficult communication scenarios drawn from oncology practice. Allied health professionals are reported to benefit from stress management training sessions.

vii. Select interventions according to the level of staff experience, for example, in-service, burnout-proofing sessions for new pediatric oncology nurses (0–3 months) might optimally include setting priorities, a review of case studies, and discussion with experienced nurses about their anxieties, whereas nurses with 12 or more months of experience in the discipline will gain more from sessions focused on social and ethical issues, the development and maintenance of professional boundaries, coping with death, and recognizing signs of burnout in themselves and colleagues.

viii. Understand that there are gender differences— both in the extent to which individuals are affected by the "vicarious" stresses of patients (women appear to be more vulnerable), and in the ways males and females use social networks versus other sources of support in times of stress. More educated women gain from the support of social networks in times of stress, whereas men are more likely to rely solely on their spouses.

   ix. Consider the interventions staff have identified and ranked as "most useful." For example, nurses endorse the following:

     (1) Peer support programs including sessions on the management of stress, strengthening nurse/manager relationships, coping with change and uncertainty, and "help lines."

     (2) Communication skills training, particularly programs addressing how to deliver a diagnosis to the child, how to help families deal with death, and how to maintain hope.

     (3) Bereavement support (e.g., conferences and workshops, and staff-parent rituals for observing patient deaths.

D. Communications programs worthy of further attention

  1. *SPIKES* interactive workshops provide oncology staff and fellows with a protocol for patient interaction and training in advanced communication skills including the breaking of bad news, techniques for patient disclosure, and the management of difficult patients and families. The acronym SPIKES summarizes six successive steps in accomplishing complex communication.

  2. *Psychological Training Programs* (PTP) in oncology. This program aims to improve skills in basic interviewing, assessment and counseling, and addresses oncology practice. The program comprises four techniques: *cognitive* (theoretical information and courses), *behavioral* (role playing), *experiential* (case discussions, staff observations) and *supportive* (staff support groups, symptom recognition).

  3. *Teaching Health-Care Providers Coping.* This multidisciplinary job stress training program consists of 1.5-hour weekly sessions over a period of 6 weeks. Sessions address actual patient scenarios using problem-focused strategies and opportunities for small group discussion. An evaluation revealed decreased

exhaustion and a significantly increased sense of personal accomplishment among staff. Booster sessions at 5, 11, and 17 months after the basic program lead to additional gains.

4. *Preventing Burnout and Building Engagement: A Complete Program for Organizational Renewal* is a theoretically sound, evidence-based, do-it yourself-version of organizational renewal, published by Leiter and Maslach (2000). Using designed tools and supportive material, a project leader and team selected from among employees execute a protocol that culminates in a "Checkup Report."

5. *Bereavement Intervention.* This program includes several components:

    a. A bereavement support group for staff;
    b. A sympathy card mailing;
    c. A calendar recording dates of patient deaths;
    d. An annual event for families in honor of loved ones; and
    e. Support group sessions that are optional and occur monthly during which suggestions are offered to prepare staff for future stressful situations.

    Research and theory in this area indicate that optimal bereavement interventions encompass individual, interpersonal, team, and organizational strategies adapted for factors that affect bereavement.

VI. CONCLUSIONS

A growing literature on the chronic stresses of health care practice identifies symptoms and risk factors and points to interventions that may be effective with different professional disciplines, ages, and levels of experience. This accumulated wisdom clearly points to two important conclusions; namely that some degree of staff discomfort is inevitable given the nature of the discipline, and that burnout may be averted or managed when staff have the right mix of skills, social support, and opportunities to control the work environment. Individual, interpersonal, and organizational characteristics of the work environment handled with insight can become important sources of job satisfaction, energy, creativity, and engagement. However, left unattended, these same factors can lead to burnout.

As pediatric oncology programs increase their skill and vigilance in the recognition of staff burnout, the factors contributing to it, and their working knowledge of promising interventions, they will become more effective in their advocacy for needed resources and more successful at achieving and maintaining an engaged, energetic, and productive staff.

Acknowledgments

The authors wish to acknowledge the contribution of Heather Shearer to literature review relevant to this chapter.

Bibliography

Baile WF, Buckman R, Lenzi R, Glober G, Beale EA, Kudkelka AP. SPIKES—A six-step protocol for delivering bad news: Application to the patient with cancer. *Oncologist* 5(4):302–11, 2000.

Grunfeld E, Whelan TJ, Zitzelsberger L, Willan AR, Montesanto B, Evans WK. Cancer care workers in Ontario: Prevalence of burnout, job stress, and job satisfaction. *Can Med Assoc J* 163(2):166–69, 2000.

Leiter MP, Maslach C. Preventing burnout and building engagement: A complete program for organizational renewal (CD ROM, survey, and workbook). San Francisco: Jossey-Bass, 2000.

Lewis AE: Reducing burnout: Development of an oncology staff bereavement program. *Oncology Nursing Forum* 26(6):1065–69, 1999.

Maslach C, Leiter MP. *The Truth about Burnout: How organizations cause personal stress, and what to do about it.* San Francisco: Jossey-Bass, 1997.

Razavi D, Delvaux N. Communication skills and psychological training in oncology. *European J Cancer* 33 (Suppl. 6):S15–21, 1997.

Rowe MM. Teaching health-care providers coping: results of a two year study. *J Behav Med* 22(5):511–27, 1999.

Spinetta JJ, Jankovic M, Arush MWB, Eden T, Epelman C, Greenberg ML, Martins AG, Mulhern RK, Oppenheim D, Masera G. Guidelines for the recognition, prevention, and remediation of burnout in health care professionals participating in the care of children with cancer: Report of the SIOP Working Committee on psychological issues in pediatric oncology. *Med and Pediatric Oncology* 35:122–25, 2000.

Whippen DA, Canellos GP. Burnout syndrome in the practice of oncology: Results of a random survey of 1000 oncologists. *J Clin Oncology* 9:1916–21, 1991.

20

Complementary and Alternative Medicine in Pediatric Oncology

Susan F. Sencer, M.D., Kara M. Kelly, M.D.,
and John Iacuone, M.D.

Parents of children with cancer are often turning to complementary or alternative medicine (CAM) treatments as part of their children's care. Recent surveys of pediatric oncology patients show that between 30–84% of families have used one or more CAM therapies. These therapies are primarily used to combat side effects of conventional therapy, but also may be used by the family to treat the cancer primarily. Historically, patients were reluctant to tell their physicians about CAM use for fear of disapproval. More recently; however, patients not only share this information, but also often have expectations that their providers will be knowledgeable about CAM and its possible interactions with standard therapy. The study of CAM and cancer is rapidly evolving, although many aspects remain controversial. The following outline reviews the primary CAM therapies; particularly those used most often by children with cancer, as well as specific potential interactions to be aware of. In addition, suggestions on discussing CAM with families are provided so that informed rational decisions regarding them can be made.

I. COMPLEMENTARY AND ALTERNATIVE MEDICINE

A. Definitions: In general, CAM refers to those medical practices that fall outside the mainstream of conventional medicine as it is practiced in the United States and Canada. While there is generally scientific theory and some scientific evidence for many CAM practices, often many questions regarding efficacy and safety remain to be examined in well designed scientific studies.

1. Complementary medicine: modalities used in addition to conventional medicine.
2. Alternative medicine: those therapies used in place of conventional medicine.
3. Integrative medicine: a combination of conventional medicine and those CAM therapies for which there is sufficient scientific evidence for safety and efficacy.

B. Framework
    The National Center for Complementary and Alternative Medicine, a center of the National Institutes of Health, has classified CAM therapies into five major groupings, although other frameworks exist.
    1. Alternative medical systems, those systems, which have evolved outside of, and often earlier than, traditional Western medicine built on a complete system of theory and practice. Among these are:
        a. Traditional Oriental/Chinese medicine: emphasizes the proper balance of energy (qi); includes acupuncture, herbal medicine, and *qi gong*. Acupuncture has been used successfully to treat the pain of sickle cell crisis and to treat chemotherapy-induced nausea in children and adults.
        b. Ayurveda: the traditional medicine of India with the goal of restoring harmony of mind, body, and spirit through the use of diet, exercise, mediation, controlled breathing, and herbs.
        c. Homeopathy: based on the principle of "like cures like," highly diluted minute amounts of plant or medicinal substances are given to stimulate the body's defenses against a symptom.
        d. Naturopathy: diseases are viewed as alterations in the body's natural healing process and can be manipulated through a combination of diet, exercise, spinal and soft-tissue manipulations, among others.
    2. Mind-body interventions: techniques designed to enhance the mind's ability to affect the body and; therefore, health. Many of these have now become mainstream such as support groups, biofeedback, hypnosis, imagery/relaxation, and cognitive and behavioral therapies. Techniques currently undergoing scientific

        inquiry and; therefore, still considered CAM include meditation, prayer, mental healing, art, music, and dance therapies.

3. Biologically based therapies: the medicinal use of substances found in nature such as herbs, vitamins, and foods. Nutraceuticals and nutritional supplements fall under this category, as do special diets and herbal therapies.

4. Manipulative and body-based methods

   a. Chiropractic care: manipulation of skeletal structures

   b. Osteopathy: manipulation of the musculoskeletal system

   c. Massage therapy: the therapeutic manipulation of soft tissues. Massage has been found to be effective in reducing pain and anxiety related to cancer in adults; studies in pediatric cancer patients are currently ongoing.

5. Energy therapies involve the use of energy fields

   a. Biofield therapies: intended to affect energy fields that are felt to surround and penetrate the human body; includes *qi gong*, Reiki, and Healing and Therapeutic Touch.

   b. Bioelectromagnetic-based therapies: the unconventional use of electromagnetic fields such as pulsed, magnetic, and alternating or direct current fields to treat disease.

II. BIOLOGICALLY BASED CAM THERAPIES IN PEDIATRIC ONCOLOGY

For most pediatric oncologists, the challenges related to CAM come primarily from patients' desire to use the biologically based therapies, either ingested or injected. These agents can be problematic because of both safety and efficacy concerns. Nutritional supplements, the category under which most CAM biological therapies fall, are not rigorously regulated in the United States, in contrast to pharmaceuticals and cancer trials. As a result, supplements may be contaminated or may not have standardized amounts of active ingredients. The potential for contamination is particularly high in products imported from developing countries. There is a danger, also, of interactions with conventional therapies, which may decrease effectiveness or increase toxicities of these therapies. Finally, there is also a danger that the lure of (perceived) more "natural" CAM therapies that promise fewer side effects will steer families away from potentially life-saving chemotherapy, radiation, and surgery.

A. Use of antioxidants during chemotherapy
    and radiation therapy
    The initiation, promotion, and progression of cancer, as well as the side effects of chemotherapy and radiation therapy, are related to an imbalance between reactive oxygen species and the antioxidant defense system. The cancer protective effects of a healthy diet are most often associated with dietary intake of fruits and vegetables. This is likely related to their roles as important sources of antioxidant micronutrients such as vitamins C and E, carotenoids, coenzyme Q_{10}, phytoestrogens, glutathione, polyphenols and other bioflavanoids, and phytonutrients such as lycopene, limonene, and allyl sulfides.

    Many patients are taking oral antioxidant supplements or herbal agents with antioxidant effects while receiving conventional chemotherapy and/or radiation therapy. Insufficient information is available to counsel patients definitively on the risks and benefits of antioxidant supplement use. The following reviews the current state of knowledge as it pertains to pediatric oncology.
    1. Antioxidant supplements commonly used by patients
        with cancer
        a. Vitamin C
        b. Vitamin E
        c. Beta carotene
        d. Selenium
        e. Coenzyme Q_{10}
        f. Blue-green algae
        g. Herbal products
    2. Estimates of antioxidant use among children with
        cancer
        a. 36% using dietary supplements (including megadose combination products, C, E, selenium, coenzyme Q_{10}, blue-green algae, pycnogenol)
        b. 27% using herbal agents (including green tea, grape seed extract)

     c. Majority were concurrently enrolled on conventional clinical trials for treatment of their cancer

     d. 50% or more of antioxidant use was not reported to the child's physician

3. Potential beneficial effects of antioxidants in cancer therapy

     a. Reduce tumor growth

     b. Reduce side effects of chemotherapy and radiation therapy

     c. Reduce risk for second malignant neoplasms and other late effects of therapy

     d. Improve quality of life

4. Anticancer therapies potentially altered by antioxidants

     a. Alkylating agents (cyclophosphamide, ifosfamide)

     b. Platinum compounds (cisplatin)

     c. Antibiotics (doxorubicin, bleomycin)

     d. Topoisomerase II inhibitors (etoposide)

     e. Radiation

5. Dietary factors also have an impact on antioxidant status:

Foods rich in antioxidants include: berries, plums, oranges, red grapes, cherries, kale, beets, red bell peppers, brussels sprouts, corn, spinach, onions, and broccoli.

Until further research is undertaken on the risks and benefits of antioxidant supplementation, recommendations for supplementation must be made with caution. Patients need to clearly understand that they may be sacrificing a long-term cure for a short-term improved tolerance of treatment. As there are limited data on the interactions of antioxidants and chemotherapy, patients should be counseled to defer high-dose antioxidant supplementation until the completion of chemotherapy or radiation to minimize the risk of adversely affecting the efficacy of chemotherapy. Consultation with a nutritionist would be appropriate. The use of a daily multivitamin should not routinely be discouraged, although the issue of folate-containing vitamins among children receiving methotrexate remains controversial. There are low folate vitamins available.

B. Specific herb—drug interactions
The following known or potential herb—drug interactions are a small fraction of the possibilities for herbal toxicities. Those documented below relate in some way to the practice of pediatric hematology/oncology.
1. Anticoagulants
   a. Agents which may increase bleeding potential: Angelica root, anise, arnica flower, black cohosh, Asafoetida, capsicum, celery, chamomiles, clove, denshen, devil's claw, dong quai, evening primrose, fenugreek, feverfew, garlic, ginkgo biloba, guarana, horse chestnut, licorice, onion, papain, parsley, passion flower, quassia, quinine, red clover, sweet clover, and sunflower seeds (vitamin E).
   b. Agents which may decrease effectiveness of anticoagulation: broccoli, ginseng, green tea, plantain, Saint John's wort, turmeric, and alfalfa (vitamin K).
2. Corticosteroids, Cyclosporine (immunosuppressive agents)
   a. Agents that may block the effectiveness of these immunosuppressive agents: alfalfa sprouts, echinacea, licorice, Saint John's wort, vitamin E, and zinc.
   b. Agents that may increase cyclosporine toxicity (increase levels): grapefruit juice.
3. Methotrexate
   Agents which may increase hepatotoxicity: echinacea, black cohosh
4. Tamoxifen
   Agents which may decrease effectiveness: black cohosh, soy.
5. Cisplatin
   Agents which may increase toxicity: selenium
6. Intraconazole
   Agents which may decrease effectiveness: grapefruit juice
7. Penicillins
   Agents which may decrease effectiveness: khat
8. Etoposide
   Agents which may increase toxicity: Saint John's wort

   Herbs that over time cause liver damage can also interfere with chemotherapy. *Germander* may cause hepatic necrosis; Comfrey (pyrrolizidine alkaloids) causes veno-occlusive liver disease; and Chaparral and Kombucha tea may cause hepatocellular damage.

C. Immunostimulants

Immunostimulants or immunomodulators refer to a broad category of agents, which purport to affect one or more elements of the immune system. Echinacea, for instance, is an herbal remedy used to treat upper respiratory tract infections. Its exact method of action is not completely understood, but it has been shown in human studies to increase phagocytosis, antibody-dependent cellular cytotoxicity, and natural killer cell activity. The majority of immunostimulants used by cancer patients generally increase either cytotoxic T cells, natural killer cells, or endogenous production of interferon, interleukins, or other cytokines. The actual antitumor effect of these possibilities has generally not been well studied. Common immunostimulants used in pediatric oncology are:

1. Mistletoe (Iscador or Iscar): widely used in Germany. Proliferation of peripheral mistletoe lectins cause both apoptosis and directly cytotoxicity in vitro.

2. Asian mushrooms (maitake, reishi, shiitake, coriolus versicolor, or PSK): widely studied in Japan; show evidence of direct tumor toxicity in the in vitro studies and lessening of chemotherapy-induced side effects. Combinations of mushrooms and other immunostimulants are commercially available in most pharmacies.

3. Astragalus: used extensively in Chinese medicine in conjunction with chemotherapy; increases LAK cell cytotoxicity. Studies from China show improved survival and attenuation of side effects of chemotherapy in adults with cancer.

There have been, to date, no well designed scientific studies of the efficacy or safety of immunostimulants in children with cancer. Their use should be discouraged in individuals with lymphopoietic malignancies, autoimmune disease, and status after bone marrow transplant or solid organ transplant.

III. HELPING FAMILIES MAKE DECISIONS ABOUT ALTERNATIVE MEDICINE

A. Some suggestions for discussing alternative medicine with families:

1. Avoid taking an authoritarian approach.
2. Use common English, avoid "medicalese."
3. Be open about discussing diet and vitamins.
4. Do not abandon your own convictions, but be open.
5. Offer to look into treatments with which you are unfamiliar.

B. Tips on evaluating CAM products, websites, or practitioners:
1. Be wary of those manufacturers who make broad general claims such as those that claim the product or modality can cure not only cancer, but also arthritis, diabetes, chronic fatigue, etc.
2. Websites are often funded by commercial operations. Follow the money. Who is promoting the website, updating it, conducting research, and what do they have to gain from it? Are there pyramid schemes, indirect commercial links, questionable distributors, or unclear supporting information? Has the site earned awards, seals of approval, or merits for conduct? Are these awards from commercial vendors?
3. Be distrustful of those promoters who emphasize how controversial their therapy is, claiming persecution from the standard medical and legal communities; or those practitioners who seek testimonials and publicity but avoid peer review.
4. Remember that many concepts can have a "plausible" scientific rationale. The job is to figure out if anyone besides the promoter thinks there is validity to the claims.

IV. CONCLUSIONS

The amazing improvements in childhood cancer survival in the last 30 years are unprecedented. Nonetheless, there is a common misperception that cancer remains an untreatable disease. In addition, some people gravely mistrust "the medical establishment." Our primary goal must be to treat patients with the most up-to-date standard of care; therefore, we must keep lines of communication open with parents who seek alternative medicine, thereby ensuring that they allow their children to be treated with proven therapies. We run the risk of alienating patients and their families, and thus driving them away from standard therapy if we rigidly refuse to consider alternative therapies. While no forms of alternative medicine have been shown scientifically to systematically cure cancer, several may indeed have a role in the quality of life and supportive care arenas.

Resources

cancer.gov/cancer_information/zem
  The NCI website has PDQ Cancer Information Summaries on a limited number of complementary and medicine.
carolann.hs.columbia.edu/
  Columbia University Pediatric Oncology and CAM website: contains comprehensive listings of articles on children with cancer and CAM modalities.
www.mcp.edu/herbal/
  Longwood Herbal Task Force: comprehensive reviews of many herbal agents with special attention to pediatrics.
www.childrensintegrativemed.org/
  Children's Hospitals and Clinics/Minneapolis–St. Paul website with pediatric oriented information and educational sheets on CAM modalities.
www.nccam.nih.gov/
  National Center for Complementary and Alternative Medicine.

Bibliography

D'Arcy PF. Adverse reactions and interactions with herbal medicines. Part 2: Drug interactions. *Toxicology Review* 12(3):147–62, 1993.

Kelly K, Jacobson JS, Kennedy DD, Braudt SM, Mallick M, Weiner MA. Use of unconventional therapies by children with cancer at an urban medical center. *J Pediatric Hematology/Oncology* 22(5):412–16, September/October 2000.

Miller L. Herbal Medicinal, Arch. *Internal Medicine* 158 (Nov. 9):2200–2211, 1998.

Pledge M. Herbal remedies: Are they safe to use in children? Children's Hospital of Denver website.

Post-White J, Sencer S, Fitzgerald M. Complementary and alternative treatments. In Baggott CR, et al., eds., *Nursing Care of Children and Adolescents with Cancer*. Philadelphia: W. B. Saunders, 2001.

The Review of Natural Products, December 2000.

Yance D. *Herbal Medicine, Healing and Cancer.* Keats Publishing, 1999.

21

Palliative Care

Sarah Friebert, M.D., and Joanne M. Hilden, M.D.

I. STATISTICS

A. Despite medical progress, approximately 25–33% of children with cancer will die. Cancer remains the leading cause of nonaccidental death in children.

B. Slightly more than half of children with cancer who die, do so at home.

C. Between 2–10% of dying children receive hospice/palliative care services.

D. Even children who don't die, and their families, can benefit from palliative care services as they negotiate life-threatening illness.

E. Access to palliative and/or supportive care programs is even less available in rural areas and for children of non-white descent.

II. DEFINITIONS

A. *Palliative care* is comprehensive, multidisciplinary care that "seeks to prevent or relieve the symptoms produced by a life-threatening medical condition or its treatment, to help patients with such conditions and their families live as normally as possible, and to provide them with timely and accurate information and support in decision-making". Palliative care is not synonymous with lack of care and may include chemotherapy, analgesics, surgery, radiation therapy, and other comfort measures. Included in the World Health Organization definition is the concept that such care is not limited to the end of life and can be provided concurrently with curative or life-prolonging treatment. In addition to focusing on impeccable assessment and holistic treatment of symptoms interfering with quality of life, palliative care also provides help with: practical issues;

restoring or maintaining functional capacity; maintaining independence; negotiating the overwhelming complexity of a health care system that contributes to fragmentation; promoting understanding of good medical information to facilitate informed decisionmaking, especially for the ill child, at his or her appropriate developmental level; addressing spiritual issues of the child and family; helping siblings; creating opportunities for growth, memory-making and closure; and bereavement.

B. *Hospice care* incorporates all of the principles of palliative care, but is more focused on patients with a terminal prognosis. Hospice is not a place; instead, it is a family-centered system or philosophy of care that focuses on patients who are likely to die by promoting quality of life, fostering choice in end-of-life decisionmaking, and supporting effective grieving for patients and families. Implemented anywhere the child is located (including the intensive care unit), such care affirms life and enables families to spend less time and energy on overwhelming medical and practical obstacles and more time on enjoying each minute with the child.

1. Hospice reimbursement is traditionally based on Medicare regulations including the proviso that a physician must consider the child's life span to be no longer than 6 months (if the illness were to follow its expected course) for the child to be formally enrolled on the benefit.

2. Hospice programs are not reimbursed well enough to provide the high technology and/or "aggressive care" that is often appropriate for pediatric patients; this currently means families must choose between hospice care and continued anticancer therapy. In some areas, transition or supportive care programs may help bridge this gap.

3. Palliative care and/or bridge programs may enable families to receive support designed to reduce suffering while receiving more disease-directed care.

III. TENETS OF PALLIATIVE CARE

The American Academy of Pediatrics set the following as a minimum standard for pediatric palliative care: "Excellence in pediatric palliative care is essential for hospitals and other facilities caring for children. Program development in pediatric palliative care, along with community outreach and public education, must be a priority of tertiary care centers serving children."

A. Essential skills: communication, ability to assist with decisionmaking, management of complications of treatment and disease, symptom control, psychosocial care of patient and family, and care of the dying.

B. Guidelines for comprehensive pediatric palliative care programs:
    1. Palliative care and respite programs need to be universally available.
    2. An integrated model of palliative care is most efficacious when introduced at diagnosis for a disease likely to be life-limiting. Such care should be continued throughout the course of the illness, regardless of whether the outcome is cure or death.
    3. Access to these services must be improved for children in need.
    4. All physicians need to be familiar and comfortable providing palliative care to children and their families.
    5. Support for research into all aspects of pediatric palliative care must be increased.
    6. Care and decisions are not directed at shortening life.

C. Universal ingredients:
    1. Care consistent with child's and family's values.
    2. Child-focused, family-oriented, relationship-centered.
    3. Must involve the primary treatment team; might include partnership with visiting nurse or home health agency, bridge programs, or hospice programs.
    4. Care coordination and streamlined communication, which includes the child at developmentally appropriate level.
    5. Better accepted by patients and families when integrated earlier in treatment course.
    6. Does not require "Do Not Resuscitate" orders.

D. Cultural issues: Efforts must be made to provide care to families and children in accordance with their cultural, religious/spiritual, ethnic, and racial identities and traditions. Families need to be involved in defining goals of care, as well as what a good death is, for their child in accordance with their preferences. Care must be taken to avoid generalizations or superimposition of provider biases and training.

IV. TEAM MEMBERS AND ROLES

A. Multidisciplinary team with the child and family at the center
B. Involves coordination with primary treatment team
C. Includes primary care provider, where appropriate, as well as all involved subspecialists and pediatric palliative care specialist or pain management specialist, where available
D. Nursing support
E. Social work support
F. Bereavement support (for as long as needed)
G. Chaplaincy services
H. Child life services
I. Expressive therapists
J. Pediatric psychology
K. PT/OT/speech therapy
L. Volunteer support

V. INTEGRATION OF PALLIATIVE CARE WITH ANTINEOPLASTIC THERAPY

The provision and receipt of palliative care is not and should not be mutually exclusive with cure-directed therapy.

A. Family perspective
Dual goals are often appropriate. Parents should not need to choose between palliative care and continued treatment of their child's underlying cancer. Further, treatment options for cancer are often appropriate for palliating symptoms of progressive disease. Risks and benefits must be carefully balanced including the burden of increased numbers of visits to, and time spent at, treatment institutions (especially daily trips back and forth for radiation). For some families, increased hospital time is actually beneficial as they receive support and nurturing from their treatment teams. For others, transportation issues and time taken away from other family activities make this choice burdensome. Each therapy decision must be weighed with

benefits and burdens in mind and with individual attention to the priorities of each family.

B. Chemotherapy
Several adult studies show improved quality of life for patients receiving palliative chemotherapy. Limited formal studies have been done on the role of palliative chemotherapy in children. As one example, oral etoposide has demonstrated antitumor effect with limited toxicity in children with refractory neuroblastoma, germ cell tumors, rhabdomyosarcoma, and other solid tumors. Common choices with low side effect profiles include:
1. Oral etoposide
2. Oral Topotecan
3. Hydroxyurea
4. Cytarabine
5. Monthly Vincristine

C. Radiation therapy
Focus in the palliative setting should be on higher fractions delivered over shorter time frames since late effects of therapy are not the primary concern.
Common indications for palliative radiation include:
1. Pain relief from bone metastases or pulmonary metastases and tumors causing nerve root and soft tissue infiltration
2. Control of bleeding
3. Control of fungation and ulceration
4. Relief of impeding or actual obstruction (for example, of the large airways)
5. Shrinkage of tumor masses causing symptoms (such as brain metastases, skin lesions, and other sites)
6. Oncologic emergencies (such as spinal cord compression, superior vena-caval obstruction)

D. Surgical intervention
1. Even when complete resection of recurrent or progressive tumor is not feasible or safe, surgical procedures to remove easily accessible painful or problematic masses may be part of the palliative plan of care.
2. Placement of epidural catheters or blocks may provide superior pain relief for recalcitrant tumors (especially those with significant nerve involvement, which may be difficult to manage medically).

3. Surgical intervention for bowel obstruction or spinal cord compression may be less morbid than medical management.
4. Incorporating the pediatric surgeon or anesthesiologist into the palliative care team can help ensure that goals are kept in concert with family preference.

E. Phase I/II clinical trials
The goal of phase I research is to determine toxicity and dose levels of investigational drugs. As many as 5% of patients may experience tumor response in these trials. Yet most families cannot accurately state the purpose of a phase I trial and are strongly motivated to participate because of hope of therapeutic benefit. Physicians, too, often overestimate the beneficial effects of phase I drugs. With these realities in mind, treatment teams should:
1. Ensure that palliative care is available in conjunction with phase I trial participation.
2. Secure the child's assent for participation (with a younger age minimum than for therapeutic trials; most investigators suggest age 7 for research assent).
3. Avoid biased presentations of risks and benefits.
4. Assess and reassess comprehension of communication regarding experimental chemotherapy.
5. For non-phase I oncology centers, benefits and burdens of therapy must include the costs (financial and otherwise) of traveling to an unfamiliar location away from family support to participate in research trials.

VI. CONTROL OF TROUBLING SYMPTOMS

A. Pain (not covered in depth here; see Chapter 11 section III) Considerations for children with recurrent or progressive disease:
1. Most pain in dying children is due to progression of disease.
2. Pain medication is most effective when given around-the-clock; avoid PRN-only administration, which necessitates that the child be in pain before meds are given.
3. Use the route most comfortable for the patient and family; avoid IM medications.
4. Pain is best treated through a multimodal approach including pharmacologic choices directed at the elicited

or likely mechanism of the pain, adjuvant pain medication, and nonpharmacologic techniques.

5. Constipation is the only side effect to which patients do not develop tolerance; therefore, bowel regimens should be instituted with pain medication.

6. Families need education about the difference between tolerance, dependence, and addiction; children with cancer *rarely* become addicted to pain medication.

7. Drowsiness/lethargy and nausea are common at the start of scheduled pain medication usage; these effects diminish in a few days. Concomitant use of antinausea medication can preempt problems.

8. Children near the end of life often have rapidly escalating pain, which requires large doses of medication. Opioid therapy should be titrated for pain relief without regard for "maximum" or "ceiling" doses.

9. Exercise caution with combination analgesics containing acetaminophen in order to avoid exceeding the daily maximum (75 mg/kg/day or 4,000 mg).

10. Pain must be assessed regularly and consistently using age-appropriate measures.

11. Treatment of underlying disease can continue while maximizing comfort.

12. Trilisate (choline magnesium salicylate) contributes NSAID profile of relief with less hematologic toxicity.

13. Appropriate use of opioid and nonopioid medication does not hasten death; in fact, adequate treatment of pain may prolong life and may increase responsiveness to disease-modifying therapy because of overall well being.

14. Difficult-to-treat neuropathic pain from extensive tumor invasion may require infusional analgesics such as ketamine, methadone, or lidocaine.

15. Anecdotally, bone pain due to metastatic disease responds to bisphosphanate therapy; phase I/II studies of these medications in children are currently underway.

B. Dyspnea/respiratory distress
    1. Subjective symptom of air hunger; often does not correlate with physiologic measurements such as pulse oxygenation.
    2. Difficult for children to describe; very frightening.

3. May be caused by disease or treatment complications concurrent infection or airway reactivity, changes in acid/base balance.
4. Oxygen, humidified air, and cool mist help subjective shortness of breath.
5. Aerosols, using normal saline (particularly for increased secretions), albuterol (for bronchospastic responses), and opioids (which decrease the subjective sense of air hunger) are anecdotally very effective.
6. Opioids and benzodiazepines administered systemically are helpful when the above listed interventions fail. See Chapter 11, Section III and Table 11.1.
7. For escalating dyspnea caused by pleural effusion or space-occupying lesions, thoracentesis, placement of an indwelling chest tube, or surgical removal may provide symptom relief.

C. Anxiety/depression
1. Anxiety and reactive depression are prevalent in children and adolescents with recurrent or progressive disease and contribute substantially to suffering.
2. Untreated anxiety and depression worsen pain and dramatically decrease quality of life.
3. Pharmacologic therapy can improve quality of life especially when symptoms are accompanied by insomnia. SSRIs are the usual starting treatment of choice for depression; *short-term use* of benzodiazepines for anxiety also may provide adjuvant pain relief and decrease insomnia.
4. Psychostimulants (ex: Ritalin) are the preferred class of drug near the end of life because they take effect within days. They may also counteract the sedative effect of opioid therapy.
5. Psychological and other nonpharmacologic interventions can facilitate coping, but the dying child may not be able to engage in psychotherapy.
6. Assessment should regularly include whole-body evaluation as untreated pain and other physical distress can contribute to anxiety and depression.

D. Fatigue/lack of energy
1. Very common symptom, difficult to measure and treat.

2. Treatable underlying causes should be excluded and/ or addressed (such as hypothyroidism, severe anemia, anxiety/depression, insomnia/sleep disturbance).

3. Appetite stimulants (megestrol acetate, cyprohepta- dine (Periactin), short courses of dexamethasone) can be useful if nutritional issues are contributing to weakness and the child has quality time remain- ing.

4. Transfusions for clinically significant anemia may be helpful provided the time and/or effort required does not detract substantially from remaining time.

5. Transfusion therapy should be guided clinically with a minimum of laboratory investigation and can be stopped at any time. Blood transfusion can often be done at home.

E. Nausea/vomiting

1. Nausea and vomiting are usually tumor-related, sec- ondary to gastrointestinal illness, or a consequence of therapy (chemotherapy or, more commonly, opioid therapy).

2. Consider constipation as an etiology!

3. In children too young to describe it, nausea may mani- fest as inactivity, weakness/lethargy, irritability, and/or poor appetite.

4. $5-HT_3$ antagonists are the mainstay of therapy for tumor-related symptoms supplemented by drugs such as lorazepam or diphenhydramine.

5. Haloperidol and other phenothiazines (e.g., chlorpro- mazine [Thorazine] or promethazine [Phenergan]) are extremely effective for N/V caused by medica- tions or combined etiology; if used regularly, diphenhy- dramine should be prescribed concomitantly to avoid extrapyramidal reactions. Prochlorperazine (Com- pazine) frequently causes dysphoria in children but may be effective for some patients.

6. Opioid-induced N/V is often aggravated by movement and may respond to scopalamine or meclizine (An- tivert).

7. Nausea due to increased intracranial pressure often responds to dexamethasone and/or acetazolamide (Diamox).

8. Nonpharmacologic approaches include TENS, acupuncture, and psychological measures (such as hypnosis and guided imagery).

F. Constipation
1. Treat the underlying cause of constipation as possible.
2. The more common causes of constipation are immobility, poor PO intake, and opioids.
3. The most effective therapy is combination treatment with stool softeners (docusate) with a stimulant (senna) or osmotic laxatives (lactulose). For refractory symptoms, Miralax is effective without causing severe cramping; its use is problematic when fluid volume is an issue.
4. Rectal therapy with suppositories should be kept to a minimum for comfort reasons. For patients who are not tolerating PO, this route may be preferable; the family will need guidance to transition to something long-forbidden during active treatment.

G. Diarrhea
1. Diarrhea can be caused by infection (viral, bacterial) or by inability to absorb nutrition.
2. With fever, cramps, and/or bloody stools, consider dysentery syndrome and treat empirically with cotrimoxazole (Bactrim, Septra).
3. Dehydration is a possibility, and discussion of hydration techniques should be undertaken proactively.
4. First attempt hydration with oral solutions such as Pedialyte in small amounts; IV or subcutaneous (hypodermoclysis) therapy can be used in selected cases.
5. Products with kaolin and pectin can be useful, as can Questran (cholestyramine).
6. If the child is near the end of life, diarrhea may signify inability to tolerate exogenous nutrition/hydration. This complication should prompt further dialogue regarding burdens and benefits of ongoing efforts to provide food and/or fluids.

H. Fever/infection
Most oncology families are conditioned to respond to fever/possible infection as an emergency. Transition to a palliative approach will need to include discussions with the family regarding goals of diagnostic testing (blood

cultures, x-rays), antibiotics, and hospitalization. When possible, empiric treatment of presumed infection with home antibiotics is often the least burdensome option for the family.

I. Bleeding
   1. Massive "bleeding out" is commonly feared by families but is an uncommon event in the dying child with cancer.
   2. Prophylactic or therapeutic platelet transfusions may be appropriate palliative care; these usually require a trip to the hospital or clinic.
   3. Goals should be decided together with the family including stopping criteria.
   4. Practical advice includes the in-home availability of sedatives and dark colored towels.

J. Seizures/neurologic symptoms
   1. May occur as a result of primary brain tumors, metastases, bleeding, or hypercoagulable states.
   2. If new-onset, it may be appropriate to do work-up to establish treatable causes.
   3. If the child is known to have a seizure disorder, increasing anticonvulsant doses and/or adding short-acting benzodiazepine may be sufficient. This usually can be done empirically without checking levels unless symptoms of toxicity develop.
   4. Children at risk for seizures should have benzodiazepines available in the home.
   5. Increased intracranial pressure can be managed with radiation and/or increasing/long-term doses of dexamethasone for children willing to withstand the side effects. Families need to understand that the benefit is time-limited. Acetazolamide (Diamox) also may be helpful temporarily.
   6. For spinal cord compression, radiation therapy, chemotherapy, and surgery may all be appropriate palliative measures for patients with remaining quality of life. Again, individual treatment goals need to be decided by the child and family.

K. Nutritional support
   1. Nutrition and hydration are extremely complex issues, both physically and emotionally/psychologically.

Open, ongoing communication with families is essential.
2. All types of medically-provided nutrition have side effects, which need to be weighed equally with potential benefits. Patients who have good quality time remaining may well benefit from additional energy and well being gained. For others, increased fluid/osmolar loads may cause more harm than good (especially when increased intracranial pressure is already a problem).
3. Frequently, families are under tremendous social, religious, and personal pressure, which must be acknowledged and worked through spiritual care providers can be only helpful with these issues.
4. When possible, the patient's opinion should be solicited.
5. In the dying child, oral intake decreases naturally and is not uncomfortable. Dying children should have open access to food and fluids should they desire them.

L. Sleep disturbance
1. For the problem to be discovered, providers must ask about this.
2. Seek and treat aggravating factors such as pain, dyspnea, and anxiety.
3. The mainstay of therapy is sedating medications including diphenhydramine, lorazepam, and chloral hydrate.
4. Low-dose antidepressant tricyclic therapy also may be helpful, especially with concomitant neuropathic pain.

M. Mucositis
1. May be caused by chemotherapy, radiation therapy, medications, or decreased oral stimulation/intake.
2. Careful attention to oral hygiene with soft toothettes and lip moisturizers is helpful.
3. Focus should be on comfort; avoid irritant solutions (such as chlorhexidine).
4. Empiric treatment with oral antifungals and acyclovir may be indicated.

N. Pruritis
1. Pruritis is commonly caused by dry skin, accumulation of toxic metabolites, and opioids.

2. Treatment depends on etiology; start with moisturizers and emollients if skin is dry.
3. Opioid-induced pruritis is treated with antihistamines or partial opioid antagonists such as nalbuphine; persistent pruritis will probably require a medication change.
4. Pruritis caused by hepatic/renal failure may respond to H2 blockers or cholestyramine.

O. Edema/anasarca
1. Most often due to venous/lymphatic obstruction, medications, or intolerance to nutrition/hydration.
2. Diuretics may be helpful even if obstruction is the cause; also try Mannitol.
3. Supportive care such as ace wraps to affected limbs may increase comfort.

VII. MEDICAL DECISION MAKING AND/OR ADVANCE DIRECTIVES

A. Assent
A child's assent is sought in research studies, which infers that we respect the child's decision-making input. Considering the rights and wishes of minors in terms of palliative care and end-of-life issues establishes a connection between caregiver and patient that transcends paternalism. Children and adolescents with cancer have usually acquired a good understanding of their disease and treatment course. Cultural, familial, and societal restrictions may prevent them from voicing their understanding or openly discussing their wishes. Palliative care providers need to form alliances with parents to create a system of care, which allows children and adolescents more input into decisions surrounding palliative care issues. A long-standing relationship between the child and a Child Life or pediatric psychology professional can be very instrumental here.

B. Withdrawal of life-sustaining treatment/DNR
Benefits and burdens of life-sustaining treatment need to be evaluated individually with the child's input when possible. While children under 18 cannot legally author advance directives, their preferences regarding life-sustaining treatment and resuscitation should be elicited when

appropriate and be documented during noncrisis times of decision making.

C. Ethical issues concerning children
1. Parents make decisions for minor children.
2. Many children with chronic illness are developmentally more mature than well children and are more capable of participating in health care decision-making.
3. The AAP supports the role of the child in decision-making as is developmentally appropriate.
4. In deciding end-of-life issues, respect the rights and wishes of minors.
5. Seek a child's assent for research participation when developmentally possible.
6. Most ethical conflict is the result of poor communication, which needs to be addressed early and in a multidisciplinary fashion.

VIII. CARING FOR THE DYING CHILD

A. Children understand death differently at different developmental levels, regardless of chronological age. Ability to understand death and dying is determined by personal experience/history with disease, previous experiences with death, and stage of emotional and cognitive development. Full understanding of death involves recognizing irreversibility, finality, inevitability, and causality; many children can grasp these concepts by age 7.
B. Children need to discover meaning and purpose in their experiences, belong to something beyond themselves, and be part of something greater just as adults do. Facilitating a child's spirituality through interaction with a spiritual care provider or through use of spiritual interventions can greatly ease a child and family's suffering.
C. The experience of serious illness often leads to maturity in understanding death and dying; however, it is worth remembering that some children may regress along the trajectory.
D. Children are often aware that they are dying long before the adults in their lives. Reluctance or refusal on the part of family or care team to discuss the issues may prevent a child from achieving life goals and may increase fear, isolation, and suffering.

E. When a child is dying, she or he might want to participate in funeral planning and memory-making with family and friends. This gives the patient the chance to leave a mark on the world and should be encouraged whenever possible.

F. Location of death also needs to be individualized to meet the needs of the family; parents who are not able to "choose home" for their terminally ill child should not be made to feel guilty. When children prefer to die at home, every effort should be made to support the family through the process.

G. During the dying process: families need to be taught what to expect; symptoms should be managed clinically/ empirically; only essential medications should be continued, and should be given through the route most comfortable for the child; the primary care team should continue to be involved (through calls and visits, even just to provide "presence") when children are dying at home; and families should be given a realistic estimate of prognosis when possible (in general terms, such as "hours to days" or "days to weeks") to facilitate their ability to anticipate and plan.

IX. CARING FOR THE WHOLE FAMILY

A. Palliative care is truly family-centered care. However, it behooves providers to remember that the dying child/adolescent is our patient. Although family members are the ones who will be left to contemplate the outcome of decisions, it is the child whose suffering is paramount.

B. Siblings are often neglected as family becomes more focused on ill or dying child. They will process illness in different ways and may have ongoing bereavement issues as they age, encountering the loss of their sibling at each new stage. They need individualized support—someone who is "theirs" to talk to, to lean on. Parents need support and guidance for spending individual quality time with well siblings. Siblings should be encouraged to make memories with and spend as much time with ill siblings as they are comfortable. Most children handle funerals well, with adequate preparation, and this enables them to have closure as well.

C. Attention must be paid to each family's spiritual, cultural, and ethnic background.

X. CARING FOR THE COMMUNITY

The "forgotten grievers" need support as well. Community bereavement resources, through local hospices or funeral homes, are appropriate for those touched by the child's illness (grandparents, extended family, school personnel and classmates, scout troops, sports teams, church groups, etc.). Primary team can assist with adjustment in the school system.

XI. SELF-CARE FOR HEALTH PROFESSIONALS

A. Caring for dying children is extremely rewarding but also incredibly stressful.

B. Inadequate self-care preparation contributes greatly to "compassion fatigue" in caregivers. (see Chapter 19 section II.C).

C. Recognition of the toll, as well as proactive strategies such as increased awareness, limit setting, delineation of team roles, and self-care can reduce stress.

D. Care providers who derive comfort from attending memorial services should be able to do so.

XII. AFTER DEATH

A. Children who die at home will need to be pronounced; this can be accomplished by a hospice or qualified home care agency nurse under the direction of the managing physician.

B. Families should be offered the opportunity for autopsy, even when the cause seems obvious.

C. Children who die in the hospital do not automatically need to be evaluated by the medical examiner unless the death is completely unanticipated.

D. Scheduling a follow-up visit with the family to answer their medical questions, review autopsy findings, and provide closure with the medical team is part of ongoing care of the family.

XIII. BEREAVEMENT CARE

A. Anticipatory bereavement may begin at diagnosis for some families as they face losses of health, well child, hopes, and dreams.

B. Families never "get over" losing a child. Bereavement follow-up should extend as long as the family needs care.

C. Grief and bereavement do not follow prescribed "stages" with defined times attached. Pathologic grief should, however, be recognized and treated by a professional.

D. The care team should be prepared to offer resources (educational, group/individual counseling) and provide ongoing support.

E. Presence by the care team at the memorial services (when possible), and afterward by remembering special occasions with cards or phone calls, are especially appreciated by families. A condolence letter should be sent from the primary care team to the family.

XIV. FINANCIAL ISSUES

A. Insurance caps on home care services may preclude care being delivered in the home.

B. Readmission to the hospital for symptom control may be denied if the patient has previously been managed in the home and outpatient setting.

C. Indirect costs to families can be quite substantial (gas/ travel, loss of income).

D. Counseling and bereavement services are generally poorly reimbursed, if at all, as are other essential "nonbillable" services provided by a palliative care team including Child Life, pharmacy, and social work. Even billable services such as psychology and occupational/physical therapies may not be covered if the child is in the home.

E. In many states, home-based palliative care services are provided by hospice agencies whose cost/reimbursement system is based on the adult Medicare model and is a poor fit for the needs of children and adolescents. When paid per diem, agencies cannot or will not cover "aggressive" therapies, which are more the norm for children with cancer than not (such as infusion services, blood transfusions, palliative chemotherapy, palliative radiation, and similar therapies). To receive hospice services to enable them to keep their dying child at home, parents who are accustomed to a very high intensity of care must accept relatively minimal services without much opportunity for transition. While many parents may not want resuscitative therapies for their child, continued comfort-directed therapies such as transfusions, IV antibiotics, and IV nutrition/hydration to treat anorexia and wasting are often desired and appropriate to maximize a child's quality of life.

Bibliography

American Academy of Pediatrics, Committee on Bioethics and Hospital Care. Palliative care for children. *Pediatrics* 106(2):351–57, 1998.

Field MJ, Behrman RE, eds. When children die: Improving palliative and end-of-life care for children and their families. *Institute of Medicine Report*, 2002. Washington, D.C.: National Academy Press.

Friebert SE, Kodish ED. Kids and cancer: Ethical issues in treating the pediatric oncology patient. In Angelos P, ed. *Ethical Issues in Cancer Patient Care*. Norwell, Mass.: Kluwer Academic Publishers, 1999; pp. 99–135.

Hilden JM, Himelstein BP, Freyer DR, Friebert S, Kane JR. Excellent end-of-life care for cancer patients: Special issues in pediatrics. In Foley KM, Gelband H, eds., *Improving Palliative Care for Cancer*. Washington, D.C.: National Academy Press, 2001.

Hilden J, Friebert S, Himelstein B, Freyer D, Wheeler J. Palliative care for the child with cancer. In Carter B, Levetown M, eds. *Palliative Care for Infants, Children, and Adolescents: A Practical Handbook*, forthcoming.

Kane JR, Himelstein BP. Palliative care in pediatrics. In Berger AM, Portenoy RK, Weissman DE, eds., *Principles and Practice of Palliative Care and Supportive Oncology*, 2nd edition. Philadelphia: Lippincott Williams & Wilkins, 2002.

Wolfe J, Friebert S, Hilden J. Caring for children with advanced cancer: Integrating palliative care. *Pediatric Clinics of North America* 49:1043–62, 2002.

Wolfe J, Grier HE. Care of the dying child. In Pizzo P, Poplack D, eds., *Principles and Practice of Pediatric Oncology*, 4th edition. Philadelphia: Lippincott Williams & Wilkins, 2002.

Index

Page numbers in *italics* denote figures; those followed by "t" denote tables